Non-Suicidal Self-Injury in Eating Disorders

Laurence Claes • Jennifer J. Muehlenkamp
Editors

Non-Suicidal Self-Injury in Eating Disorders

Advancements in Etiology and Treatment

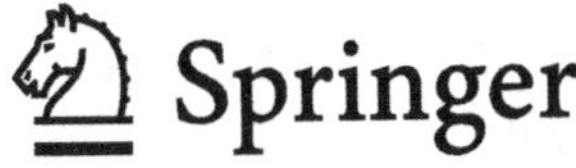

Editors
Laurence Claes
Department of Psychology
KU Leuven
Leuven
Belgium

Jennifer J. Muehlenkamp
Department of Psychology
University of Wisconsin-Eau Claire
Eau Claire
WI, USA

ISBN 978-3-662-52297-4 ISBN 978-3-642-40107-7 (eBook)
DOI 10.1007/978-3-642-40107-7
Springer Heidelberg New York Dordrecht London

Softcover reprint of the hardcover 1st edition 2014

Printed on acid-free paper

Springer is part of Springer Science+Business Media (www.springer.com)

Contents

Part I

Background and General Aspects

Non-suicidal Self-Injury and Eating Disorders: Dimensions of Self-Harm

1

Laurence Claes and Jennifer J. Muehlenkamp

Abstract

Both non-suicidal self-injury (NSSI) and eating disorders (ED) are considered to be harmful behaviors falling within a behavioral spectrum ranging from self-care to self-harm. The high degree of co-occurrence of these behaviors, along with their shared body focus has motivated researchers to investigate and theorize about the potential shared factors driving their comorbidity. In this chapter, we present a conceptual model based upon the current empirical literature depicting distal and proximal psychosocial risk factors shared by NSSI and ED. This model provides a framework for understanding the co-occurrence of NSSI and ED, with the different components being further elaborated on and discussed with regards to treatment recommendations across the different chapters included in this volume. The chapter concludes with a short introduction and summary of each of the chapters within this book.

1.1 Self-Harm Spectrum

Many behaviors that an individual chooses to engage in can be placed along a general continuum ranging from "normal/healthy" self-care to serious self-harm. Normal self-care consists of behaviors which are socially prescribed or accepted and are engaged in to attain or maintain health and/or a norm of physical attractiveness. A self-harm behavior is viewed as socially unacceptable and typically serves the idiosyncratic purpose of coping with a personal problem or subjective distress (Claes & Vandereycken, 2007). Both NSSI and ED are considered to be self-harming behaviors

L. Claes (✉)
Faculty of Psychology and Educational Sciences, University of Leuven, Leuven, Belgium
e-mail: Laurence.Claes@psy.kuleuven.be

J.J. Muehlenkamp
Psychology Department, University of Wisconsin Eau Claire, Eau Claire, WI, USA
e-mail: MUEHLEJJ@uwec.edu

L. Claes and J.J. Muehlenkamp (eds.), *Non-Suicidal Self-Injury in Eating Disorders*, DOI 10.1007/978-3-642-40107-7_1, © Springer-Verlag Berlin Heidelberg 2014

lying within this spectrum. While from the patient's perspective, the ED or NSSI behaviors may represent a type of self-care (e.g., reducing distress, improved feeling of control); most professionals will conceptualize these behaviors as existing in the self-harm dimension of the continuum but acknowledge the varying severity the behaviors can pose even within the self-harm dimension. Self-harm behaviors can be broadly categorized as including both direct and indirect modes of self-damaging acts such as NSSI, suicide attempts, particular habits of eating, drinking, and smoking (Lloyd-Richardson, Perrine, Dierker & Kelley, 2007; St. Germain & Hooley, 2012). Behaviors such as eating disorders, substance abuse, and sexual risk taking are conceptualized as indirect forms of self-harm because the damage caused to the body may be more diffuse and/or may not manifest until later after multiple engagements in the behavior. Furthermore, the primary motivation behind the indirect forms of self-harm may be secondary to inflicting pain or visible tissue damage. NSSI, on the contrary, is characterized by the directness of the act, often resulting in immediately visible tissue damage. Thus, the link between the behavior and the physical consequence is often instantaneous and unequivocal (Claes & Vandereycken, 2007).

1.2 Definitions of NSSI and ED

We define NSSI as any socially unaccepted behavior causing intentional and direct injury to one's own body tissue without suicidal intent, such as cutting, skin abrading, or burning oneself, that is engaged in to help regulate internal or interpersonal states (see also Nock, 2009). Although NSSI and suicidal behavior are distinct in many ways including their primary motivation and medical severity (Muehlenkamp & Kerr, 2010), they are not unrelated (e.g., Claes et al., 2010). The presence of NSSI is associated with an increased risk of suicide (Andover & Gibb, 2010; Whitlock et al., 2013), possibly due to the fact that NSSI helps one habituate to self-inflicted violence (Joiner, 2005). The severity of NSSI can range from mild to severe, depending on the actual behavior one engages in, the frequency of the behavior, the number of methods used, as well as the severity of the wounds created (Claes & Vandereycken, 2007). Individuals who engage in NSSI are often found to have a high rate of other adverse mental health conditions, including depression, anxiety disorders, PTSD, and personality disorder features (Jacobson, Muehlenkamp, Miller & Turner, 2008; Lofthouse, Muehlenkamp & Adler, 2009; Nock, Joiner, Gordon, Lloyd-Richardson & Prinstein, 2006).

An ED is a condition defined by abnormal eating habits that may involve either insufficient or excessive food intake to the detriment of an individual's physical and mental health. Anorexia nervosa (AN) and bulimia nervosa (BN) are the most common specific types of eating disorders according to the DSM-5 (American Psychological Association, 2013), but the general eating disorder not otherwise specified category is the most frequently diagnosed and captures a broad range of disordered eating practices. *Anorexia nervosa* is characterized by food restriction; intense, irrational fears of gaining weight; and an unrealistic perception of current body weight. Two subtypes of AN are described within the DSM-5: AN of the restrictive type and AN of the binge eating/purging type. *Bulimia nervosa* is a disorder characterized by binge eating followed by purging behaviors (e.g., self-induced vomiting, excessive use of laxatives/diuretics, or excessive exercise) as well as weight and body concerns. *Binge eating disorder* is defined as uncontrolled binge eating without purging or compensatory behaviors. It is often, but not always, associated with obesity. The *eating disorder not otherwise specified* diagnosis captures maladaptive eating patterns co-occurring with significant weight/body concerns that do not meet the DSM-5 criteria for anorexia, bulimia, or binge eating disorder. Consistent with a spectrum model, mild forms of disordered eating consist of using unhealthy weight management behaviors typically characterized by temporary food or fat/sugar restriction combined with increased physical exercise in individuals who want to diet, whereas severe eating disorders are characterized by behaviors that may involve significant starvation (e.g., only eating salad or yogurt), extreme binge eating (i.e., consuming large quantities of food in a very short period of time), and/or dangerous compensatory behaviors (such as extreme exercising, vomiting, laxative abuse). The consequences of these eating disorder behaviors can be severe, including death caused by direct medical complications (e.g., electrolyte imbalances, cardiac arrhythmias) or from comorbid conditions such as depression with suicidal ideation.

1.3 Prevalence of NSSI and ED

Most individuals who engage in NSSI begin to do so during early to middle adolescence with the average age of onset for NSSI ranging between 12 and 16 years of age (Rodham & Hawton, 2009). A recent systematic review of empirical studies reporting on the prevalence of NSSI in adolescent samples across the globe found a mean lifetime prevalence of 18 % and an average 12-month prevalence of 19 % (Muehlenkamp, Claes, Havertape & Plener, 2012). More focused epidemiological studies suggest a 12-month prevalence estimate of 7.3 % among US adolescents (Taliaferro et al., 2013). The prevalence estimates of NSSI in young adults (aged 18–25 years) have centered around 17 %, with individual studies reporting rates ranging between 5 and 35 % (Gratz, 2001; Nada-Raja, Skegg, Langley, Morrison & Sowerby, 2004; Whitlock et al., 2011). In the US current rates of NSSI among adults (typically including ages 25 and older) are estimated to be around 5 % (Klonsky, 2011). Although researchers and clinicians have been suggesting that the rates of self-injury are significantly increasing among adolescence in particular, results reported by Muehlenkamp, Claes et al. (2012), Muehlenkamp et al. (2009) suggest that they may have stabilized. However, there continues to be considerable variability in the reported prevalence rates of NSSI which is likely the result of assessment and sample-size biases. Early research on NSSI suggested that this behavior was predominantly displayed by females, whereas more recent research has shown that males and females may differ less than previously assumed (Whitlock et al., 2011). However, different features of NSSI, such as frequency of NSSI, types of NSSI, places on the body that are injured, and motivations appear to vary across genders (e.g., Whitlock, Eckenrode & Silverman, 2006, Whitlock et al., 2011).

Eating disorders are relatively rare among the general population (for a detailed overview see Smink, van Hoeken & Hoek, 2012); however, engagement in unhealthy weight management behaviors are more common particularly among adolescents (Croll, Neumark-Sztainer, Story & Ireland, 2002). Based on a large representative sample of US adolescents, the lifetime prevalence of AN was estimated to be 0.3 % in females as well as males; the lifetime prevalence of BN was 1.3 % for females and 0.5 % for males, and the lifetime prevalence of BED ranged from 0.8 % in males to 2.3 % in female adolescents (Swanson, Crow, LeGrange, Swendsen & Merikangas, 2011). Based on population-based studies in the USA (Hudson et al., 2007) and Europe (Preti et al., 2009), the lifetime prevalence of AN was 0.9 % among *adult* females and 0.3 % among *adult* males. The lifetime prevalence of BN varied between 0.9 and 1.5 % among women and between 0.1 and 0.5 % among men. For BED, international differences in prevalence have been observed with life prevalence of BED in Europe estimated at 1.9 % for women and 0.3 % for men, whereas in the USA the lifetime prevalence rates were significantly higher at 3.5 % for women and 2.0 % for men (Smink et al., 2012). While the overall rate of AN has remained stable over the past decades, there has been an increase observed within the high-risk group of 15–19-year-old girls. The occurrence of BN in general appears to have decreased during the late 1990s of the last century (Smink et al., 2012).

Concerning the co-occurrence of both NSSI and ED, studies show that up to 72 % of those with eating disorders also engage in NSSI (Claes, Klonsky, Muehlenkamp, Kuppens & Vandereycken, 2010; Claes, Vandereycken & Vertommen, 2001, 2003; Muehlenkamp, Peat, Claes & Smits, 2012); and between 25 and 54 % of people who engage in NSSI report comorbid disordered eating (Gollust, Eisenberg & Golberstein, 2008; Heath, Toste, Nedechava & Charlebois, 2008; Muehlenkamp, Peat et al., 2012). The prevalence of NSSI appears to be higher in patients with BN (26–55.2 %) or AN-BP (27.8–68.1 %) than in the restrictive subtype of AN (13.6–42.1 %) (Claes et al., 2001, 2003; Svirko & Hawton, 2007). The relationship between gender and risk for engaging in NSSI among patients with ED and vice versa is unclear (e.g., Gollust et al., 2008; Peebles, Wilson & Lock, 2011).

1.4 Reasons for the Co-occurrence of NSSI and Eating Disorders

Given that both NSSI and ED are body-focused disorders, researchers have begun to investigate and theorize about the potential shared factors driving their co-occurrence. In Fig. 1.1, we present a model depicting distal and proximal as well as individual, social, and cultural risk factors shared by NSSI and eating disorders. Individual distal risk factors include temperament and personality traits, whereas cultural, family, and traumatic interpersonal experiences are included on the social

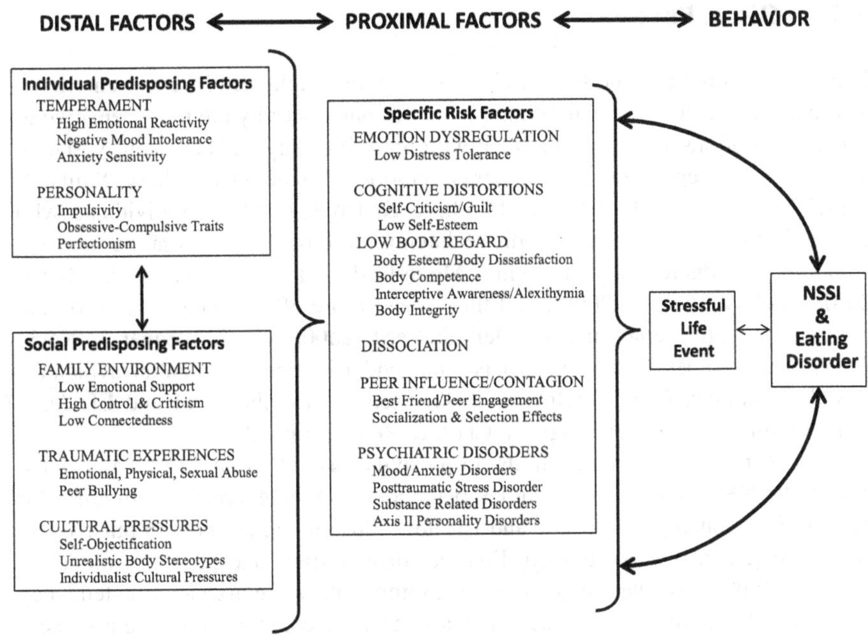

Fig. 1.1 Conceptual model of the interactive risk factors for both NSSI and ED

level. Proximal risk factors include emotion dysregulation, cognitive distortions, low body regard, dissociation, peer pressure/contagion, and comorbid psychiatric disorder(s). Within this theoretical model, it is assumed that interactions among the risk factors occur both within categories (e.g., among the distal factors) and across categories (e.g., select distal factors interact with select proximal factors) to increase an individual's vulnerability to developing the behavior of NSSI, ED, or their co-occurrence. Also depicted within the model is how these distal and proximal risk factors interplay with stressful events that can increase internal distress, which is then regulated by the behaviors of NSSI and/or ED, which in turn can again influence or reinforce the proximal risk factors. This reciprocal interplay between the behaviors and risk factors are believed to contribute to the cyclical and repetitive pattern of the NSSI and ED behavior typically observed among clients. In what follows, we briefly discuss select studies supporting the inclusion of, and associations between, the distal and proximal risk factors for both NSSI and ED. It is important to note that we emphasize only those factors that have shown similar associations to *both* NSSI and ED. We recognize other factors may pose unique risk to the development ED or NSSI but these elements are not the focus of this volume. More elaborate discussions of many of the risk factors within our proposed model are included in the subsequent chapters of the current volume.

1.5 Distal Factors

Individuals with NSSI and ED are characterized by heightened levels of emotional reactivity. Individuals who are higher in emotional reactivity are more sensitive to negative emotions, experiencing them with more intensity and persistence relative to those who report low or moderate emotional reactivity (Claes, Smits & Bijttebier, 2013; Nock, Wedig, Holmberg & Hooley, 2008). Individuals who engage in these behaviors also indicate having more difficulty tolerating negative emotions and distress (Corstorphine, Mountford, Tomlinson, Waller & Meyer, 2007; Nock & Mendes, 2008), and they spend more effort trying to control and minimize negative emotions (Ghaderi & Berit, 2000; Najmi, Wegner & Nock, 2007). This temperamental pattern is what underlies the experiential avoidance model (Chapman, Gratz & Brown, 2006) used to describe NSSI and ED (e.g., Corstorphine et al., 2007; Kingston, Clark & Remington, 2010).

With respect to personality traits, impulsivity has been found to be associated with both NSSI and eating disorder behaviors. Drawing upon the Five-Factor Model of personality, Whiteside and Lynam (2001) identified how impulsiveness is represented in three of the Big Five personality traits and present a model of impulsivity based on these elements. For example, negative urgency (the tendency to act rashly in the face of negative affect) is a component of Neuroticism; sensation-seeking tendencies stem from Extraversion, and a lack of premeditation and/or perseverance—both facets of Conscientiousness—refers to the inability to delay action/acting without thinking and to stay with a task until completion. Several studies (Claes & Muehlenkamp, 2013; Glenn & Klonsky, 2010, 2011) have shown that NSSI is positively related to negative urgency and lack of premeditation. Similar results have been found in eating disorders (e.g., Cassin & Von Ranson, 2005; Claes, Vandereycken & Vertommen, 2005); specifically, patients with BN tend to score significantly higher on negative urgency and sensation seeking, as well as significantly lower on lack of perseverance/premeditation compared to restrictive AN patients.

Also, obsessive-compulsive and perfectionistic characteristics have been noted in both NSSI (Claes, Soenens, Vansteenkiste & Vandereycken, 2012; Hoff & Muehlenkamp, 2009) and ED samples (Boone, Soenens, Braet & Goossens, 2010; Serpell, Livingstone, Neiderman & Lask, 2002). Obsessive-compulsive characteristics may be demonstrated among individuals with more chronic and repetitive NSSI due to the reinforcing effects of the behavior, and individual's report that urges to self-injure can come on suddenly and be hard to resist (Washburn, Juzwin, Styer & Aldridge, 2010). Similarly, individuals who are diagnosed with the restrictive subtype of AN tend to show high comorbidity with OC(P)D (Claes, Vandereycken & Vertommen, 2002; Halmi et al., 2005; Serpell et al., 2002).

On the social dimension of distal risk factors, the cultural pressure on individuals to be physically "perfect" is an important factor for the development of both ED and NSSI. The sexual objectification of the female body, and more recently the male body as well, has perpetuated an unrealistic stereotype of what constitutes the ideal, attractive body (Calogero, Tantleff-Dunn & Thompson, 2010). These unrealistic body stereotypes are portrayed and reinforced by the media, fashion, and entertainment industries, which subsequently have a strong influence on an individual's body dissatisfaction. Furthermore, studies have indicated that these sociocultural messages can become internalized contributing to an individual's tendency of viewing one's own body from an outsider, or "others," perspective. Such self-objectifying practices have been associated with increased bodily disconnection, which has been linked to both NSSI and ED (Calogero et al., 2010; Muehlenkamp & Saris-Baglama, 2002; Nelson & Muehlenkamp, 2012; Peat & Muehlenkamp, 2011).

The family context of individuals with ED and NSSI show some similar characteristics. Research finds that the family environment of individuals with ED and/or NSSI tend to be characterized by low levels of emotional support and high levels of psychological (e.g., critique) and behavioral control compared to individuals without NSSI or ED (e.g., Claes et al., 2012; Soenens et al., 2008). Additionally, Claes, Vandereycken and Vertommen (2004) compared the family context in ED patients with and without NSSI, finding that eating disorder patients with NSSI described their family environment as less cohesive and expressive and more conflictual than patients without NSSI. A recent study by Claes et al. (2012) showed that the relationship between parental criticism and NSSI in ED patients was mediated by high self-criticism.

Theorists have also proposed that experiencing childhood trauma, often in the form of abuse, plays a central role in the etiology of both NSSI and ED (e.g., Neumark-Sztainer, Story, Hannan, Beuhring & Resnick, 2000; Yates, Carlson & Egeland, 2008). Some research has suggested that the association between abuse experiences and NSSI/ED is more complex than previously assessed (Muehlenkamp, Kerr, Bradley & Larsen, 2010). For example, some have reported that the association between sexual abuse and NSSI/ED is attenuated or becomes nonsignificant when other clinically relevant variables are controlled (Klonsky & Moyer, 2008; Smolak & Murnen, 2002). Yet, the relationship between physical abuse and NSSI/ED remains when those same variables are controlled (Muehlenkamp et al., 2010; Treuer, Koperdak, Rozsa & Füredi, 2005; Yates et al., 2008). The relationships between abuse and NSSI or ED may be better understood from meditational models, in which intervening variables (such as emotion regulation, dissociation, attachment style) are taken into account while investigating the associations between abuse and NSSI/ED (Heath et al., 2008; Muehlenkamp et al., 2010; Ward, Ramsay & Treasure, 2000; Wonderlich, 2007; Yates et al., 2008).

1.6 Proximal Risk Factors

It is useful to view disordered eating as well as NSSI as disorders of emotion dysregulation (Haynos & Fruzetti, 2011; Klonsky, Muehlenkamp, Lewis & Walsh, 2011). Several studies suggest that self-injurers and ED patients experience more frequent and intense negative emotions than individuals without NSSI and ED. Intense emotions such as anxiety, frustration, and anger often precede specific acts of NSSI and ED practices, and both behaviors cause a quick decrease in the intensity of the emotions as a result of engaging in the NSSI/ED (Crosby et al., 2009; Klonsky et al., 2011; Muehlenkamp et al., 2009). Additionally, individuals report that engaging in NSSI and ED increases feelings such as calm and relaxation (Claes, Klonsky et al., 2010; Crosby et al., 2009; Klonsky, 2007, 2009). Moreover, those who report the greatest reductions in negative emotions appear to be the ones who engage in these behaviors more frequently (Klonsky, 2009).

Recent studies suggest that low self-esteem and self-criticism may also be important factors in understanding ED and NSSI (Baetens, Claes, Muehlenkamp, Grietens & Onghena, 2012; Shafran, Cooper & Fairburn, 2002). Both, NSSI and eating disorder symptoms (e.g., excessive exercise, purging) have been reported by patients as means of self-punishment, which might be another indication of a self-criticizing cognitive style (Svirko & Hawton, 2007). Claes et al. (2003) also found that self-injuring ED patients showed significantly more self-criticism and guilt than non-injuring ED patients. Additionally, several authors (e.g., Glassman, Weierich, Hooley, Deliberto & Nock, 2007; Soenens et al., 2008; Wedig & Nock, 2007) have reported that self-criticism mediated the relationship between (emotional) abuse and NSSI/ED.

Also commonly studied as a correlate of ED and NSSI are symptoms of dissociation. Studies have reported significant associations between dissociation and both ED (Vanderlinden, Vandereycken & Claes, 2007) and NSSI (Muehlenkamp, Claes, Peat, Smits & Vandereycken, 2011). Additionally, studies have shown an indirect path from childhood traumatic experiences to NSSI via dissociation in general patient populations (e.g., Low, Jones, MacLeod, Power & Duggan, 2000; Vanderlinden et al., 2007) as well as in ED patients (Claes et al., 2001, 2003; Muehlenkamp et al., 2011), although it is important to note that not all individuals will experience dissociation. Mild aspects of dissociation may also contribute to some of the bodily disturbances observed among individuals with NSSI and ED. Some researchers acknowledge that a negative attitude toward the body and disconnection from bodily experiences (e.g., alexithymia) may be a critical component in both NSSI and ED (Muehlenkamp, Swanson & Braush, 2005; Walsh, 2012) because dissatisfaction may promote devaluing of the body alongside views of the body as a hated object, which make it easier to harm. The increased rates of body dissatisfaction among those who engage in NSSI are even notable within ED patients, who conceptually already suffer from high levels of body dissatisfaction (Muehlenkamp et al., 2011).

Empirical evidence suggests that NSSI and disordered eating are related to peer relationships. NSSI, for example, is more common among young adolescent girls with a best friend who has engaged in NSSI (Claes, Houben, Vandereycken, Bijttebier & Muehlenkamp, 2010; Diliberto & Nock, 2008; Hilt, Nock, Lloyd-Richardson & Prinstein, 2008, in this volume), and body image and weight loss behaviors are more similar among friends within a group than among peers in different groups (Paxton, Schutz, Wertheim & Muir, 1999). Much of the peer influence literature focuses on the idea that peers who affiliate tend to share similar attributes, and this may be due to selection and/or socialization (e.g., contagion via modeling) effects (Hutchinson & Rapee, 2007; Prinstein, Guerry, Browne & Rancourt, 2009, Prinstein et al., 2010).

Finally, a survey of the literature indicates that NSSI as well as disordered eating can co-occur with multiple Axis I psychiatric disorders, including major depression, anxiety disorders, posttraumatic stress disorder, and alcohol/substance-related disorders as well as Axis II personality disorders (Baetens et al., 2012; Jacobson et al., 2008; Nock et al., 2006). The study of Nock et al. (2006) revealed that 87.6 % of adolescents engaging in NSSI met criteria for a DSM-IV Axis I diagnosis, and 63.6 % met criteria for an Axis II personality disorder. Swanson et al. (2011) reported that a sizable majority of adolescents with AN, BN, or BED endorsed 1 or more comorbid Axis I disorders across the life-span, whereas Rosenvinge, Martinussen and Ostensen (2000) found a higher proportion of eating-disordered patients being diagnosed with any personality disorder compared to comparison groups.

Based on the findings of this brief overview, we can conclude that NSSI and disordered eating share many individual, social, and culture risk factors that likely account for their high comorbidity. The interacting influences of these risk factors need to be taken into consideration when conducting future studies and designing treatment or prevention programs. Many of the components just described will be discussed in greater depth and detail, including direct links to assessment and treatment recommendations, in each of the following chapters.

1.7 Content of the Book

The purpose of this book is to provide comprehensive, state-of-the-art information on the origins, assessment, and treatment of NSSI in eating disorders. The chapters are empirically grounded, providing a clear overview of the current knowledge, practical applications for intervention, and avenues for future research. A broad range of chapters are presented by researchers, scholars, and clinicians who are experts in the field of NSSI and/or eating disorders. The book was written to be useful for researchers, clinicians, scholars, and students in mental health professions such as clinical/counseling psychology, social work, and psychiatry.

The chapters of this book have been organized into three parts. *Part I*, Background and General Aspects of NSSI and ED, provides an overview of the definitions, epidemiology, development, and etiological and functional models of NSSI and ED as well as their co-occurrence. Within this first chapter (Chap. 1), we (L.C. and J.J.M) have presented NSSI and ED as body-focused disorders, falling within a spectrum of self-care and self-harm that can vary across individuals and behaviors. We discuss the definitions of NSSI and ED and developed a comprehensive theoretical model depicting the interactive nature of common risk factors shared by both NSSI and eating disorders. Colleen Jacobson and colleagues (Chap. 2) give us a comprehensive overview of the epidemiological and sociocultural aspects contributing to the overlap between NSSI and ED behaviors.

Specifically, they report on the demographic (including gender, age, ethnic, psychiatric profile) and sociocultural (including cultural values, family structure, and life experiences) characteristics of people with ED who also engage in NSSI and conversely with the ultimate goal of providing an initial understanding of the mechanisms underlying the co-occurrence of these two behaviors. Barrocas, Holm-Denoma, and Hankin (Chap. 3) provide a developmental perspective on the factors that impact the onset, maintenance, and treatment of ED and NSSI. This chapter briefly reviews the epidemiological data on NSSI and ED in youth and examines several specific developmental vulnerabilities for both outcomes. Kathryn Gordon and colleagues (Chap. 4) present a comprehensive review of etiological models and their supporting data, designed to explain why NSSI and EDs occur. In addition, models relevant for explaining the high rate of comorbidity between NSSI and EDs are presented with direct implications for treatment. In the final chapter of *Part I*, Michelle Wedig (Chap. 5) focuses on the psychological meanings and functions believed to motivate and underlie NSSI and eating-disordered behaviors. Empirical literature describing the functions of NSSI and eating-disordered behaviors individually are reviewed, followed by a discussion of the differences and shared functions of these two behaviors.

Part II provides information about the assessment and treatment of NSSI and ED, with each chapter highlighting recommendations and approaches for treating the simultaneous occurrence of NSSI and ED behavior. It will be of interest and great value to anyone conducting clinical work with individuals engaging in NSSI and/or ED. Andover and colleagues (Chap. 6) describe how to utilize a functional assessment of both behaviors to directly inform the treatment planning and selection of interventions with one's patients, ensuring an individualized yet empirically grounded approach to therapy. The chapter clearly demonstrates how functional assessment is useful at the beginning of treatment to inform case conceptualization treatment planning for a given client as well as being a therapeutic tool on its own. In Chap. 7, Christine Peat describes how Cognitive Behavioral Therapy (CBT) can be applied when treating NSSI and/or ED. CBT addresses the connections among dysfunctional emotions, cognitive processes, and maladaptive behaviors, and has consistently been considered the gold standard for the treatment of ED and of NSSI. Practical suggestions of how to utilize CBT in alleviating both NSSI and ED behaviors simultaneously are presented. Barent Walsh and Jennifer Eaton (Chap. 8) review the basics of Dialectical Behavior Therapy (DBT) as applied in the treatment of co-occurring NSSI and eating disorders. The four major components of DBT are discussed, and these authors provide an easily accessible description of DBT using a case example to depict the critical components of the treatment throughout the chapter. Paul Robinson (Chap. 9) discussed the application and effectiveness of using Mentalization-Based Therapy (MBT) in reducing NSSI in patients with Borderline Personality Disorder and suggests it is likely to be effective when used with patients presenting with both ED and NSSI. Hughes, Allan, and LaGrange (Chap. 10) describe Family-Based Treatment (FBT), which currently has the strongest evidence base for effective treatment of adolescents with AN. In FBT, the family is perceived as a resource for recovery and problematic family relationships are treated without blame and typically only when they present barriers to recovery. Given some of the familial risk and protective factors shared by NSSI and ED, the application of FBT is likely to produce positive results and be useful as an adjunctive or main treatment approach particularly for those presenting with AN and NSSI. In Chap. 11, Arcelus, Baggott, and Bouman describe how to use Interpersonal Psychotherapy (IPT), highlighting the need for identifying and addressing the interpersonal factors most closely associated with the unhealthy behavior. This chapter describes a modified version of IPT specifically designed for treating eating disorders and also makes suggestions on how IPT may be used to address NSSI behavior within patients with eating disorders, viewing both behaviors as markers of distress. In the final chapter of *Part II*, Paul Plener and Ulrike Schulze (Chap. 12) deal with the complexities of treating NSSI, ED, and their comorbidity with pharmacological agents. Drawing upon the most current research, these authors discuss how different pharmacological options may impact NSSI and eating disorder behavior both separately and in combination. The authors aim to help readers develop an understanding about when pharmacological interventions might be warranted and also when they are not.

Part III of the book reviews special topics and populations that have received increased attention among researchers and clinicians and represent some of the newest developments in the field pertaining to the coexistence of NSSI and ED. For example, NSSI and ED frequently co-occur with other health-risk behaviors among youth and young adults. Jamie Duggan and Nancy Heath (Chap. 13) review the prevalence of various health-risk behaviors from clinical and community samples of youth and young adults, presenting trends and patterns of both the scope and nature of co-occurring health-risk behaviors in NSSI/ED. Given that both NSSI and eating disorders are body-focused behaviors, Brausch and Muehlenkamp (Chap. 14) provide a comprehensive discussion pertaining to the experiences of the body in both populations. Empirical data is infused with innovative theoretical explanations for why bodily experiences are essential to understanding and treating both behaviors. Treatment suggestions focusing on body-related aspects are also offered. The next two chapters focus on the social influence of peers, which can play a role in the development and maintenance of both NSSI and ED behaviors, via direct and/or indirect contact (e.g., media, internet). Lori Hilt and Emily Hamm (Chap. 15) show that peer relationships can influence both NSSI and disordered eating via mechanisms of social selection and socialization/contagion via modeling. In Chap. 16, Stephen Lewis discusses how online communities and material regarding NSSI and ED are abundant, easily accessible, and may influence the behaviors. He shows that online activities can be positive in a number of ways (e.g., providing support to otherwise isolated individuals) but that they may be detrimental in others (e.g., contributing to continued and unhealthy self-destructive behaviors). Useful suggestions for what therapists need to know and how to address use of online content related to ED and NSSI as part of treatment are also provided. While much of the current literature emphasizes understanding risk factors and developing effective interventions, Lara Cox and Michael Levine (Chap. 17) provide a seminal contribution focused on the prevention and postvention of NSSI and ED. The chapter offers a conceptual and empirical foundation for reducing the incidence of NSSI and eating disorders among adolescents. Specific guidelines for developing integrated interventions at various points along the spectrum of prevention are provided, in addition to offering strategies to consider when addressing postvention for families and friends supporting adolescents who are struggling with disordered eating and/or NSSI. In Chap. 18, Jason Washburn and colleagues focus on the role of primary care practitioners in the treatment of ED and NSSI. Practical guidance is provided for identifying and assessing the severity of ED and NSSI for the primary care practitioners as well as determining the best level of care for someone with these complex conditions. To round out the special topics, Fernando Fernandez-Aranda and colleagues present an overview of NSSI and ED among males, a frequently overlooked and understudied population. Their chapter focuses upon the prevalence and particular features of NSSI and ED in male populations.

It is clear from the chapters of this book that the study of NSSI, ED, and their behavioral co-occurrence is gathering momentum and advancing scientific knowledge designed to address these large public health problems through empirically informed and practical applications. Various mental health professionals and scholars are invested in the theoretical and clinical issues related to the study and treatment of the co-occurrence of NSSI and ED. We hope that this book will not only convey current knowledge and inform current treatment practices but will also provide a framework and stimulus for future research in theory development and the treatment of NSSI and ED.

References

American Psychological Association. (2013). *Diagnostic and statistical manual of mental disorders* (5th ed.). Washington, DC: APA.

Andover, M. S., & Gibb, B. E. (2010). Non-suicidal self-injury attempted suicide, and suicidal intent among psychiatric inpatients. *Psychiatry Research, 178*, 101–105.

Baetens, I., Claes, L., Muehlenkamp, J., Grietens, H., & Onghena, P. (2012). Differences in psychological symptoms and self-competencies in non-suicidal self-injurious Flemish adolescents. *Journal of Adolescence, 35*, 753–759.

Boone, L., Soenens, B., Braet, C., & Goossens, L. (2010). An empirical typology of perfectionism in early-to-mid adolescents and its relation with eating disorder symptoms. *Behaviour Research and Therapy, 48*, 686–691.

Calogero, R. M., Tantleff-Dunn, S., & Thompson, J. K. (Eds.). (2010). *Self-objectification in women. Causes, consequences, and counteractions*. Washington, DC: American Psychological Association.

Cassin, S. E., & Von Ranson, K. M. (2005). Personality and eating disorders. A decade in review. *Clinical Psychology Review, 25*, 895–916.

Chapman, A. L., Gratz, K. L., & Brown, M. Z. (2006). Solving the puzzle of deliberate self-harm: The experiential avoidance model. *Behaviour Research and Therapy, 44*, 371–394.

Claes, L., Houben, A., Vandereycken, W., Bijttebier, P., & Muehlenkamp, J. (2010). Brief report: The Association between non-suicidal self-injury, self-concept and acquaintance with self-injurious peers in a sample of adolescents. *Journal of Adolescence, 33*, 775–778.

Claes, L., Klonsky, E. D., Muehlenkamp, W., Kuppens, P., & Vandereycken, W. (2010). The affect-regulation function of non-suicidal self-injury in eating- disordered patients: Which affect states are regulated? *Comprehensive Psychiatry, 51*, 386–392.

Claes, L., & Muehlenkamp, J. (2013). The relationship between the UPPS-P impulsivity dimensions and non-suicidal self-injury characteristics in male and female high school students. *Hindawi Psychiatry Journal, Special Issue NSSI.*

Claes, L., Muehlenkamp, J., Vandereycken, W., Hamelinck, L., Martens, H., & Claes, S. (2010). Comparison of non-suicidal self-injurious behavior and suicide attempts in patients admitted to a psychiatric crisis unit. *Personality and Individual Differences, 48*, 83–87.

Claes, L., Smits, D., & Bijttebier, P. (2013). The Dutch version of the Emotion Reactivity Scale: Validation and relation with temperament, coping and self-harming behaviors in a sample of high school students. *European Journal of Psychological Assessment.*

Claes, L., Soenens, B., Vansteenkiste, M., & Vandereycken, W. (2012). The scars of the inner critic: Perfectionism and nonsuicidal self-injury in eating disorders. *European Eating Disorders Review, 20*, 196–202.

Claes, L., & Vandereycken, W. (2007). Self-injurious behavior: Differential diagnosis and functional differentiation. *Comprehensive Psychiatry, 48*, 137–144.

Claes, L., Vandereycken, W., & Vertommen, H. (2001). Self-injurious behaviors in eating-disordered patients. *Eating Behaviors, 2*, 263–272.

Claes, L., Vandereycken, W., & Vertommen, H. (2002). Impulsive and compulsive traits in eating disordered patients compared with controls. *Personality and Individual Differences, 32*, 707–714.

Claes, L., Vandereycken, W., & Vertommen, H. (2003). Eating-disordered patients with and without self-injurious behaviors: A comparison of psychopathological features. *European Eating Disorders Review, 11*, 379–396.

Claes, L., Vandereycken, W., & Vertommen, H. (2004). Family environment of eating-disordered patients with and without self-injurious behaviors. *European Psychiatry, 19*, 494–498.

Claes, L., Vandereycken, W., & Vertommen, H. (2005). Impulsivity-related traits in eating disorder patients. *Personality and Individual Differences, 39*, 739–749.

Corstorphine, E., Mountford, V., Tomlinson, S., Waller, G., & Meyer, C. (2007). Distress tolerance in eating disorders. *Eating Behaviors, 8*, 91–97.

Croll, J., Neumark-Sztainer, D., Story, M., & Ireland, M. (2002). Prevalence and risk and protective factors related to disordered eating behaviors among adolescents: Relationship to gender and ethnicity. *Journal of Adolescent Health, 31*, 166–175.

Crosby, R. D., Wonderlich, S. A., Engel, S., Simonich, H., Smyth, J., & Mitchell, J. E. (2009). Daily mood patterns and bulimic behaviors in the natural environment. *Behaviour Research and Therapy, 47*, 181–188.

Diliberto, T. L., & Nock, M. K. (2008). An exploratory study of correlates, onset, and offset of non-suicidal self-injury. *Archives of Suicide Research, 12*, 219–231.

Ghaderi, A., & Berit, S. (2000). Coping in dieting and eating disorders: A population-based study. *Journal of Nervous & Mental Disease, 188*, 273–279.

Glassman, L. H., Weierich, M. R., Hooley, J. M., Deliberto, T. L., & Nock, M. K. (2007). Child maltreatment, non-suicidal self-injury, and the mediating role of self-criticism. *Behaviour Research and Therapy, 45*, 2483–2490.

Glenn, C. R., & Klonsky, E. D. (2010). A multimethod analysis of impulsivity in nonsuicidal self-injury. *Personality Disorders: Theory, Research, and Treatment, 1*, 67–75.

Glenn, C. R., & Klonsky, E. D. (2011). Prospective prediction of nonsuicidal self-injury. A I-year longitudinal study in young adults. *Behavior Therapy, 42*, 751–762.

Gollust, S., Eisenberg, D., & Golberstein, E. (2008). Prevalence and correlates of self-injury among University Students. *Journal of American College Health, 56*, 491–498.

Gratz, K. L. (2001). Measurement of deliberate self-harm: Preliminary data on the Deliberate Self-Harm Inventory. *Journal of Psychopathology and Behavioral Assessment, 23*, 253–263.

Halmi, K. A., et al. (2005). The relation among perfectionism, obsessive-compulsive personality disorder and obsessive-compulsive disorder in individuals with eating disorders. *International Journal of Eating Disorders, 38*, 371–374.

Haynos, A., & Fruzetti, A. (2011). Anorexia nervosa as a disorder of emotion dysregulation: Evidence and treatment implications. *Clinical Psychology: Science & Practice, 18*, 183–202.

Heath, N. L., Toste, J. R., Nedechava, T., & Charlebois, A. (2008). An examination of nonsuicidal self-injury among college students. *Journal of Mental Health Counseling, 30*, 137–156.

Hilt, L. M., Nock, M. K., Lloyd-Richardson, E. E., & Prinstein, M. J. (2008). Longitudinal study of an interpersonal model of non-suicidal self-injury among young adolescents. *Journal of Early Adolescence, 28*, 455–469.

Hoff, E. R., & Muehlenkamp, J. J. (2009). Nonsuicidal self-injury in college students: The role of perfectionism and rumination. *Suicide and Life-Threatening Behavior, 39*, 576–587.

Hudson, J. I., et al. (2007). The prevalence and correlates of eating disorders in the National Comorbidity Survey Replication. *Biological Psychiatry, 61*, 348–358.

Hutchinson, D. M., & Rapee, R. M. (2007). Do friends share similar body image and eating problems? The role of social networks and peer influences in early adolescence. *Behaviour Research and Therapy, 45*, 1557–1577.

Jacobson, C. M., Muehlenkamp, J. J., Miller, A. L., & Turner, E. B. (2008). Psychiatric impairment among adolescents engaging in different types of deliberate self-harm. *Journal of Clinical Child and Adolescent Psychology, 37*, 363–375.

Joiner, T. E. (2005). *Why people die by suicide*. Cambridge, MA: Harvard University Press.

Kingston, J., Clark, S., & Remington, B. (2010). Experiential avoidance and problem behavior: A mediational analysis. *Behavior Modification, 34*, 145–163.

Klonsky, E. D. (2007). The functions of deliberate self-injury: A review of the evidence. *Clinical Psychology Review, 27*, 226–239.

Klonsky, E. D. (2009). The functions of self-injury in young adults who cut themselves: Clarifying the evidence for affect-regulation. *Psychiatry Research, 260–268*.

Klonsky, E. D. (2011). Non-suicidal self-injury in United States adults: Prevalence, socio-demographics, topography and functions. *Psychological Medicine, 41*, 1981–1986.

Klonsky, E. D., & Moyer, A. (2008). Childhood sexual abuse and non-suicidal self-injury: Meta-analysis. *British Journal of Psychiatry, 192*, 166–170.

Klonsky, E. D., Muehlenkamp, J. J., Lewis, S. P., & Walsh, B. (2011). *Nonsuicidal self-injury*. Canada: Hogrefe.

Lloyd-Richardson, E. E., Perrine, N., Dierker, L., & Kelley, M. L. (2007). Characteristics and functions of non-suicidal self-injury in a community sample of adolescents. *Psychological Medicine, 37*, 1183–92.

Lofthouse, N., Muehlenkamp, J., & Adler, R. (2009). Non-suicidal self-injury and co-occurrence. In M. K. Nixon & N. L. Heath (Eds.), *Self-injury in youth: The essential guide to assessment and treatment* (pp. 59–78). New York: Routledge.

Low, G., Jones, D., MacLeod, A., Power, M., & Duggan, C. (2000). Childhood trauma, dissociation and self-harming behavior: A pilot study. *British Journal of Medical Psychology, 73*, 269–278.

Muehlenkamp, J. J., Claes, L., Havertape, L., & Plener, P. L. (2012). International prevalence of adolescent non-suicidal self-injury and deliberate self-harm. *Child and Adolescent Psychiatry and Mental Health, 6*(10), 1–9.

Muehlenkamp, J. J., Claes, L., Peat, C., Smits, D., & Vandereycken, W. (2011). Non-suicidal self-injury in eating disordered patients: A test of a conceptual model. *Psychiatry Research, 188*, 102–108.

Muehlenkamp, J. J., Engel, S. G., Wadeson, A., Crosby, R., Wonderlich, S. A., Simonich, H., et al. (2009). Emotional states preceding and following acts of non-suicidal self-injury in bulimia nervosa patients. *Behaviour Research and Therapy, 47*, 83–87.

Muehlenkamp, J. J., & Kerr, P. L. (2010). Untangling a complex web: How non-suicidal self-injury and suicide attempts differ. *Prevention Researcher, 17*, 8–10.

Muehlenkamp, J. J., Kerr, P. L., Bradley, A. R., & Larsen, M. A. (2010). Abuse subtypes evidence and non-suicidal self-injury. Preliminary evidence of complex emotion regulation patterns. *Journal of Nervous and Mental Disease, 198*, 258–263.

Muehlenkamp, J. J., Peat, C., Claes, L., & Smits, D. (2012). Self-injury and disordered eating: Expressing emotion dysregulation through the body. *Suicide & Life-Threatening Behavior, 42*, 416–425.

Muehlenkamp, J. J., & Saris-Baglama, R. N. (2002). Self-objectification and its psychological outcomes for college women. *Psychology of Women Quarterly, 26*, 371–379.

Muehlenkamp, J. J., Swanson, J. D., & Braush, A. (2005). Self-objectification, risk taking, and self-harm in college women. *Psychology of Women Quarterly, 29*, 24–32.

Nada-Raja, S., Skegg, K., Langley, J., Morrison, D., & Sowerby, P. (2004). Self-harmful behaviors in a population-based sample of young adults. *Suicide and Life-Threatening Behavior, 34*, 177–186.

Najmi, S., Wegner, D. M., & Nock, M. K. (2007). Thought suppression and self-injurious thoughts and behaviors. *Behavior Research and Therapy, 45*, 1957–1965.

Nelson, A., & Muehlenkamp, J. J. (2012). Body attitudes and objectification in non-suicidal self-injury: Comparing males and females. *Archives of Suicide Research, 16*, 1–12.

Neumark-Sztainer, D., Story, M., Hannan, P. J., Beuhring, T., & Resnick, M. D. (2000). Disordered eating among adolescents: Associations with sexual/physical abuse and other familial/psychosocial factors. *International Journal of Eating Disorders, 28*, 249–258.

Nock, M. K. (2009). *Understanding nonsuicidal self-injury. Origins, assessment and treatment.* Washington, DC: American Psychological Association.

Nock, M. K., Joiner, T. E., Gordon, K. H., Lloyd-Richardson, E., & Prinstein, M. J. (2006). Non-suicidal self-injury among adolescents: Diagnostic correlates and relation to suicide attempts. *Psychiatry Research, 144*, 65–72.

Nock, M. K., & Mendes, W. B. (2008). Physiological arousal, distress tolerance, and social problem solving deficits among adolescent self-injurers. *Journal of Consulting and Clinical Psychology, 76*, 28–38.

Nock, M. K., Wedig, M. M., Holmberg, E. B., & Hooley, J. M. (2008). The emotion reactivity scale: Development, evaluation, and relation to self-injurious thoughts and behaviors. *Behavior Therapy, 39*, 107–116.

Paxton, S. J., Schutz, H. K., Wertheim, E. H., & Muir, S. L. (1999). Friendship clique and peer influences on body image concerns, dietary restraint, extreme weight-loss behaviors, and binge eating in adolescent girls. *Journal of Abnormal Psychology, 108*, 255–266.

Peat, C., & Muehlenkamp, J. J. (2011). Objectification, disordered eating, and depression: A test of mediational pathways. *Psychology of Women Quarterly, 35*, 441–450.

Peebles, R., Wilson, J. L., & Lock, J. D. (2011). Self-injury in adolescents with eating disorders: Correlates and provider bias. *Journal of Adolescent Health, 48*(3), 310–313.

Preti, A., Girolamo, G., Vilagut, G., Alonso, J., Graaf, R., Bruffaerts, R., et al. (2009). The epidemiology of eating disorders in six European Countries: Results of the ESEMeD-WMH project. *Journal of Psychiatric Research, 43*, 1125–1132.

Prinstein, M. J., Guerry, J. D., Browne, C. B., & Rancourt, D. (2009). Interpersonal models of nonsuicidal self-injury. In M. K. Nock (Ed.), *Understanding nonsuicidal self-injury: Origins, assessment, and treatment* (pp. 79–98). Washington, DC: American Psychological Association.

Prinstein, M. J., Heilbron, N., Guerry, J. D., Franklin, J. C., Rancourt, D., Simon, V., et al. (2010). Peer influence and nonsuicidal self-injury: Longitudinal results in community and clinically-referred adolescent samples. *Journal of Abnormal Child Psychology, 38*, 669–682.

Rodham, K., & Hawton, K. (2009). Epidemiology and phenomenology of nonsuicidal self-injury. In M. K. Nock (Ed.), *Understanding non-suicidal self-injury: Origins, assessment, and treatment*. Washington, DC: American Psychological Association.

Rosenvinge, J. H., Martinussen, M., & Ostensen, E. (2000). The comorbidity of eating disorders and personality disorders: A meta-analytic review of studies published between 1983 and 1998. *Eating and Weight Disorders, 5*, 52–61.

Serpell, L., Livingstone, A., Neiderman, M., & Lask, B. (2002). Anorexia nervosa: Obsessive–compulsive disorder, obsessive–compulsive personality disorder, or neither? *Clinical Psychology Review, 22*, 647–669.

Shafran, R., Cooper, Z., & Fairburn, C. G. (2002). Clinical perfectionism: A cognitive-behavioural analysis. *Behaviour Research and Therapy, 40*, 773–791.

Smink, F. R. E., van Hoeken, D., & Hoek, H. W. (2012). Epidemiology of eating disorders: Incidence, prevalence and mortality rates. *Current Psychiatry Reports, 14*, 406–414.

Smolak, L., & Murnen, S. K. (2002). A meta-analytic examination of the relationship between sexual abuse and eating disorders. *International Journal of Eating Disorders, 31*, 136–150.

Soenens, B., Vansteenkiste, M., Vandereycken, W., Luyten, P., Sierens, E., & Goossens, L. (2008). Perceived parental psychological control and eating-disordered symptoms. Maladaptive perfectionism as a possible intervening variable. *The Journal of Nervous and Mental Disease, 196*, 144–152.

St. Germain, S. A., & Hooley, J. M. (2012). Direct and indirect forms of non-suicidal self-injury: Evidence for a distinction. *Psychiatry Research, 197*, 78–84.

Svirko, E., & Hawton, K. (2007). Self-injurious behavior and eating disorders: The extent and nature of the association. *Suicide and Life-Threatening Behavior, 37*, 409–421.

Swanson, S. A., Crow, S. J., LeGrange, D., Swendsen, J., & Merikangas, K. R. (2011). Prevalence and correlates of eating disorders in adolescents in the National Comorbidity Survey Replication, Adolescent Supplement. *Archives of General Psychiatry, 68*, 714–23.

Taliaferro, L.A., Muehlenkamp, J.J., Borowsky, I.W., McMorris, B.J., & Kugler, K.C. (2013). Risk factors, protective factors, and co-occurring health-risk behaviors distinguishing self-harm groups: A population-based sample of adolescents. *Academic Pediatrics.*

Treuer, T., Koperdak, M., Rozsa, S., & Füredi, J. (2005). The impact of physical and sexual abuse on body image in eating disorders. *European Eating Disorders Review, 13*, 106–111.

Vanderlinden, J., Vandereycken, W., & Claes, L. (2007). Trauma, dissociation, and impulse dyscontrol: Lessons from the eating disorder field. In E. Vermetten, M. Dorahy, & D. Spiegel (Eds.), *Traumatic dissociation: Neurobiology and treatment* (pp. 317–333). Arlington: American Psychiatric Publishing.

Walsh, B. W. (2012). *Treating self-injury: A practical guide* (2nd ed.). New York, NY: Guilford.

Ward, A., Ramsay, R., & Treasure, J. (2000). Attachment research in eating disorders. *British Journal of Medical Psychology, 73*, 35–51.

Washburn, J. J., Juzwin, K. R., Styer, D. M., & Aldridge, D. (2010). Measuring the urge to self-injury: Preliminary data from a clinical sample. *Psychiatry Research, 178*, 540–544.

Wedig, M. M., & Nock, M. K. (2007). Parental expressed emotion and adolescent self-injury. *Journal of the American Academy of Child and Adolescent Psychiatry, 46*, 1171–1178.

Whiteside, S. P., & Lynam, D. R. (2001). The five-factor model and impulsivity: Using a structural model of personality to understand impulsivity. *Personality and Individual Differences, 30*, 669–689.

Whitlock, J. L., Eckenrode, J., & Silverman, D. (2006). Self-injurious behaviors in a college population. *Pediatrics, 117*, 1939–1948.

Whitlock, J., Muehlenkamp, J., Eckenrode, J., Purington, A., Abrams, G.B., Barreira, P., et al. (2013). Non-suicidal self-injury as a gateway to suicide in young adults. *Journal of Adolescent Health, 52*, 486–492.

Whitlock, J., Muehlenkamp, J., Purington, A., Eckenrode, J., Barreira, J., Abrams, G. B., et al. (2011). Non-suicidal self-injury in a college population: General trends and sex differences. *Journal of American College Health, 59*, 691–698.

Wonderlich, S. (2007). The effects of childhood trauma on daily mood lability and comorbid psychopathology in bulimia nervosa. *Journal of Traumatic Stress, 20*, 77–87.

Yates, T. M., Carlson, E. A., & Egeland, B. (2008). A prospective study of child maltreatment and self-injurious behaviour in a community sample. *Development and Psychology, 20*, 651–671.

Epidemiology and Sociocultural Aspects of Non-suicidal Self-Injury and Eating Disorders

2

Colleen M. Jacobson and Cynthia C. Luik

Abstract

Eating disorders (ED), including anorexia nervosa, bulimia nervosa, and binge-eating disorder, and non-suicidal self-injury (NSSI) are significant public health problems among adolescents and young adults. This chapter reviews the overlap between these behaviors, focusing on epidemiological and sociocultural characteristics that may be related to the high degree of comorbidity within patients. Eating disorders and NSSI fall along the continuum of self-harm, and up to 72 % of people with an ED also engaging in NSSI and up to 54 % of people who engage in NSSI report comorbid eating pathology. The likelihood of engaging in NSSI is greater among patients with purging-type EDs than those with non-purging-type EDs, suggesting an etiological link between purging and NSSI. Those engaging in ED and NSSI are at an increased risk for suicidal behaviors and are likely to have certain comorbidities including Borderline Personality Disorder, depressive symptoms, and substance use. Further, people with comorbid ED and NSSI are at an increased risk for experiencing traumatic events and having negative attitudes toward their bodies. Clinical implications for assessment and treatment of individuals with ED and NSSI are discussed throughout the chapter.

2.1 Introduction

Eating disorders (ED), including bulimia nervosa (BN), anorexia nervosa (AN), and binge-eating disorder (BED), and non-suicidal self-injurious (NSSI) behaviors, including self-cutting and burning, are significant public health problems among adolescents and young adults. Each of these behaviors falls along the continuum of self-harm. Eating disorders may be conceptualized as the less direct, although not

C.M. Jacobson (✉) • C.C. Luik
Department of Psychology, Iona College, New Rochelle, NY, USA
e-mail: cjacobson@iona.edu

L. Claes and J.J. Muehlenkamp (eds.), *Non-Suicidal Self-Injury in Eating Disorders*, DOI 10.1007/978-3-642-40107-7_2,

less severe, form of self-harm characterized by engagement in aberrant eating patterns that may include restricting food intake and/or purging behaviors. NSSI is defined as direct and purposeful damage to body tissue intended to inflict harm but not death to oneself (Jacobson & Gould, 2007). While they seem to fall along the same behavioral continuum, there may be a "dimensional link" between certain types of direct NSSI and purging behaviors common to eating disorders (Favaro, Ferrara & Santonastaso, 2007). Neither eating disorders nor NSSI are suicidal in nature; however, people who suffer from EDs are at increased risk for premature death, both due to all-cause mortality (especially for anorexia nervosa) and suicide (Button, Chadalavada & Palmer, 2010; Crow et al., 2009; Rosling, Sparén, Norring & Knorring, 2011), and those who engage in NSSI are at an elevated risk of suicidal behaviors, and therefore, death, as well (Asarnow et al., 2011).

Although the 12-month prevalence rate of diagnosed eating disorders among adolescents and young adults is relatively low, between 0.3 and 1.6 % for adolescents (Swanson, Crow, LeGrange, Swendsen & Merikangas, 2011) and between 0.5 and 2.15 % for adults (Preti et al., 2009), up to 22 % of adolescents report engaging in some type of disordered eating each year (Jones, Bennett, Olmsted, Lawson & Rodin, 2001). With regard to specific types of eating disorders, estimates suggest a lifetime prevalence rate of 0.5 % for anorexia nervosa, 0.5 % for bulimia nervosa, and 1.12 % for binge-eating disorder among adults (Preti et al., 2009). Among adolescents the lifetime prevalence rate for anorexia nervosa is suggested to be 0.3 %, for bulimia nervosa 0.9 %, and for binge-eating disorder 1.6 % (Swanson et al., 2011). Additionally, up to 27 % of adolescents and 7 % of young adults report engaging in some form of NSSI each year (Lloyd-Richardson, Perrine, Dierker & Kelley, 2007; Whitlock et al., 2011), with between 4 and 12 % of high school students and young adults cutting themselves annually (Gratz, Conrad & Roemer, 2002; Lloyd-Richardson et al., 2007; Whitlock et al., 2011). However, it is important to note that there is a significant amount of overlap between these two behaviors as reported in several empirical research reports. Specifically, up to 72 % of those with eating disorders also engage in NSSI (Claes, Vandereycken & Vertommen, 2001, 2004; Favaro & Santonastaso, 1998; Tobin & Griffing, 1995; see Svirko & Hawton, 2007 for review), and between 25 and 54 % of people who engage in NSSI report comorbid disordered eating (Gollust, Eisenberg & Golberstein, 2008; Herpertz, 1995; Whitlock, Eckenrode & Silverman, 2006).

Due to the high degree of overlap between these two distinct types of behaviors that result in physical harm to oneself, it is likely that there is a common underlying etiology, and it is apparent that they share some phenomenological components linked to epidemiological and sociocultural factors (Svirko & Hawton, 2007). The current chapter will provide a comprehensive overview of the epidemiological and sociocultural aspects of the overlap between eating disorders and non-suicidal self-injurious behaviors. Specifically, we report on the demographic (including gender, age, ethnic, psychiatric profile) and sociocultural (including cultural values, family structure, and life experiences) characteristics of people with eating disorders who also engage in NSSI, and then, conversely, of people who engage in NSSI, who also engage in disordered eating, with the ultimate goal of providing an initial understanding of the mechanisms underlying the overlap and providing implications for clinicians in terms of assessment and treatment for clients engaging in NSSI and/or disordered eating behaviors. To achieve this goal, we reviewed three types of studies: (1) large epidemiological, community-based surveys that assess the presence of both ED and NSSI and report on the overlap and predictors of the different possible combinations of the two (strongest design for purposes of this chapter), (2) general population and clinically based studies that focus on patients with eating disorders primarily and then assess presence of comorbid NSSI, and, finally, (3) general population and clinically based studies that focus primarily on NSSI and also assess comorbidity of ED. The search terms included Eating Disorder, non-suicidal self-injury, self-injurious behaviors, and self-harm behavior. For NSSI, we included only articles that differentiated between NSSI and suicidal behaviors when possible, although some of the earlier articles and/or those conducted in Europe used a definition of NSSI that did not specifically denote absence of suicidal intent within the definition.

2.2 Eating Disorders and NSSI

To most accurately examine the overlap and shared demographic and cultural features of ED and NSSI, a community-based sample in which both behaviors are assessed and reported on separately AND together is needed. To our knowledge only one such study exists. Wright, Bewick, Barkham, House and Hill (2009) assessed the presence of both ED and NSSI among a large sample ($n = 5860$) of university students in the UK over the course of several years using two different questionnaires. For the first questionnaire, the overall recent ("during the current semester") prevalence rate of eating problems fell around 13 %, while the overall presence of recent NSSI was 7.4 %. There were no differences based on gender for either NSSI or ED; however, females were more likely to indicate more extreme problems with eating than males. In terms of overlap, 4.5 % ($n = 227$) of those who completed the first questionnaire endorsed both recent ED and NSSI. Among those who completed the second questionnaire (which included a more in-depth assessment of disordered eating behaviors), 24.7 % of females and 8 % of males had elevated ED symptoms associated with a potential ED, whereas 9.7 % of females and 7 % of males had recently engaged in NSSI. Among the 805 participants who completed the second questionnaire, 4.9 % had a likely ED and recent NSSI. Among the females, there was a significant relationship between engagement in NSSI and disordered eating; however, this was not the case for males, as only one male with an ED also reported NSSI. Interestingly, half of those with a history of NSSI also had a likely ED, whereas 20 % of those with likely ED also engaged in NSSI, suggesting the likelihood of comorbidity is higher among those who self-injure than those with ED. Further, those who had ED and NSSI had an earlier age of onset of their ED symptoms than those with only ED symptoms. This study provides important information regarding the likelihood of comorbidity of NSSI and ED within a large, community sample; however, it fails to answer questions regarding shared or unique risks factors and correlates of engaging in one versus both behaviors.

2.3 The Occurrence of NSSI Among People with Eating Disorders

Prevalence. Quite a large body of research exists that examines the epidemiologic and sociocultural characteristics of people with eating disorders who also engage in self-injurious behaviors. Among people with an eating disorder, the prevalence rates for co-occurring engagement in NSSI range from 12.5 to 72 % (e.g., Anderson, Carter, Mcinstosh, Joyce & Bulik, 2002; Claes, Klonsky, Muehlenkamp, Kuppens & Vandereycken, 2010; Favaro & Santonastaso, 1998; Ruuska, Kaltiala-Heino, Rantanen & Koivisto, 2005; Svirko & Hawton, 2007). There is a large amount of variability across studies that is likely due to a variety of factors including, but not limited to, differing definitions and assessments of ED and NSSI, largely different samples sizes, and use of prospective versus retrospective (i.e., chart review) designs. For example, the study that found the smallest amount of co-occurrence (12.5 %) had 152 participants and only 19 of those participants had BN (Anderson et al., 2002) and the other participants were utilized as controls, whereas the largest amount of co-occurrence (72 %) was found in the study that had over 125 participants with BN (Favaro & Santonastaso, 1998). Peebles, Wilson and Lock (2011) conducted a chart review of 1,432 10–21-year-olds being treated for an eating disorder at an outpatient clinic. NSSI was identified in 40.8 % of patients, although only 50 % of the charts had documented that NSSI was assessed; therefore, this prevalence rate may be an underestimation.

When examining the different subtypes of eating disorders and comorbid NSSI, the ranges in prevalence across studies are also quite large. The prevalence of people who are diagnosed with anorexia and also engage in NSSI ranges from 14.7 to 63.6 % (e.g. Ahrén-Moonga, Holmgren, Von Knorring & Af Klinteberg, 2008; Favaro & Santonastaso, 1996; Ruuska et al., 2005; Wiederman & Pryor, 1995). The prevalence of people who are diagnosed with bulimia and also engage in NSSI ranges from 22.9 to 55.6 % (e.g., Ahrén-Moonga et al., 2008; Claes et al., 2001; Ruuska et al., 2005). The prevalence of people who are diagnosed with ED-NOS, including BED, and also engage in NSSI ranges from 15.8 to 35.8 % (i.e., Favaro & Santonastaso, 1996; Paul, Schroeter, Dahme & Nutzinger, 2002).

Some evidence suggests that bulimic and purging-type eating behaviors are associated with an increased risk for engaging in NSSI compared to having a history of only engaging in restrictive or binge-eating behaviors with no purging. In one of the earlier studies to assess NSSI within ED, Favaro and colleagues (1996) found that NSSI is more common within the patients who engaged in purging behaviors regardless of whether they had anorexia or bulimia. Specifically, approximately one quarter of those with anorexia purging subtype also engaged in NSSI, whereas only 7 % of those who did not purge engaged in NSSI. For those with bulimia, approximately 33 % of those who purged also engaged in NSSI, whereas only 8.6 % of those with bulimia non-purging subtype reported NSSI. Paul et al. (2002) completed a study utilizing 378 female inpatients who were either diagnosed with Eating Disorder-Not Otherwise Specified (ED-NOS), AN, or BN. They found that there are higher rates of NSSI in those with BN and ED-NOS than in those with AN. Ruuska et al. (2005) studied 57 female outpatients who were diagnosed with either AN or BN. They found that both suicidal ideation and NSSI were more common in individuals with BN than individuals with AN. Further, among a group of 422 females being treated on an inpatient unit for ED, those with binge-purging subtypes of ED engaged in NSSI using more methods than those with the other ED types (non-purging), although eating disorder subtype was not significantly associated with frequency or duration of NSSI (Muehlenkamp, Claes, Smits, Peat & Vandereycken, 2011). Finally, in the large chart review study, risk factors for engaging in NSSI included female gender, history of bulimia nervosa, binge-eating disorder with purging, comorbid psychiatric diagnosis, and abuse (Peebles et al., 2011). The stronger link between purging-type EDs and NSSI in comparison to non-purging EDs suggests that purging and NSSI fall close to one another on the self-harm continuum as purging requires more proactive, deliberate action on one's body, similar to NSSI, in comparison to the more passive action of restricting food intake (Favaro et al., 2007). Further, these findings suggest that clinicians should routinely assess for NSSI among patients with ED, especially those who are engaging in purging behaviors.

Age of Onset. Engagement in each type of self-harm behavior (ED and NSSI) is associated with an age of onset in the teen years (NSSI: Jacobson & Gould, 2007; Swanson et al., 2011; ED: American Psychiatric Association, 2000; Kimura, Tonoike, Muroya, Yoshida & Ozaki, 2007; Stice, Killen, Hayward & Taylor, 1998). It is unclear whether there is a difference in age between those who engage in NSSI and those who do not among people with eating disorders; however, there is some evidence to suggest that those who eventually engage in both disordered eating and NSSI may have an earlier age of onset of symptoms than those who only engage in disordered eating (Wright et al., 2009). With regard to "which comes first," some research indicates that the disordered eating is more likely to precede the self-injury than the other way around. For example, Paul et al. (2002) studied 376 female inpatients all with a diagnosis of either AN, BN, or BED. They found that the onset of NSSI occurred after the onset of ED in 49.2 % ($n = 64$) of their participants and the onset of NSSI occurred before the onset of ED in 25.4 % ($n = 33$) of their participants. For the remaining participants the behaviors co-occurred. This study suggests that it is more common for the self-injuring to begin after the development of the eating disorder; however, it is also common that they develop simultaneously. This suggests that clinicians treating patients with eating disorders should not only assess for NSSI at the start of treatment but should continue to do so throughout the course of treatment.

Gender. Eating disorders are more prevalent among women across several studies and meta-analyses (Preti et al., 2009; Swanson et al., 2011), though not all studies find a gender difference (i.e., Wright et al., 2009). A large epidemiological study conducted in the UK did not find a difference based on gender in eating disorder status (Wright et al., 2009); however, this was a self-report study in which no formal assessment of ED was used, and this study did find that females were more likely to report a severe eating problem than males. Conversely, whether NSSI is more common in females, as many believe, is very uncertain with approximately 50 % of empirical studies finding a gender difference, including a large-scale epidemiological study of young adults that found that females were more likely to report lifetime NSSI; however, there was no difference between males and females in past year NSSI (Whitlock et al., 2011). In a recent paper, Latzman et al. (2010) concluded that findings suggest the prevalence of NSSI within the USA seems equal among males and females, whereas data point to a higher rate among females than males outside of the USA (e.g., Europe). However, again, it should be noted that NSSI was equally prevalent among males and females in the large study conducted in the UK by Wright et al. (2009).

The relationship between gender and risk for engaging in NSSI among patients with ED is unclear. One study found that males with ED were more likely than females to also engage in NSSI than females with ED (Gollust et al., 2008). Conversely, in another study being female was associated with a greater risk for engaging in NSSI in a multivariate model predicting NSSI among 1,432 patients in treatment for ED (Peebles et al., 2011).

Ethnicity. Data from large-scale epidemiologic studies within the USA (such as the national comorbidity adolescent replication study) suggest Hispanic adolescents are at elevated risk for bulimia nervosa and possibly BED, while Whites are at increased risk for anorexia (Swanson et al., 2011). The Wright et al. (2009) study found no difference in eating pathology based on ethnicity; however, in this study a very large majority of the participants were White. Regarding NSSI, recent research indicates that the association between ethnicity and NSSI may be quite complex (Gratz et al., 2012; Latzman et al., 2010). When evaluating a main effect of ethnicity on NSSI, some studies of high school students (e.g., Lloyd-Richardson et al., 2007) found a higher rate of NSSI reported by White children, whereas one study of middle school students (Hilt, Nock, Lloyd-Richardson & Prinstein, 2008) and another study of young adults (Wright et al., 2009) did not find a difference in NSSI based on ethnicity. One group of researchers (Gratz et al., 2012; Latzman et al., 2010) identified an interaction between ethnicity and gender in predicting NSSI with African American (AA) boys reporting higher rates of NSSI overall than AA girls, White boys, and White girls among a sample of low SES adolescents. However, it is very interesting to note that while the rate of NSSI was higher among AA boys in middle school, this flipped in high school with White youth engaging in NSSI more frequently. Further, while there was no gender difference in NSSI overall, boys were more likely than girls to engage in burning and hitting.

Very few studies have assessed whether the overlap of NSSI and ED among ED patients varies based upon ethnicity; clearly much more research is needed in this area. Dohm et al. (2002) conducted a study utilizing both Black and White women all with BED ($n = 162$) or BN, purging type ($n = 53$). Nearly 12 % of the White women with bulimia engaged in NSSI and 9.1 % of the Black women with bulimia engaged in NSSI. Of those with BED, 19.6 % of the White women also engaged in NSSI, whereas only 1.7 % ($n = 1$) of the Black women engaged in NSSI. Although this difference in prevalence of comorbid NSSI by ethnicity in the BED group seems very large, it was not significant, likely due to the small sample size and low power.

Psychiatric Comorbidity/Overall Severity. The comorbid psychiatric diagnoses of people with eating disorders and NSSI are similar and include Obsessive Compulsive Disorder (OCD), drug and alcohol abuse, Borderline Personality Disorder (BPD), and depression and anxiety (NSSI: Jacobson, Muehlenkamp, Miller & Turner, 2008; Nock, Joiner, Gordon, Lloyd-Richardson & Prinstein, 2006; ED: Halmi, Marchi, Sampungnaro, Apple & Cohen, 1991; Garfinkel et al., 1995; Wildman, Lilenfeld & Marcus, 2004).

A fair amount of research has addressed whether specific comorbid diagnoses are associated with engagement in NSSI among people with eating disorders (Ahrén-Moonga et al., 2008; Claes, Vandereycken & Vertommen, 2003; Favaro et al., 2008; Lacey, 1993; Peebles et al., 2011; Welch & Fairburn, 1996; Wildman et al., 2004). Findings indicate that the likelihood of having comorbid Borderline Personality Disorder (BPD) among those with eating disorders may be greater if the patient also engaged in NSSI (Claes et al., 2003; Favaro et al., 2008). Although, it is important to note that not all studies have confirmed the association of BPD in people with ED and NSSI in comparison to ED only (i.e., Ahrén-Moonga et al., 2008). There is also some evidence to suggest that the presence of comorbid substance/alcohol abuse is increased in those with eating disorders and NSSI in comparison to those with only ED (Favaro et al., 2008; Lacey, 1993; Peebles et al., 2011). Finally, some evidence suggests rates of mood disorder, including depression and anxiety, may be elevated in people who engage in both NSSI and disordered eating in comparison to those with only ED (Claes et al., 2003; Peebles et al., 2011).

With regard to suicide attempts and completed suicide, although limited research studies have empirically assessed the relationship, it is likely that the risk for engaging in suicidal behaviors is greater among those with comorbid ED and NSSI than in people with ED with no history of self-injurious behaviors. There is a considerable amount of within-person overlap of NSSI and suicide attempts (Jacobson & Gould, 2007). Additionally, NSSI is a risk factor for future suicide attempts (e.g., Asarnow et al., 2011). One study that directly assessed this relationship supports this assumption: among a sample of 95 patients with bulimia nervosa, those who reported impulsive NSSI behaviors, such as cutting, burning, and self-hitting, were at an increased risk for also having engaged in suicide attempts than those who did not (Favaro et al., 2008).

Finally, one unique study examined the comorbidity pattern, including age of onset of different Axis I disorders, among a group of 54 women with eating disorders, half of whom had a history of NSSI and suicide attempts (this group was called the parasuicidal group in this study; Wildman et al., 2004). While we comment on the findings of this study, it is important to note the methodological limitation as suicidal behaviors and NSSI were grouped together. Results indicated that while all women experienced comorbid major depression, an anxiety diagnosis was significantly more common in the suicide/NSSI group. Substance abuse was present in about half of the participants, and the likelihood of this did not differ based on self-harm status. Interestingly, those in the suicide/NSSI group were more likely to have been diagnosed with major depression before the eating disorder than those not in the suicide/NSSI group, while there were no differences based on self-harm status in onset of anxiety or substance use. The implications of this study suggest that clinicians working with patients who are suffering from anxiety and eating disorders should closely monitor for NSSI as well.

Cultural Factors. Both disordered eating behavior and self-injurious behaviors involve an attack on the body that may be driven by a dislike for oneself and one's own body. Both people who engage in NSSI and those with eating disorders seem to have a negative impression of and relationship toward their own bodies that may be related to our cultural values and proclivity toward thinness (e.g., ED: Stice & Shaw, 1994; Striegel-Moore & Bulik, 2007; NSSI: Muehlenkamp, Swanson & Braush, 2005).

Several reports have identified a link between the cultural value of "thin as beautiful" and disordered eating (e.g., Stice & Shaw, 1994; Striegel-Moore & Bulik, 2007). It is hypothesized and supported empirically that internalization of the thin ideal leads to dissatisfaction with one's body which then leads to disordered eating, including bulimia and anorexia (Griffiths et al., 1999, 2000; Stice & Agras, 1998). Additionally, several investigations have noted a link between body dissatisfaction or objectification and risk for engagement in NSSI (Favaro et al., 2007; Muehlenkamp et al., 2005; Nelson & Muehlenkamp, 2012; Ross, Heath & Toste, 2009). Although not yet studied empirically, it is likely that the body dissatisfaction and objectification experienced by those who self-injure may also be linked to the cultural value of thinness. With regards to the co-occurrence of NSSI behaviors within people with eating disorders, a growing body of research suggests that body disgust and dissatisfaction are even more elevated among those with ED who also self-injure than people with ED only (Claes et al., 2003; Muehlenkamp et al., 2011; Solano, Fernandez-Aranda, Lopez & Vallejo, 2005). Thus, clinicians may want to consider assessing and treating body dissatisfaction as part of their work with clients who report both NSSI and ED.

Family Environment. Research indicates that people who engage in disordered eating behaviors or NSSI report increased interpersonal difficulties and poor interpersonal relationships compared to healthy controls (e.g., NSSI: Hankin & Abela,

2011; Hilt et al., 2008; ED: Hartmann, Zeeck & Barrett, 2010; Mcintosh, Bulik, Mckenzie & Jordan, 2000). The interpersonal difficulties experienced may be associated with familial relationships. There are few studies that speak of the effects of family environment in relation to engaging in NSSI among people with eating disorders. Claes et al. (2004) studied 131 female ED patients diagnosed with anorexia restrictive subtype (AN-R), anorexia purging subtype (AN-P), bulimia nervosa purging subtype (BN-P), or bulimia nervosa non-purging subtype (BN-NP), 47.3 % of whom also engaged in NSSI. The patients who self-injured described their family environment as "less cohesive, expressive, and more conflictual (p. 496)" than patients who did not self-injure. These results are quite interesting in light of the fact that there is a growing body of evidence showing that people who engage in NSSI tend to be less emotionally expressive than their non-self-injuring peers (e.g., Gratz, 2006). Living in a family environment where expression of emotions is not encouraged or modeled may lead individuals to internalize the value that expressing oneself to others is not appropriate. Furthermore, in another study completed by Claes, Soenens, Vansteenkiste & Vandereycken (2012), which included 95 women with various eating disorders, 38.9 % of whom engaged in NSSI, those with comorbid NSSI and EDs scored higher on scales of evaluative concerns perfectionism and perceived parental criticism. It was found that evaluative concerns perfectionism partially mediates the relationship between perceived parental concern and NSSI. The authors conclude that women with ED who perceive their parents as critical may internalize that view and become more critical of themselves leaving them at an increased risk for NSSI. This conclusion is consistent with previous research among adolescent self-injurers that found that internalized criticism indeed mediated the relationship between abuse and NSSI (Glassman, Weirich, Hooley, Deliberto & Nock, 2007). As self-criticism appears to play an important role with regard to both ED and NSSI, treatment strategies should target negative cognitions about oneself and aim to increase positive self-talk and feelings of self-worth.

Trauma and Abuse. Difficult experiences during childhood are integral to the development of both eating disorders and NSSI. For example, a history of trauma, specifically, physical and sexual abuse, is associated with increased risk for developing an ED (e.g., Schmidt, Humfress & Treasure, 1997; Steiger et al., 2010; Wonderlich, Brewerton, Jocic, Dansky & Abbott, 1997) and engagement in NSSI (e.g., Klonksy & Moyer, 2008; Lipschitz et al., 1999; Muehlenkamp, Kerr, Bradley & Adams-Larson, 2010; Zoroglu et al., 2003).

There is a growing body of research that has identified a link between experiencing abuse as a child and engagement in NSSI among people with ED. Various studies conducted in both the USA and Europe indicate that abuse of various types (emotional, sexual, and physical) predicts engagement in NSSI among people with ED (Claes et al., 2003; Claes & Vandereycken, 2007; Dohm et al., 2002; Favaro & Santonastaso, 1998; Paul et al., 2002; Tobin & Griffing, 1995). In one study that examined the link between abuse and NSSI within 70 women with severe eating disorders, results indicated that the strength of the relationship between abuse and NSSI varied as a function of specific type of abuse (Claes et al., 2003). Emotional abuse was the least strongly associated with NSSI (although this link was significant and relatively robust) and sexual intimidation was the most strongly associated with NSSI. Additionally, the women who engaged in two or more forms of NSSI reported experiencing more traumatic experiences compared to those who engaged in only one form of NSSI. Finally, there is some evidence to suggest that the association between abuse and NSSI may be indirect in that childhood trauma has an indirect link to NSSI that is expressed via body dissatisfaction, low self-esteem, psychopathology, and dissociation (Muehlenkamp et al., 2011). The apparent link between abuse and NSSI and ED highlights the need for clinicians working with people with ED and NSSI to assess for history of abuse and, if present, assess for PTSD and provide relevant treatment when needed.

2.4 Eating Disorders Within People Who Engage in NSSI

As described above, there is a relatively large body of research that hones in on the presence of NSSI within samples of people with ED. In comparison, there is a small amount of research that has assessed the predictors or correlates of engaging in disordered eating among samples of people who self-injure. This section will review this literature base that dates back to Favazza and Conterio's (1989) early report. Of the studies mentioned in the following section, three include a sample in which the entire sample engaged in NSSI (i.e., Favazza & Conterio, 1989; Herpertz, 1995; Murray, MacDonald & Fox, 2008) and five assessed community samples with a focus on NSSI and examined whether NSSI was a risk for eating pathology (Favaro et al., 2007; Gollust et al., 2008; Hilt et al., 2008; Ross et al., 2009; Whitlock et al., 2006).

The prevalence of eating pathology among those who engage in NSSI ranges from 24 to 61 % (Favazza & Conterio, 1989; Favaro et al., 2007; Gollust et al., 2008; Herpertz, 1995; Whitlock et al., 2006). The large degree of variability across studies is due partially to differences in participant groups, with clinical samples of adults (i.e., Herpertz, 1995) reporting greater comorbidity than samples of university students (e.g., Gollust et al., 2008; Whitlock et al., 2006) or women in the community (Favaro et al., 2007). The type of eating pathology associated with people who engage in NSSI seems to range fairly consistently across anorexia, bulimia, binge eating, and even obesity (Favazza & Conterio, 1989; Hilt et al., 2008; Ross et al., 2009); however, only a few studies have noted formal psychiatric diagnoses of specific eating disorders and most used self-report methods. The one study that assessed NSSI and eating pathology among junior high students confirmed an association between NSSI and aberrant body perception and eating behavior (Hilt et al., 2008). Specifically, among a sample of 508 junior high students, engagement in NSSI was associated with an increased risk for fasting, bingeing, and perception of being overweight, even though those who engaged in NSSI and those who did not were equivalent with regard to actual height and weight. The same is true for a sample of high school students, in which reporting a history of NSSI was associated with an increased risk for bulimia, body dissatisfaction, and desire for thinness (Ross et al., 2009). Interestingly, in that study, frequency of NSSI behaviors was not associated with severity of ED symptoms.

Age of Onset. As noted above, the typical age of onset of NSSI and ED falls in the teen years. Using retrospective methods, Favazza and Conterio (1989) concluded that among the women who engaged in both NSSI and ED, the average age of onset of the ED was 16 years whereas the age of onset for NSSI was 14 years indicating the NSSI preceded the eating pathology in this group.

Gender. Whether gender is associated with likelihood of engaging in eating pathology among those who self-injure is unclear as little research has addressed this question. Interestingly, as referenced above, in one large study of young adults that focused on risk factors for engaging in NSSI, having an eating disorder increased the likelihood of engaging in NSSI for male participants but not female participants (Gollust et al., 2008).

Ethnicity. We are unaware of any studies that have specifically assessed whether people of certain ethnic backgrounds are at increased risk for eating pathology compared to others among people who engage in NSSI. This is another area in need of further research.

Psychiatric Comorbidity/Overall Severity Pathology. Very little research has addressed whether people who self-injure and engage in disordered eating are at elevated risk for certain psychiatric diagnoses and/or suicidal behaviors compared to those who self-injure but do not have co-occurring eating pathology. Herpertz's early investigation of 54 women with severe self-injury concluded that risk for engaging in disordered eating behavior was higher among the women with NSSI and Borderline Personality Disorder than women with NSSI only (Herpertz, 1995). This finding is consistent with the research reviewed in the previous section that found a greater risk for NSSI among women with BPD and eating disorder compared to those with only an eating disorder.

Cultural Factors. As noted in the previous section, dissatisfaction with one's body is associated with engagement in NSSI and disordered eating (e.g., Griffiths et al., 2000; Muehlenkamp et al., 2005). To our knowledge no research has assessed whether body dissatisfaction is elevated among those who self-injure if they also engage in disordered eating; however, it is the case that among those with eating disorders, those who also self-injure have elevated dislike toward their bodies than those who do not self-injure (Claes et al., 2003; Muehlenkamp et al., 2011).

Family Environment. Similarities and/or differences in the family environment among people who engage in NSSI and disordered eating compared to those who only self-injure has not been formally assessed to our knowledge. This is yet another area that is in need of empirical investigation.

Trauma and Abuse. Very little research has specifically focused on whether child abuse or trauma leaves some people who engage in NSSI at risk for engagement in eating disorders as well. Among a sample of 113 young adults with a history of NSSI, having a history of sexual abuse indicated higher eating pathology than no history of sexual abuse (Murray et al., 2008).

2.5 Summary and Concluding Remarks

Both non-suicidal self-injury and disordered eating, in the form of bingeing, purging, and/or restricting, involve harm to one's own body, whether passive or active. Thus, it is not surprising that these two behaviors overlap within people and share many similarities. Among people with eating disorders, up to 72 % may also engage in NSSI (Favaro & Santonastaso, 1998), whereas among people with NSSI, approximately 50 % have been reported to also engage in disordered eating (Herpertz, 1995; Wright et al., 2009). However, as noted throughout the chapter, the prevalence rates of each behavior within the other range greatly due to methodological differences. Further, a fair amount of evidence suggests that among people with eating disorders, those who engage in purging behaviors in general are an increased likelihood of comorbid NSSI than those who do not (i.e., Favaro & Santonastaso, 1996; Peebles et al., 2011), and this may be because purging and self-injury fall closer to one another on the self-harm continuum compared to restricting and self-injury. Additionally, impulsive NSSI, such as cutting, may be more likely to be comorbid with eating pathology than compulsive NSSI, such as hair pulling (Favaro et al., 2007). The high degree of comorbidity of these two self-harm behaviors has clear clinical implications for mental health practitioners. Clinicians are advised to routinely assess for engagement in NSSI behaviors throughout the course of treatment among their ED patients. Conversely, clinicians working with patients who engage in NSSI should assess for comorbid eating pathology.

While it is unclear whether men or women or people of certain ethnicities are more likely to engage in both NSSI and eating disorders, it does seem that there are certain psychiatric diagnoses that are associated with engagement in both forms of these self-harm behaviors, including Borderline Personality Disorder; mood disorders, including depression; and Substance Use Disorder (Claes et al., 2003; Favaro et al., 2008; Peebles et al., 2011). Further, while both NSSI and having a diagnosis of an eating disorder each uniquely leave one at risk for suicide attempts, engaging in NSSI may leave people with ED at an even greater risk than those with ED in the absence of comorbid self-injury (Favaro et al., 2008). Therefore, presence of suicidal ideation and suicidal behaviors should be frequently assessed among patients with comorbid ED and NSSI.

Finally, there are specific cultural values and traumatic experiences that seem to be involved in the development of NSSI and ED individually, in addition to leaving one at risk for both. Internalization of the thin ideal is associated with elevated body dissatisfaction which is associated with increased risk for NSSI among people with eating disorders (Claes et al., 2003; Muehlenkamp et al., 2011). The findings suggest that treatments for patients with comorbid NSSI and ED who express negative attitudes toward their bodies should target the patient's relationship with his/her body and perhaps include cognitive restructuring for negative body distortions. With regard to traumatic experiences, childhood abuse, especially sexual abuse, is associated with increased risk for comorbid NSSI and ED (Claes et al., 2003: Murray et al., 2008). Clinicians should assess for a history of abuse, as well as the psychological sequelae of abuse, within their ED and NSSI patients. Treatments for people who are affected by trauma, ED, and NSSI should be multifaceted and not only target the self-harm behaviors but the symptoms related to the trauma as well.

Both NSSI and eating pathology are detrimental to functioning and associated with increased risk for morbidity and death and represent a significant public health concern, especially among our youth and young adults. Engagement in these two behaviors together is even more concerning. Understanding the demographic, health, and sociocultural factors that are associated with the overlap of these two behaviors is paramount to our efforts to continue to improve understanding, diagnosis, and treatment efforts.

References

Ahrén-Moonga, J., Holmgren, S., Von Knorring, L., & Af Klinteberg, B. (2008). Personality traits and self-injurious behaviour in patients with eating disorders. *European Eating Disorders Review, 16*, 268–275.

American Psychiatric Association. (2000). *Diagnostic and statistical manual for mental disorders, 4th ed, text revision*. Washington, DC: American Psychiatric Association.

Anderson, C. B., Carter, F. A., Mcinstosh, V. V., Joyce, P. R., & Bulik, C. M. (2002). Self-harm and suicide attempts in individuals with bulimia nervosa. *Eating Disorders, 10*, 227–243.

Asarnow, J. R., Porta, G., Spirito, A., Emslie, G., Clarke, G., Wagner, K. D., et al. (2011). Suicide attempts and nonsuicidal self-injury in the treatment of resistant depression in adolescents: Findings from the TORDIA study. *Journal of the American Academy of Child and Adolescent Psychiatry, 50*, 772–781.

Button, E. J., Chadalavada, B., & Palmer, R. L. (2010). Morality and predictors of death in a cohort of patients presenting to an eating disorder service. *International Journal of Eating Disorders, 43*, 387–389.

Claes, L., Klonsky, D., Muehlenkamp, J., Kuppens, P., & Vandereycken, W. (2010). The affect-regulation function of non-suicidal self-injury in eating-disordered patients: Which affect states are regulated? *Comprehensive Psychiatry, 51*, 386–392.

Claes, L., Soenens, B., Vansteenkiste, M., & Vandereycken, W. (2012). The scars of the inner critic: Perfectionism and non-suicidal self-injury in eating disorders. *European Eating Disorders Review, 20*, 196–202.

Claes, L., & Vandereycken, W. (2007). Is there a link between traumatic experiences and self-injurious behaviors in eating-disordered patients? *Eating Disorders, 15*, 305–315.

Claes, L., Vandereycken, W., & Vertommen, H. (2001). Self-injurious behavior in eating-disordered patients. *Eating Behaviors, 2*, 263–272.

Claes, L., Vandereycken, W., & Vertommen, H. (2003). Eating-disordered patients with and without self-injurious behaviours: A comparison of psychopathological features. *European Eating Disorders Review, 11*, 379–396.

Claes, L., Vandereycken, W., & Vertommen, H. (2004). Family environment of eating disordered patients with and without self-injurious behaviors. *European Psychiatry, 19*, 494–498.

Crow, S. J., Peterson, C. B., Swanson, S. C., Raymond, N. E., Specker, S., Eckert, E. D., et al. (2009). Increased mortality in bulimia nervosa and other eating disorders. *American Journal of Psychiatry, 166*, 1342–1346.

Dohm, F., Striegel-Moore, R. H., Wiley, D. E., Pike, K. M., Hook, J., & Fairburn, C. G. (2002). Self-harm and substance use in a community sample of Black and White women with binge and eating disorder or bulimia nervosa. *International Journal of Eating Disorders, 32*, 389–400.

Favaro, A., Ferrara, S., & Santonastaso, P. (2007). Self-injurious behavior in a community sample of young women: Relationship with childhood abuse and other types of self-damaging behaviors. *Journal of Clinical Psychiatry, 68*, 122–130.

Favaro, A., & Santonastaso, P. (1996). Purging behaviors, suicide attempts, and psychiatric symptoms in 398 eating disorder subjects. *International Journal of Eating Disorders, 20*, 99–103.

Favaro, A., & Santonastaso, P. (1998). Impulsive and compulsive self-injurious behavior in bulimia nervosa: Prevalence and psychological correlates. *The Journal of Nervous and Mental Disease, 186*, 156–165.

Favaro, A., Santonastaso, P., Monteleone, P., Bellodi, L., Mauri, M., Rotondo, A., et al. (2008). Self-injurious behavior and attempted suicide in purging bulimia nervosa: Associations with psychiatric comorbidity. *Journal of Affective Disorders, 105*, 285–289.

Favazza, A. R., & Conterio, K. (1989). Female habitual self-mutilators. *Acta Psychiatrica Scandinavia, 79*, 283–289.

Garfinkel, P. E., Lin, E., Goering, P., Spegg, C., Goldbloom, D. S., Kennedy, S., et al. (1995). Bulimia nervosa in a Canadian community sample: Prevalence and comparison of subgroups. *American Journal of Psychiatry, 152*, 1052–1058.

Glassman, L. H., Weirich, M. R., Hooley, J. M., Deliberto, T. L., & Nock, M. K. (2007). Child maltreatment, non-suicidal self-injury, and the mediating role of self-criticism. *Behaviour Research and Therapy, 45*, 2483–2490.

Gollust, S., Eisenberg, D., & Golberstein, E. (2008). Prevalence and correlates of self-injury among university students. *Journal of American College Health, 56*, 491–498.

Gratz, K. L. (2006). Risk factors for deliberate self-harm among female college students: The role and interaction of childhood maltreatment, emotional inexpressivity, and affect intensity/reactivity. *American Journal of Orthopsychiatry, 76*, 238–250.

Gratz, K. L., Conrad, S. D., & Roemer, L. (2002). Risk factors for deliberate self-harm among college students. *American Journal of Orthopsychiatry, 72*, 128–140.

Gratz, K. L., Latzman, R. D., Young, J., Heiden, L. J., Damon, J., Hight, T., et al. (2012). Deliberate self-harm among underserved adolescents: The moderating roles of gender, race, and school-level and association with borderline personality features. *Personality Disorders: Theory, Research, and Treatment, 3*, 39–54.

Griffiths, R. A., Beumont, P. J., Russell, J., Schotte, D., Thornton, C., Touyz, S., et al. (1999). Sociocultural attitudes towards appearance in dieting disordered and non-dieting subjects. *European Eating Disorder Review, 7*, 193–203.

Griffiths, R. A., Mallia-Blanco, R., Boesenburg, E., Ellis, C., Fischer, K., Taylor, M., et al. (2000). Restrained eating and sociocultural attitudes to appearance and general dissatisfaction. *European Eating Disorder Review, 8*, 394–402.

Halmi, K. A., Marchi, P., Sampungnaro, V., Apple, R., & Cohen, J. (1991). Comorbidity of psychiatric diagnoses in anorexia nervosa. *Archives of General Psychiatry, 48*, 712–718.

Hankin, B. L., & Abela, J. R. (2011). Non-suicidal self-injury in adolescence: Prospective rates and risk factors in a 2½ year longitudinal study. *Psychiatry Research, 186*, 65–70.

Hartmann, A., Zeeck, A., & Barrett, M. S. (2010). Interpersonal problems in eating disorders. *International Journal of Eating Disorders, 43*, 619–627.

Herpertz, S. (1995). Self-injurious behavior: Psychopathological and nosological characteristics in subtypes of self-injurers. *Acta Psychiatrica Scandinavica, 91*, 57–68.

Hilt, L. M., Nock, M. K., Lloyd-Richardson, E. E., & Prinstein, M. J. (2008). Longitudinal study of non-suicidal self-injury among young adolescents, rates, correlates, and preliminary test of an interpersonal model. *Journal of Early Adolescence, 28*, 455–469.

Jacobson, C. M., & Gould, M. (2007). The epidemiology and phenomenology of non-suicidal self-injurious behavior among adolescents: A critical review of the literature. *Archives of Suicide Research, 11*, 129–147.

Jacobson, C. M., Muehlenkamp, J. J., Miller, A. L., & Turner, E. B. (2008). Psychiatric impairment among adolescents engaging in different types of deliberate self-harm. *Journal of Clinical Child and Adolescent Psychology, 37*, 363–375.

Jones, J. M., Bennett, S., Olmsted, M. P., Lawson, M. L., & Rodin, G. (2001). Disordered eating attitudes and behaviors in teenaged girls: A school-based study. *Canadian Medical Association Journal, 165*, 547–552.

Kimura, H., Tonoike, T., Muroya, T., Yoshida, K., & Ozaki, N. (2007). Age of onset has Limited association with body mass index at time of for Anorexia Nervosa: Comparison of peak-onset and late-onset Anorexia Nervosa groups. *Psychiatry and Clinical Neurosciences, 61*, 646–650.

Klonksy, E. D., & Moyer, A. (2008). Childhood sexual abuse and non-suicidal self-injury: Meta-analysis. *British Journal of Psychiatry, 192*, 166–170.

Lacey, J. H. (1993). Self-damaging and addictive behaviour in bulimia nervosa. *The British Journal of Psychiatry, 163*, 190–194.

Latzman, R. D., Gratz, K. L., Young, J., Heiden, L. J., Damon, J. D., & Hight, T. L. (2010). Self-injurious thoughts and behaviors among youth in an underserved area of the Southern United States: Exploring the moderating roles of gender, racial/ethnic background, and school-level. *Journal of Youth Adolescence, 39*, 270–280.

Lipschitz, D. S., Winegar, R. K., Nicolaou, A. L., Hartnick, E., Wolfson, M., & Southwick, S. (1999). Perceived abuse and neglect as risk factors for suicidal behaviors in adolescent inpatients. *The Journal of Nervous and Mental Disease, 187*, 32–39.

Lloyd-Richardson, E. E., Perrine, N., Dierker, L., & Kelley, M. L. (2007). Characteristics and functions of non-suicidal self-injury in a community sample of adolescents. *Psychological Medicine, 37*, 1183–1192.

Mcintosh, V. V., Bulik, C. M., Mckenzie, J. M., & Jordan, S. E. (2000). Interpersonal psychotherapy for anorexia nervosa. *International Journal of Eating Disorders, 27*, 125–139.

Muehlenkamp, J. J., Claes, L., Smits, D., Peat, C. M., & Vandereycken, W. (2011). Non-suicidal self-injury in eating disordered patients: A test of a conceptual model. *Psychiatry Research, 188*, 102–108.

Muehlenkamp, J. J., Kerr, P. L., Bradley, A., & Adams-Larson, M. (2010). Abuse subtypes and non-suicidal self-injury: Preliminary evidence of complex emotion regulation patterns. *Journal of Nervous and Mental Disease, 198*, 258–263.

Muehlenkamp, J. J., Swanson, J. D., & Braush, A. (2005). Self-objectification, risk taking, and self-harm in college women. *Psychology of Women Quarterly, 29*, 24–32.

Murray, C., MacDonald, S., & Fox, J. (2008). Body satisfaction, eating disorders and suicide ideation in an internet sample of self-harmers reporting and not reporting childhood sexual abuse. *Psychology Health Medicine, 13*, 29–42.

Nelson, A., & Muehlenkamp, J. J. (2012). Body attitudes and objectification in non-suicidal self-injury: Comparing males and females. *Archives of Suicide Research, 16*, 1–12.

Nock, M., Joiner, T. E., Gordon, K. H., Lloyd-Richardson, E., & Prinstein, M. J. (2006). Non-suicidal self-injury among adolescents: Diagnostic correlates and relation to suicide attempts. *Psychiatry Research, 144*, 65–72.

Paul, T., Schroeter, K., Dahme, B., & Nutzinger, D. (2002). Self-injurious behavior in women with eating disorders. *American Journal of Psychiatry, 159*, 408–411.

Peebles, R., Wilson, J. L., & Lock, J. D. (2011). Self-injury in adolescents with eating disorders: Correlates and provider bias. *Journal of Adolescent Health, 48*, 310–313.

Preti, A., Girolamo, G., Vilagut, G., Alonso, J., Graaf, R., Bruffaerts, R., et al. (2009). The epidemiology of eating disorders in six European countries: Results of the ESEMeD-WMH project. *Journal of Psychiatric Research, 43*, 1125–1132.

Rosling, A. M., Sparén, P., Norring, C., & Knorring, A. (2011). Morality of eating disorders: A follow-up study of treatment in a specialist unit 1974–2000. *International Journal of Eating Disorders, 44*, 304–310.

Ross, S., Heath, N. L., & Toste, J. R. (2009). Non-suicidal self-injury and eating pathology in high school students. *American Journal of Orthopsychiatry, 79*, 83–92.

Ruuska, J., Kaltiala-Heino, R., Rantanen, P., & Koivisto, A. (2005). Psychopathological distress predicts suicidal ideation and self-harm in adolescent eating disorder outpatients. *Europe Child Adolescent Psychiatry, 14*, 276–281.

Schmidt, U., Humfress, H., & Treasure, J. (1997). The role of general family environment and sexual and physical abuse in the origins of eating disorders. *European Eating Disorder Review, 5*, 184–207.

Solano, R., Fernandez-Aranda, A., Lopez, C., & Vallejo, J. (2005). Self-injurious behavior in people with eating disorders. *European Eating Disorder Review, 13*, 3–10.

Steiger, H., Richardson, J., Schmitz, N., Israel, M., Bruce, K. R., & Gauvin, L. (2010). Trait-defined eating-disorder subtypes and history of childhood abuse. *International Journal of Eating Disorders, 43*, 428–432.

Stice, E., & Agras, W. S. (1998). Predicting onset and cessation of bulimic behaviors during adolescence: A longitudinal group analysis. *Behavior Therapy, 29*, 257–276.

Stice, E., Killen, J. D., Hayward, C., & Taylor, C. B. (1998). Age of onset for binge eating and purging during late adolescence: A 4-year survival analysis. *Journal of Abnormal Psychiatry, 107*, 671–675.

Stice, E., & Shaw, H. E. (1994). Adverse effects of the media portrayed thin-ideal on women and linkages to bulimic symptomatology. *Journal of Social and Clinical Psychology, 13*, 288–308.

Striegel-Moore, R. H., & Bulik, C. M. (2007). Risk factors for eating disorders. *American Psychologist, 62*, 181–198.

Svirko, E., & Hawton, K. (2007). Self-injurious behavior and eating disorders: The extent and nature of the association. *Suicide and Life-Threatening Behavior, 37*, 409–421.

Swanson, S. A., Crow, S. J., LeGrange, D., Swendsen, J., & Merikangas, K. R. (2011). Prevalence and correlates of eating disorders in adolescents: Results from the national co-morbidity survey replication adolescent sample. *Archives of General Psychiatry, 68*, 714–723.

Tobin, D. L., & Griffing, A. S. (1995). Coping, sexual abuse, and compensatory behavior. *International Journal of Eating Disorders, 20*, 143–148.

Welch, S. L., & Fairburn, C. G. (1996). Impulsive or comorbidity in bulimia nervosa: A controlled study of deliberate self-harm and alcohol and drug misuse in a community sample. *The British Journal of Psychiatry, 169*, 451–458.

Whitlock, J., Eckenrode, J., & Silverman, D. (2006). Self-injurious behaviors in a college population. *Pediatrics, 117*, 1939–1948.

Whitlock, J., Muehlenkamp, J., Purington, A., Eckenrode, J., Barreira, P., Abrams, G. B., et al. (2011). Nonsuicidal self-injury in a college population: General trends and sexual differences. *Journal of American College Health, 59*, 691–698.

Wiederman, M. W., & Pryor, T. (1995). Multi-impulsivity among women with bulimia nervosa. *International Journal of Eating Disorders, 20*, 359–365.

Wildman, P., Lilenfeld, L. R., & Marcus, M. D. (2004). Axis I comorbidity onset and parasuicide in women with Eating Disorders. *International Journal of Eating Disorders, 35*, 190–197.

Wonderlich, S. A., Brewerton, T. D., Jocic, Z., Dansky, B., & Abbott, D. W. (1997). Relationship of childhood sexual abuse and eating disorders. *Journal of the American Academy of Child and Adolescent Psychiatry, 36*, 1107–1115.

Wright, F., Bewick, B. M., Barkham, M., House, A. O., & Hill, A. J. (2009). Co-occurrence of self-reported disordered eating and self-harm in UK university students. *British Journal of Clinical Psychology, 48*, 397–410.

Zoroglu, S. S., Tuzun, U., Sar, V., Tutkin, H., Savas, H. A., et al. (2003). Suicide attempt and self-mutilation among Turkish high school students in relation with abuse, neglect, and dissociation. *Psychiatry and Clinical Neurosciences, 57*, 119–126.

Developmental Influences in NSSI and Eating Pathology

3

Andrea L. Barrocas, Jill M. Holm-Denoma, and Benjamin L. Hankin

Abstract

Developmental psychopathology perspectives can help in formulating better conceptualizations of the origins of factors that impact the onset, maintenance, and treatment of EDs and NSSI. This chapter examines several specific vulnerabilities for both outcomes. The broader literature on developmental psychopathology theories is explored, including the importance of temporal order of variables, transactional associations, and concepts such as equifinality and multifinality that may be important for understanding the development of NSSI and/or EDs in youth. In addition, this chapter reviews several specific methodological issues (e.g., design, sampling) that are important to consider when studying NSSI and EDs among youth. Finally, a clinical vignette helps to demonstrate how NSSI and EDs can co-occur as a result of similar risks and vulnerabilities during childhood and adolescence. Throughout this chapter, there are suggested areas for future research (e.g., comorbidity rates between NSSI and EDs among youth) that will be important to assess using a developmental lens in the coming years as well as suggestions for clinicians wanting to practice in a developmentally sensitive manner.

3.1 Introduction

Of those individuals who have been diagnosed with an eating disorder (ED) and who have engaged in nonsuicidal self-injury (NSSI) during their lifetime, many report that they first became symptomatic during youth (e.g., Rodham & Hawton, 2009; Swanson, Crow, Le Grange, Swendsen, & Merikangas, 2011). Additionally, vulnerabilities for engaging in NSSI or developing an ED typically appear early in life even for those who do not develop symptoms until adulthood (e.g., Hoek & Van

A.L. Barrocas (✉) • J.M. Holm-Denoma • B.L. Hankin
Department of Psychology, University of Denver, Denver, CO, USA
e-mail: andrea.barrocas@du.edu

L. Claes and J.J. Muehlenkamp (eds.), *Non-Suicidal Self-Injury in Eating Disorders*, DOI 10.1007/978-3-642-40107-7_3, © Springer-Verlag Berlin Heidelberg 2014

Hoeken, 2003). Given the high comorbidity rate between EDs and NSSI (e.g., Muehlenkamp, Claes, Smits, Peat, & Vandereycken, 2011), the fact that they both often co-occur with certain other syndromes (e.g., borderline personality disorder; Linehan, 1993), and the knowledge that there are many common risk and vulnerability factors for EDs and NSSI, taking a developmental psychopathology approach to understanding the overlap between EDs and NSSI may be valuable. Specifically, developmental psychopathology perspectives can help in formulating better conceptualizations of the origins of factors that impact the onset, maintenance, and treatment of EDs and NSSI.

This chapter takes a developmental psychopathology approach to understanding NSSI and EDs, as well as their vulnerability and protective factors. First, we briefly add to the epidemiological data on NSSI and EDs in youth already presented elsewhere in this book (Chap. 2). Second, we examine several specific vulnerabilities for NSSI and EDs. However, we do not discuss vulnerabilities for co-occurring NSSI and EDs among youth samples because there is very little research examining this topic at the current time (see Ohmann & Popow, 2012 for a review of exceptions). Third, we consider the broader literature on developmental psychopathology theories, including the importance of temporal order of variables, transactional associations, and concepts such as equifinality and multifinality that may be important for understanding the development of NSSI and/or EDs in youth. Fourth, we discuss several specific methodological issues (e.g., design, sampling) that are important to consider when studying NSSI and EDs among youth. Fifth, we explore how developmental psychopathology researchers studying NSSI can learn from the ED literature to expand upon what is already known in a developmentally sensitive manner. Finally, a clinical vignette helps to demonstrate how NSSI and EDs can co-occur as a result of similar risks and vulnerabilities during childhood and adolescence. Throughout this chapter, we include suggestions for how clinicians can enhance a developmentally sensitive practice to treating clients in their youth with NSSI and/or ED.

3.2 Epidemiology of NSSI and EDs in Youth

Whereas rates of diagnosed EDs are relatively low among adolescents, in contrast, NSSI engagement appears to increase across development and affects many youth and adolescents (Rodham & Hawton, 2009). Rates of EDs are about less than 1 % in adolescence (Swanson et al., 2011), yet 13.9–21.4 % of high school adolescents report NSSI (grades 9–12, mean age 16; Muehlenkamp & Gutierrez, 2004). Rates of both behaviors are even lower in samples of younger youth. In addition, diagnosed EDs tend to have their onset around the teenage and emerging adulthood years (American Psychiatric Association, 2000) and NSSI seems to emerge earlier (middle childhood to adolescence; see Barrocas, Hankin, Abela, & Young, 2012). A more extensive review of the epidemiology of NSSI can be found in Chap. 2 of this book.

Results from research on gender differences in NSSI in youth have been mixed, with some studies suggesting that girls engage in NSSI more than boys (Guerry & Prinstein, 2010; Muehlenkamp & Gutierrez, 2007; Ross & Heath, 2002) and other research showing no gender differences (Hilt, Nock, Lloyd-Richardson, & Prinstein, 2008; Muehlenkamp & Gutierrez, 2004). Recent research by Barrocas et al. (2012) found that older adolescent girls reported higher rates of NSSI engagement than boys of the same age; however, younger youth in this community sample showed no gender differences. Thus, it seems likely that the gender difference in NSSI engagement changes over the course of development. In contrast, research has consistently shown that females exhibit symptoms of EDs and receive ED diagnoses more commonly than males (e.g., Croll, Neumark-Sztainer, Story, & Ireland, 2002; Johnson & Connors, 1987; Swanson et al., 2011). However, the little research on clinically significant EDs in males has demonstrated that males with EDs have similar clinical presentations to females with EDs (e.g., Darcy et al., 2012; Geist, Heinmaa, Katzman, & Stephens, 1999).

3.3 Factors That Confer Vulnerability for NSSI and ED

To date, no epidemiological data on the comorbidity rate of NSSI and EDs among youth has been published. Further, most of the literature on correlates, risks, vulnerabilities, and treatment for both NSSI and EDs has used late adolescent, young adult (i.e., college age), or adult samples. However, emerging literature has consistently identified certain vulnerability factors for NSSI and EDs. Figure 3.1 shows a non-exhaustive list of vulnerabilities for NSSI and EDs that have been investigated in youth and adult samples and the significant overlap between vulnerabilities for these two outcomes. Space considerations do not permit a comprehensive summary of all of these vulnerabilities; therefore we focus our literature review on those factors for which empirical research has established these vulnerabilities for NSSI and EDs in *youth* (i.e., child and adolescent) samples (as opposed to only adult samples).

3.3.1 Vulnerabilities for NSSI in Youth

3.3.1.1 Parenting and Family Influences

Parenting behaviors and styles exert a significant role in child and adolescent development, and youths' views about their self and the world are greatly impacted by their parents (Darling & Steinberg, 1993). Children raised with insensitive and inconsistent parenting are at elevated risk for engaging in NSSI later in life. In fact, Sim, Adrian, Zeman, Cassano, and Friedrich (2009) found that adolescents who engaged in NSSI reported higher levels of invalidation from caregivers than adolescents who did not engage in NSSI.

Similarly, abused children often use avoidant emotional responses (Eisenberg, Cumberland, & Spinrad, 1998; Krause, Mendelson, & Lynch, 2003). These

Fig. 3.1 Vulnerabilities for NSSI and ED in youth. *Note*: This list of vulnerabilities for NSSI and ED is not exhaustive, although encompasses many of the known vulnerabilities in children, adolescents, and adults. We chose to depict what is unknown as a question mark in order show that these may still be vulnerabilities, yet those which are not yet established by empirical research

Vulnerability	NSSI	ED
Trauma	√	√
Parenting	√	√
Peer Influences	√	√
Negative Emotions	√	√
Emotion Regulation	√	√
Cognitive Vulnerability	√	?
Body Dissatisfaction	√	√
Genes	?	√
Culture	?	√
Gender	√	√
Early Puberty	?	√

children are punished for whatever emotion regulation strategy they choose and, as a result, may oscillate back and forth between suppressing emotional responses and having intense emotional responses (Linehan, 1993). They also lack the proper tools to identify, evaluate, and communicate emotional states to others (Yates, 2009). Consequently, sexual abuse, physical abuse, parental emotional neglect, parental overprotection, and control have been shown to be significant predictors of the frequency of NSSI (Gratz, 2003, 2006; Gratz, Conrad, & Roemer, 2002). Of note, Klonsky and Moyer (2008) caution to not overestimate the role of sexual abuse with NSSI, given that when other psychiatric risk factors are controlled for in statistical analyses, sexual abuse no longer predicts NSSI engagement.

3.3.1.2 Peer Influences

The increase in significance of peer relationships that characterizes the transition to adolescence occurs during the same developmental time frame as the rise of NSSI (Kessler, Berglund, Borges, Nock, & Wang, 2005). Several theories suggest that peer relationships during adolescence play an important role in the etiology, maintenance, and exacerbation of NSSI (e.g., Heilbron & Prinstein, 2008, see Prinstein, Guerry, Browne, & Rancourt, 2009). In addition, research suggests that interpersonal events may be especially relevant for NSSI. For example, interpersonal problems (e.g., peer conflict, peer rejection) are concurrently and longitudinally associated with suicidal ideation and behaviors and frequently precipitate suicidal behavior (Prinstein, Boegers, & Spirito, 2001; Rigby & Slee, 1999). Peer victimization has also been shown to be a correlate of NSSI in youth (Heilbron & Prinstein, 2010).

Heilbron and Prinstein (2008) have also offered a framework for the mechanisms of peer influence and peer contagion on NSSI. They suggest the possibility that youth may observe peers obtaining positive social reinforcement (e.g., high status, attention) when engaging in NSSI, which may lead to emulating NSSI behavior (i.e., through social learning; Bandura, 1973). Several studies demonstrate that NSSI enacted by one patient in a psychiatric treatment facility is associated with increases in other patients' NSSI behavior (e.g., Ghaziuddin, Tsai, Naylor, & Ghaziuddin, 1992; Rosen & Walsh, 1989). Additional detail about peer influences is included in Chap. 15.

3.3.1.3 Emotion Regulation Difficulties

Individuals typically engage in NSSI behaviors to alleviate emotional distress or negative affect (Brown, Comtois, & Linehan, 2002; Chapman, Gratz, & Brown, 2006). Theoretical models propose that individuals who engage in NSSI are more emotionally dysregulated and are more likely to use NSSI as a means of coping than their peers who do not engage in NSSI (Chapman et al., 2006; Darche, 1990; Suyemoto & MacDonald, 1995). For example, adolescents report having strong feelings of sadness and anger prior to engaging in NSSI (Nock, Prinstein, & Sterba, 2009) and perceiving these emotions as being overwhelming and uncontrollable (Chapman et al., 2006).

3.3.1.4 Body Dissatisfaction

An emerging body of evidence suggests that body dissatisfaction may confer vulnerability for NSSI in youth and young adults (Claes, Houben, Vandereycken, Bijttebier, & Muehlenkamp, 2010; Muehlenkamp et al., 2011, 2012, Muehlenkamp, Peat, Claes, & Smits, 2012). For example, adolescents who report engaging in NSSI also report higher rates of ED pathology (Ross et al., 2009). Further, Muehlenkamp and Brausch (2012) have shown that body image significantly mediates the association from negative affect to NSSI engagement in adolescents, suggesting the importance of assessing for and focusing clinically on body regard and body dissatisfaction in, specifically, older youth seeking treatment for NSSI.

3.3.2 Vulnerabilities for EDs in Youth

3.3.2.1 Parenting and Family Influences

One's family of origin may impact their likelihood of developing an ED. First, from a biological standpoint, women with EDs are much more likely to have first-degree female relatives who are also symptomatic than those without EDs (Strober et al., 2001). Further, twin studies have uncovered a significant genetic vulnerability for AN (Jacobi et al., 2004) and BN (e.g., Silberg & Bulik, 2005).

Second, families may impact the onset of EDs through modeling and/or interpersonal patterns. For instance, children of moms with EDs show elevated ED symptoms (Stein et al., 2006), and moms of children with EDs exhibit increased rates of eating pathology (Pike & Rodin, 1991). Longitudinal research has also shown that young girls whose moms were overly concerned with their own body image restricted their daughters' food intake and made verbal requests for their daughters to lose weight (Francis & Birch, 2005). The daughters were consequently observed to engage in restrictive eating practices (Francis & Birch, 2005).

3.3.2.2 Peer Influences

Peer influences are also known to place youth at risk for disordered eating and body dissatisfaction, and much research has established this relationship in adolescent females (e.g., Jones, 2004; Jones et al., 2004; Schutz & Paxton, 2007). For example, Schutz and Paxton (2007) assessed tenth grade girls' perceptions of their friendships, finding that higher conflict and alienation were related to greater dissatisfaction with one's body and more disordered eating. Further, peer appearance culture (Jones, 2004), defined as the peer norms that shape how groups of friends view the importance of their appearance which is then internalized by individuals in the group (see Clark & Tiggeman, 2006), has emerged as an important vulnerability for body dissatisfaction and EDs in youth. When peers value thinness and discuss this among members of the peer group at high rates, there tends to be a relatively high amount of body dissatisfaction among both male and female youth (Clark & Tiggeman, 2006).

3.3.2.3 Negative Affect and/or Depression

Past studies have also demonstrated that high rates of negative affect give rise to eating pathology among youth (e.g., Stice et al., 2002). For instance, one longitudinal study of a community sample demonstrated that among both boys and girls, symptoms of depression at age 10 predicted ED symptoms at age 14 (Gardner et al., 2000). Further, a study of a community sample of adolescent girls ages 12–19 suggested that initial depression predicted increased eating pathology over time, but not vice versa (Measelle et al., 2006). It is worth noting that although negative affect and depression confer increased risk for EDs, they are not specific risk factors (i.e., negative affect predicts other negative psychological outcomes as well; Clark et al., 1994).

3.3.2.4 Early Puberty

Early onset of puberty is another risk factor for ED development, at least among girls (Graber et al., 1997; Stice et al., 2001). In fact, age of puberty onset is more important than chronological age in the prediction of disordered eating among female youth (Killen et al., 1992). This may be because postpubertal girls typically experience declines in self-esteem and increases in body dissatisfaction as physical maturation occurs (Siegel et al., 1999), perhaps as a result of the normative increase in body fat that occurs during this period of maturation that leads girls to believe that they are moving away from the western thin-ideal. The link between pubertal status and EDs among boys has been less consistent, with some researchers finding no link between pubertal timing and EDs (Keel et al., 1997) and others finding that early puberty is predictive of heightened ED pathology (e.g., Field et al., 1999).

3.3.2.5 Body Dissatisfaction

Body dissatisfaction is a well-replicated risk factor for the development of ED symptoms and EDs, especially among girls. For instance, researchers have documented that body dissatisfaction among girls at ages 5 and 7 predicts higher rates of dietary restraint and maladaptive eating attitudes at age 9 (Davison et al., 2003). Prospective studies have also shown that body dissatisfaction predicts increases in ED symptoms during junior high (Ferreiro et al., 2012) and high school (Leon et al., 1993). Finally, one prospective study demonstrated that high levels of body dissatisfaction predicted the onset of clinically significant disordered eating among adolescent girls (Stice et al., 2011). The literature regarding body dissatisfaction as a risk for EDs among male youth is less abundant; however, one prospective study demonstrated that poor body image among fifth and sixth grade boys predicted heightened eating pathology 1 year later (Keel et al., 1997).

3.4 How Developmental Psychopathology Can Inform Knowledge of NSSI and EDs

A developmental psychopathology approach can provide many different avenues for understanding NSSI, EDs, and the overlap between these two outcomes. The study of developmental psychopathology includes learning about the origins, onset, and course of psychopathological outcomes as well as how other factors, such as age and time, may influence such outcomes (Sroufe & Rutter, 1984). In this section of the chapter, we introduce developmental psychopathology concepts and models, although it is not possible to go into an extensive discussion of these concepts. We hope to illuminate not only the importance of considering this approach when researching and treating youth with NSSI and EDs but also how this approach can lead to novel ideas for future research on the relationship between these outcomes.

3.4.1 The Temporal Order of Risks and Outcomes: Timing Matters

Temporal order refers to the arrangement of two or more factors in time or, in other words, the notion of "what comes first." There are several ways in which temporal order may play a role in a developmental psychopathology approach to understanding NSSI and EDs. First, it is important to understand which risk and vulnerability factors precede the onset of a psychopathological outcome and in what order (i.e., using longitudinal research). Second, we can learn if there is a typical pattern in the development of different outcomes in youth (e.g., AN develops before BN). To best understand how factors lead to the onset or recurrence of an outcome, it is imperative that longitudinal research establishes that the risk factor precedes the outcome.

Risk and vulnerability factors can be distal or proximal to the outcome of interest. For example, Nock et al. (2009) have shown that negative emotions, such as feeling sad, overwhelmed, and worthless, immediately precede engagement in NSSI. This would be considered a proximal risk factor. Risk factors may also be more distal or farther away in time. For example, Hankin and Abela (2011) found that low social support prospectively predicted NSSI 2½ years later among youth ages 11–14. Finally, research on risks in early childhood, such as sexual abuse or other experiences of trauma, constitutes another example of distal risks for NSSI engagement and ED pathology (see Linehan, 1993). It is possible that temporal associations between risks and outcomes change over development as well. For instance, the role of a traumatic experience may impact the onset of NSSI or EDs one way if the trauma occurs in early childhood and differently if it occurs in adolescent years.

To date, no research has examined the temporal order of both NSSI and ED in youth. Are NSSI and EDs sequential, such that youth reliably exhibit symptoms of one outcome before the other? Further, if the temporal order of NSSI and EDs do not reliably occur in one direction, what are some specific risk factors that may predispose youth to develop one before the other? Future researchers should examine these questions.

As research progresses, it will become easier for clinicians to use knowledge about proximal and distal risks to inform intervention. For instance, clinicians who know that children who have experienced trauma are at an increased risk for developing NSSI and/or EDs could use empirically based prevention methods (e.g., Stice et al., 2000). It is also possible that treatments that have shown efficacy in decreasing disordered eating and NSSI (e.g., Dialectical Behavior Therapy; DBT; Linehan, 1993) would be useful in treating proximal and/or distal risk factors for NSSI and EDs.

3.4.2 The Course of an Outcome: Developmental Pathways

A developmental pathway differs from the simple notion of temporal order in that one factor not only precedes another in time, but also is partly responsible for the ontogeny and development of the next. The most commonly used approach to developmental pathway models consists of conceptualizing a chain of factors, which can be comprised of both risks and outcomes. For example, researchers may look at a succession of factors over time in the following manner; a history of abuse (distal risk) may lead to an individual experiencing higher levels of low self-worth and rumination (distal vulnerabilities), which might then lead to NSSI and/or EDs (outcomes of interest) in the face of specific stressors (proximal factors).

Thinking about developmental pathways can also mean observing the course of an outcome over time, as well as specific risk factors that may serve as predictors of these courses. This can also be done by establishing the course, continuity, and desistance of one outcome over time or by assessing diagnostic crossover patterns. Research using adult samples has begun to establish the rate of diagnostic crossover in ED samples. For example, Eddy et al. (2008) found that women with AN at baseline were likely to crossover between restricting and binge/purging subtypes of

AN and to BN over a 7-year time frame, but women with BN at baseline were not likely to crossover.

To best understand the developmental unfolding of both EDs and NSSI, it is necessary to establish the course of these outcomes (i.e., continuity, desistance, crossover) beginning in childhood and adolescence when the onset of these outcomes is especially high. Research-based investigations of this nature will likely help clinicians identify the best intervention strategies (e.g., if a teen presents with NSSI engagement and eating pathology following a childhood trauma and recent interpersonal distress, would Trauma-Focused Cognitive Behavior Therapy (TF-CBT; Cohen et al., 2001) or DBT be preferable?). Clinicians may also aim to assess the timing and succession of NSSI and ED symptoms to determine if one outcome may have propagated the presence of the other, in order to guide treatment efforts.

3.4.3 Individuals Take Different Courses: Equifinality and Multifinality

The idea of psychopathological heterogeneity imparts that not all individuals with the same outcome follow the same course. In addition, individuals who experience the same risk or vulnerability factor may not all develop the same outcome. As such, it is important to consider equifinality and multifinality for NSSI and EDs in youth.

Equifinality would suggest that not all individuals who both engage in NSSI and have an ED exhibit the same risk factors. More specifically, some youth with NSSI and EDs may have experienced a significant trauma earlier in their lifetime and report high levels of dissociating compared to others, whereas other youth may report high levels of negative affect without any childhood trauma. This fact highlights the importance of clinicians assessing a variety of risk factors for NSSI and/or EDs, as the case conceptualization for a given client will vary with the risk factors she/he has experienced.

Further, multifinality suggests that a group of individuals may experience the same risk factors but develop different outcomes (i.e., some youth who experience a given risk factor may develop EDs, whereas others may engage in NSSI, and others still may not show signs of any psychopathology). For example, high levels of interpersonal stress and negative affect may be vulnerability factors that lead to different pathological outcomes, including various forms of EDs and NSSI. As such, clinicians who become aware that a given client has experienced a risk factor for either EDs or NSSI should routinely assess both outcomes, even if only one is mentioned as the presenting problem.

Figure 3.1 suggests that both equifinality and multifinality exist for NSSI and EDs in youth. There seem to be a preponderance of overlapping, or shared, risk and vulnerability factors for NSSI and EDs (e.g., trauma, parenting, peers, negative emotions, emotion regulation, gender) as well as specific risks and vulnerabilities that may exist for each separately (e.g., cognitive vulnerability for NSSI, culture, puberty, and culture for EDs). Future research should begin to determine which specific risks and vulnerabilities explain the co-occurrence and overlapping trajectories of NSSI and EDs in youth, specifically which factors maintain their predictability above and beyond the others.

3.5 Research Design Concerns: Specific Methodological and Sample Characteristics

3.5.1 Developmental Influences Change as Youth Get Older: Age

Developmental psychopathology research highlights the importance of changes that occur as individuals age and mature. At times, some psychopathology research has tended to overlook the developmental changes that occur as youth get older, such as how the role of peers changes over time or the impact pubertal changes may have on biological influences for behavior. Failing to consider these developmental changes is a mistake, however, as they have implications for understanding the onset, course, and treatment of psychopathology outcomes.

Conceptualizing vulnerability for NSSI and EDs can change as individuals age; the biological, interpersonal, and intrapersonal influences for the onset and course of NSSI and EDs may be different due to changes that occur in body and changes on social patterns. For example, we may think of the mechanisms behind a school-age child developing ED symptoms (e.g., influences within the family) differently than those that might lead a teenager to develop the same symptoms (e.g., early puberty for a female youth). Further, the same notion has implications for treatment of NSSI and ED. For example, a young boy who hits his head against the wall when angry would require a different treatment approach than a teenage girl who cuts herself. The clinical approach one would take working with a young boy engaging in NSSI is likely to be more behavioral in nature due to the limited cognitive abilities in younger children, whereas a teenage girl who frequently cuts herself would probably entail a more cognitively based therapy approach to help her understand what emotions she is trying to regulate with her NSSI engagement. Therefore, considering the age and developmental stage one is in is imperative when taking a developmental psychopathology approach to understanding the onset and course of NSSI and EDs and symptoms of these outcomes.

3.5.2 Clinical vs. Community Samples

Much of the extant research on NSSI and EDs in youth has been conducted with inpatient and outpatient psychiatric samples. Information on the risk and vulnerability factors, correlates, consequences, and functions of these outcomes in clinical samples of youth is extremely important. Yet, research with clinical samples exhibits known and problematic biases. For example, Goodman et al. (1997) showed that adolescents using outpatient mental health services had greater severity of psychiatric disorder and higher rates of comorbidity compared to peers not using these services. Moreover, research employing clinical samples is more prone to Berkson's bias (Goodman et al., 1997), a specific selection bias with clinical samples where some individuals with a certain outcome may use clinical services at greater rate than others and, therefore, be observed with this outcome at a greater rate. Effect sizes also tend to be less accurate and appropriate (both with regard to over and underestimation of effect sizes) in clinical samples (Cohen & Cohen, 1984). Using community samples for clinical outcomes has risks as well. Rates of psychiatric outcomes are lower in community samples, which makes the power for studying these outcomes difficult at times, and risks and vulnerabilities for psychiatric outcomes can sometimes vary for those with more severe symptoms and diagnoses vs. those with less severe and only sub-threshold symptoms (which is often more common in community samples). Given these known biases in psychiatric clinical samples and risks associated with community samples, it is equally as important to investigate NSSI and EDs using both clinical and community samples.

3.5.3 Gender

There are many different factors related to gender that need to be considered when thinking about NSSI and EDs from a developmental psychopathology approach, such as theoretical reasons that gender differences exist for certain types of psychopathology and methodological considerations that impact our understanding of the role of gender on these outcomes. We have briefly discussed general gender differences in NSSI and EDs, showing that for the most part, both outcomes seem to have greater prevalence among females. Similar trends have been found in other epidemiological studies of mental health outcomes in youth, and the broader developmental epidemiological literature shows a greater preponderance of emotional disorders for girls, compared to boys, starting with the adolescent transition (Kessler, 2003; Rodham et al., 2004). Theorists have proposed two types of models to understand the role of gender in developmental psychopathology. First, some theorists (e.g., Hankin & Abramson, 2001) suggest models whereby general pathways to psychopathology outcomes may be similar for males and females. According to this type of model, gender differences exist because being of a specific gender places certain individuals at greater risk to develop a given condition due to risks associated with this gender. In contrast to a general model, others have argued that gender-specific pathways exist in the emergence of psychopathology (e.g., Zahn-Waxler, 2000). According to these models, people of one gender take a distinct path from those of the other gender (i.e., the processes underlying the development of an outcome differs for males compared with females).

It is also important for research to use mixed-gender samples, even when the outcome is found mostly in females. This allows researchers and clinicians to understand what risks and protective factors may influence these outcomes in both males and females. For example, although EDs are much more common in females relative to males, it is faulty to assume we do not need to know about risks and protective factors for EDs in males. It is important to examine participants of both genders to determine whether risk factors, explanatory processes, and interventions are the same for youth of each gender group. Research has yet to establish if different pathways, as well as prevention and intervention strategies, to EDs and NSSI exist for boys vs. girls. Although not conducted with a youth sample, recent research by Claes et al. (2012) on NSSI engagement in male inpatients with EDs showed that males report similar functions of NSSI as previous research has shown for female-only samples. Further, other recent research (e.g., Barrocas et al., 2012; Taliaferro et al., 2012) has also begun to use samples consisting of both male and female participants, which allows for examination of differences and/or similarities in findings by gender. This initial descriptive research on gender differences is important, yet more is needed. It is important for developmental psychopathologists to now begin to examine if vulnerabilities for NSSI and EDs (e.g., peer influences, puberty, emotion regulation) and trajectories of these outcomes differ by gender. This cannot be done in samples of only female youth. Future research should continue to assess NSSI and EDs and explore known associations in these literatures in samples of both males and females.

3.6 Developmental Psychopathology of NSSI Can Learn From ED Literature

The field of NSSI research is still young and has room to grow. Researchers studying NSSI in children and adolescents have only agreed upon a definition of NSSI in the past 5 years and are still working to establish replicated research on risks and vulnerabilities for NSSI in youth samples. We want to make the case that the lack of developmentally sensitive research on NSSI poses problems for our understanding of the development of NSSI. As a response, we believe research on the developmental psychopathology of NSSI can learn substantially from the ED literature.

The ED field has used fairly consistent definitions for various ED presentations over the last several decades; however, until recently, not all research published on NSSI defined and measured the construct of interest the same way. For example, some research still uses the term deliberate self-harm (DSH). Thus, despite recent efforts to establish a research definition for NSSI, work still needs to be done in this area. Further, measurement of NSSI is still not consistent across studies, with some research utilizing different interview measures and others utilizing questionnaires with as little as one item. By not utilizing the same, or similar, measurements tools for NSSI, as the ED literature does, it is difficult to enable replication and cross-study examination of vulnerabilities, risks, patterns, and outcomes of NSSI. Greater progress in knowledge can be made if researchers studying NSSI began to utilize the same measurement tools consistently.

Next, NSSI and EDs are similar in their conceptualization of a diagnosis. Research on EDs, especially in youth samples (e.g., Stice et al., 2009), nicely examines sub-threshold symptoms of ED as an outcome in addition to a clinical diagnosis of ED as defined by the DSM, as well as specific risks and vulnerabilities for each level of ED pathology. With more recent proposals to think of continued NSSI engagement as a specific psychiatric disorder, it would be useful for researchers and clinicians to begin to think of youth who engage in NSSI at both the sub-threshold and clinically diagnosable pathology levels. NSSI research has begun to establish that different levels of distress exist in individuals engaging in NSSI on numerous occasions vs. just a few (Klonsky & Olino, 2008). Still, the field could learn more by beginning to disentangle what leads someone to engage in sub-threshold vs. clinically diagnosable levels. Further, since there is more empirical data on the developmental aspects of EDs, one might draw from that literature to also inform developmentally sensitive practice given some of the shared and overlapping vulnerabilities among threshold and sub-threshold NSSI and ED presentations.

In addition, the literature has just begun to touch the surface on the influence of culture on NSSI engagement. Initial empirical work (Giletta et al., 2012; Plener et al., 2009) has emerged to suggest that NSSI is a cross-cultural phenomenon. However, it is yet to be established if NSSI is more common in industrialized nations, like with EDs (American Psychiatric Association, 2000), or if NSSI engagement has similar rates in developing countries. Further, research on EDs has established that there are aspects of industrialized countries (e.g., value of thinness, peer culture around appearance, role of media attention) that impart significant influence on the degree to which individuals are dissatisfied with their body and have diagnosed EDs. To date, no research has attempted to understand, in a similar manner, how specific cultures and the values, thereof, influence why and how youth begin to engage in NSSI.

In summary, literature on the developmental psychopathology of EDs is "older and wiser" than that on NSSI. Thus, researchers studying the developmental psychopathology of NSSI can learn from ED research and grow to better understand this outcome in more depth. In addition, clinical practice can also benefit by drawing from known risks, vulnerabilities, and treatment outcomes in the research literature to inform developmentally sensitive practice with children and adolescents.

3.7 A Vignette

The following vignette exemplifies many of the concepts discussed in this chapter. Specifically, it illustrates the distal and proximal vulnerability factors that may impact the emergence of NSSI and/or EDs, the functional mechanisms that NSSI and/or EDs may serve for youth, and the transactional nature between NSSI and EDs.

Jen is a Caucasian girl who lives with her mother, father, and brother in a suburban, middle class home. Jen feels "somewhat" close with her brother, but distant from her parents. Her parents fight with each other a lot and seem too wrapped up in their own problems to pay much attention to Jen and her brother. Jen has just a couple of good friends at school, but she is a strong student and is the first-chair flutist in a local youth orchestra.

Jen started dieting when she was in the fourth grade after being called chubby by a couple of male peers. Following the teasing, she began to compare her body to that of her female peers; this pattern of comparison left her feeling unhappy with how she looked. Specifically, she felt that she had "too much flub everywhere," whereas her female peers seemed to be "thin and pretty." Although Jen tried to restrict her food intake in an effort to lose weight, she often strayed from her diet plan and always felt like a failure as a result.

As Jen approached junior high, she had a growth spurt that left her taller than most of her classmates. She also got her first period at the beginning of sixth grade, which made her feel ashamed and embarrassed. After gym class one day, Jen stealthily looked at some of her female classmates' clothes and confirmed that she was wearing larger sizes than they were. She felt disgusted with her body and vowed to redouble her efforts towards weight loss.

Jen engaged in extreme caloric restriction for 2 days. On the third day, she found out that a boy she liked was interested in one of her "skinny and beautiful" friends, and she felt crushed. That evening, she ate dinner with her family and then secretly went on to consume half a bag of pretzels, two leftover slices of pizza, two Snickers bars, and big bowl of mashed potatoes and gravy. Even as she was eating, she berated herself for being so out of control, stupid, and weak. As soon as she finished eating, she rushed to the bathroom where she clumsily attempted to make herself vomit. Despite her efforts, she was unable to make herself sick, which further reinforced her feelings of failure. Feeling helpless and alone, Jen impulsively grabbed a metal hair clip and began to scratch the underside of her forearm with it. Somehow, focusing on the tangible, physical pain seemed to momentarily distract her from her emotional tailspin.

In the months that followed, Jen often felt alienated from her friends. For instance, a girl with whom she had been friends with for 3 years seemed to spend more and more time with the popular crowd and less time with Jen. One day at school, she heard about a party that her friends were all going to that weekend, but Jen had not been invited. She felt lonely, left out, and hurt. That Friday night, while her friends were at the party, Jen cried alone in her room for almost 2 h. She felt desperate for some relief and, as a result, used a safety pin to scratch her arm until it bled. She didn't know why, but hurting herself made it easier to deal with her feelings of loneliness and self-hatred that night.

However, in the following weeks, Jen constantly thought about how isolated she felt, how "gross" her body was, and how much she disliked herself. She also continued to alternate between periods during which she restricted her food intake and those during which she binged. She learned how to make herself vomit after her binges. She expected that self-induced vomiting would make her feel successful and in control, but rather, it made her feel gross and ashamed. She often found herself scratching her arms until they bled with her hair clips, safety pins, or paper clips after she binged and purged in hopes that doing so would decrease the intensity of her negative emotions. Although she hated herself the next day for having left visible scratches and felt guilty for being emotionally out of control after her binge/purge episode, she experienced a brief sense of relief from her negative emotions when engaging in the self-harming behavior.

Jen's case exemplifies many of the concepts discussed in this chapter. She experienced some distal (e.g., being teased) and some proximal (e.g., interpersonal triggers, early puberty, feelings of sadness) risks for EDs and NSSI. She also illustrated a developmental pathway defined by early ED risk factors (body dissatisfaction) that led to eating pathology (e.g., bingeing) that resulted in negative affect (i.e., as she felt out of control with regard to her eating) that led to NSSI engagement. Further, a bidirectional developmental pathway ensued such that NSSI engagement increased negative affect which led to additional eating pathology, and so on. Disentangling the ED and self-injurious behaviors becomes almost impossible over time, which is why exploring interventions that may be effective for both concerns (e.g., DBT) may be most fruitful.

References

American Psychiatric Association. (2000). *Diagnostic and statistical manual of mental disorders* (4th ed., text rev.). Washington, DC: American Psychiatric Association.

Bandura, A. (1973). *Aggression: A social learning analysis*. Englewood Cliffs, NJ: Prentice Hall.

Barrocas, A. L., Hankin, B. L., Abela, J. R. Z., & Young, J. F. (2012). Rates of nonsuicidal self-injury in youth: Age, gender, and behavioral methods in a general community sample. *Pediatrics, 130*(1), 39–45.

Brown, M. Z., Comtois, K. A., & Linehan, M. M. (2002). Reasons for suicide attempts and nonsuicidal self-injury in women with borderline personality disorder. *Journal of Abnormal Psychology, 111*, 198–202.

Chapman, A. L., Gratz, K. L., & Brown, M. Z. (2006). Solving the puzzle of deliberate self-harm: The experiential avoidance model. *Behaviour Research and Therapy, 44*, 371–394.

Claes, L., Houben, A., Vandereycken, W., Bijttebier, P., & Muehlenkamp, J. (2010). Brief Report: The association between non-suicidal self-injury, self-concept and acquaintance with self-injurious peers in a sample of adolescents. *Journal of Adolescence, 33*, 775–778.

Claes, L., Jiménez-Murcia, S., Agüera, Z., Castro, R., Sánchez, I., Menchón, J. M., et al. (2012). Male eating disorder patients with and without non-suicidal self-injury: A comparison of psychopathological and personality features. *European Eating Disorders Review, 20*, 335–338.

Clark, L., & Tiggeman, M. (2006). Appearance culture in nine- to 12-year-old girls: Media and peer influences on body dissatisfaction. *Social Development, 15*, 628–643.

Clark, L., Watson, D., & Mineka, S. (1994). Temperament, personality, and the mood and anxiety disorders. *Journal of Abnormal Psychology, 103*, 103–116.

Cohen, P., & Cohen, J. (1984). The clinician's illusion. *Archives of General Psychiatry, 41*, 1178–1182.

Cohen, J. A., Mannarino, A. P., & Deblinger, E. (2001). *Treating trauma and traumatic grief in children and adolescents*. New York, NY: The Guilford.

Croll, J., Neumark-Sztainer, D., Story, M., & Ireland, M. (2002). Prevalence and risk and protective factors related to disordered eating behaviors among adolescents: relationship to gender and ethnicity. *Journal of Adolescent Health, 31*, 166–175.

Darche, M. (1990). Psychological factors differentiating self-mutilating and non-self-mutilating adolescent inpatient females. *The Psychiatric Hospital, 21*, 31–35.

Darcy, A. M., Doyle, A. C., Lock, J., Peebles, R., Doyle, P., & Le Grange, D. (2012). The eating disorders examination in adolescent males with anorexia nervosa: How does it compare to adolescent females? *International Journal of Eating Disorders, 45*, 110–114.

Darling, N., & Steinberg, L. (1993). Parenting style as context: An integrative model. *Psychological Bulletin, 113*, 487–496.

Davison, K., Markey, C., & Birch, L. (2003). A longitudinal examination of patterns in girls' weight concerns and body dissatisfaction from ages 5 to 9 years. *International Journal of Eating Disorders, 33*, 320–332.

Eddy, K. T., Celio Doyle, A., Rienecke Hoste, R., Herzog, D. B., & Le Grange, D. (2008). Eating disorder not otherwise specified in adolescents. *Journal of the American Academy of Child and Adolescent Psychiatry, 47*, 156–164.

Eisenberg, N., Cumberland, A., & Spinrad, T. L. (1998). Parental socialization of emotion. *Psychological Inquiry, 9*, 241–273.

Ferreiro, F., Seoane, G., & Senra, C. (2012). Gender-related risk and protective factors for depressive symptoms and disordered eating in adolescence: A 4-year longitudinal study. *Journal of Youth and Adolescence, 41*, 607–622.

Field, A., Camargo, C., Barr Taylor, C., Berkey, C., Frazier, L., Gillman, M., et al. (1999). Overweight, weight concerns, and bulimic behaviours among girls and boys. *Journal of the American Academy of Child and Adolescent Psychiatry, 38*, 754–760.

Francis, L., & Birch, L. (2005). Maternal influences on daughters' restrained eating behavior. *Health Psychology, 24*, 548–554.

Gardner, R., Stark, K., Freidman, B., & Jackson, N. (2000). Predictors of eating disorder scores in children ages 6 through 14: A longitudinal study. *Journal of Psychosomatic Research, 49*, 199–205.

Geist, R., Heinmaa, M., Katzman, D., & Stephens, D. (1999). A comparison of male and female adolescents referred to an eating disorder program. *Canadian Journal of Psychiatry, 44*, 374–378.

Ghaziuddin, M., Tsai, L., Naylor, M., & Ghaziuddin, N. (1992). Mood disorder in a group of self-cutting adolescents. *Acta paedopsychiatrica, 55*, 103.

Giletta, M., Scholte, R. H., Engels, R. C., Ciairano, S., & Prinstein, M. J. (2012). Adolescent non-suicidal self-injury: A cross-national study of community samples from Italy, the Netherlands and the United States. *Psychiatry Research*. doi:10.1016/j.psychres.2012.02.009.

Goodman, S. H., Lahey, B. B., Fielding, B., Dulcan, M., Narrow, W., & Regier, D. (1997). Representativeness of clinical samples of youths with mental disorders: A preliminary population-based study. *Journal of Abnormal Psychology, 106*, 3–14.

Graber, J., Lewinsohn, P., Seeley, J., & Brooks-Gunn, J. (1997). Is psychopathology associated with the timing of pubertal development? *Journal of the American Academy of Child and Adolescent Psychiatry, 36*, 1768–1776.

Gratz, K. (2003). Risk factors for and functions of deliberate self-harm: An empirical and conceptual review. *Clinical Psychology: Science and Practice, 10*, 192–205.

Gratz, K. (2006). Risk factors for deliberate self-harm among female college students: The role and interaction of childhood maltreatment, emotional inexpressivity, and affect intensity/reactivity. *The American Journal of Orthopsychiatry, 76*, 238–250.

Gratz, K., Conrad, S. D., & Roemer, L. (2002). Risk factors for deliberate self-harm among college students. *The American Journal of Orthopsychiatry, 72*, 128–140.

Guerry, J. D., & Prinstein, M. J. (2010). Longitudinal prediction of adolescent nonsuicidal self-injury: Examination of a cognitive vulnerability-stress model. *Journal of Clinical Child and Adolescent Psychology, 39*, 77–89.

Hankin, B. L., & Abela, J. R. Z. (2011). Nonsuicidal self-injury in adolescence: Prospective rates and risk factors in a 2 ½ year longitudinal study. *Psychiatry Research, 186*, 65–70.

Hankin, B. L., & Abramson, L. Y. (2001). Development of gender differences in depression: An elaborated cognitive vulnerability–transactional stress theory. *Psychological Bulletin, 127*, 773–796.

Heilbron, N., & Prinstein, M. J. (2008). Peer influence and adolescent nonsuicidal self-injury: A theoretical review of mechanisms and moderators. *Applied and Preventative Psychology, 12*, 169–177.

Heilbron, N., & Prinstein, M. J. (2010). Adolescent peer victimization, peer status, suicidal ideation, and nonsuicidal self-injury: Examining concurrent and longitudinal associations. *Merrill-Palmer Quarterly, 56*, 388–419.

Hilt, L. M., Nock, M. K., Lloyd-Richardson, E. E., & Prinstein, M. J. (2008). Longitudinal study of nonsuicidal self-injury among young adolescents. *The Journal of Early Adolescence, 28*, 455–469.

Hoek, H. W., & Van Hoeken, D. (2003). Review of the prevalence and incidence of eating disorders. *International Journal of Eating Disorders, 34*, 383–396.

Jacobi, C., Hayward, C., de Zwaan, M., Kraemer, H., & Agras, S. (2004). Coming to terms with risk factors for eating disorders: Applications of risk terminology and suggestions for a general taxonomy. *Psychological Bulletin, 130*, 19–65.

Johnson, C., & Connors, M. E. (1987). *The etiology and treatment of bulimia nervosa: A biopsychosocial perspective*. New York, NY: Basic Books.

Jones, D. C. (2004). Body image among adolescent girls and boys: A longitudinal study. *Developmental Psychology, 40*, 823.

Jones, D. C., Vigfusdottir, T. H., & Lee, Y. (2004). Body image and the appearance culture among adolescent girls and boys an examination of friend conversations, peer criticism, appearance magazines, and the internalization of appearance ideals. *Journal of Adolescent Research, 19*, 323–339.

Keel, P., Fulkerson, J., & Leon, G. (1997). Disordered eating precursors in pre- and early adolescent girls and boys. *Journal of Youth and Adolescence, 26*, 203–216.

Kessler, R. C. (2003). Epidemiology of women and depression. *Journal of Affective Disorders, 74* (1), 5–13.

Kessler, R. C., Berglund, P., Borges, G., Nock, M. K., & Wang, P. S. (2005). Trends in suicide ideation, plans, gestures, and attempts in the United States, 1990–1992 to 2001–2003. *Journal of the American Medical Association, 293*, 2487–2495.

Killen, J., Hayward, C., Litt, I., Hammer, L., Wilson, D., Miner, B., et al. (1992). Is puberty a risk factor for eating disorders? *Archives of Pediatrics and Adolescent Medicine, 146*, 323–325.

Klonsky, E. D., & Moyer, A. (2008). Childhood sexual abuse and non-suicidal self-injury: Meta-analysis. *The British Journal of Psychiatry, 192*, 166–170.

Klonsky, E. D., & Olino, T. M. (2008). Identifying clinically distinct subgroups of self-injurers among young adults: A latent class analysis. *Journal of Consulting and Clinical Psychology, 76*, 22.

Krause, E. D., Mendelson, T., & Lynch, T. R. (2003). Childhood emotional invalidation and adult psychological distress: The mediating role of emotional inhibition. *Child Abuse and Neglect, 27*, 199–213.

Leon, G., Fulkerson, J., Perry, C., & Cudeck, R. (1993). Personality and behavioral vulnerabilities associated with risk status for eating disorders in adolescent girls. *Journal of Abnormal Psychology, 102*, 438–444.

Linehan, M. M. (1993). *Cognitive-behavioral treatment of borderline personality disorder*. New York, NY: The Guilford.

Measelle, J., Stice, E., & Hogansen, J. (2006). Developmental trajectories of co-occurring depressive, eating, antisocial, and substance abuse problems in female adolescents. *Journal of Abnormal Psychology, 115*, 524–538.

Muehlenkamp, J. J., & Brausch, A. M. (2012). Body regard and non-suicidal self-injury in adolescents. *Journal of Adolescence, 35*, 1–9.

Muehlenkamp, J. J., Claes, L., Smits, D., Peat, C. M., & Vandereycken, W. (2011). Non-suicidal self-injury in eating disordered patients: A test of a conceptual model. *Psychiatry Research, 188*, 102–108.

Muehlenkamp, J. J., & Gutierrez, P. M. (2004). An investigation of differences between self-injurious behavior and suicide attempts in a sample of adolescents. *Suicide and Life-Threatening Behavior, 34*, 12–23.

Muehlenkamp, J. J., & Gutierrez, P. M. (2007). Risk for suicide attempts among adolescents who engage in non-suicidal self-injury. *Archives of Suicide Research, 11*, 69–82.

Muehlenkamp, J. J., Peat, C. M., Claes, L., & Smits, D. (2012). Self-injury and disordered eating: Expressing emotion dysregulation through the body. *Suicide and Life-Threatening Behavior, 42*, 416–425.

Nock, M. K., Prinstein, M. J., & Sterba, S. K. (2009). Revealing the form and function of self-injurious thoughts and behaviors: A real-time ecological assessment study among adolescents and young adults. *Journal of Abnormal Psychology, 118*, 816–827.

Ohmann, S., & Popow, C. (2012). Self injurious behavior in adolescent girls with eating disorders. In I. J. Lobera (Ed.), *Relevant topics in eating disorders.* http://www.intechopen.com/books/relevant-topics-in-eating-disorders/self-injurious-behavior-inadolescent-girls-with-eating-disorders

Pike, K., & Rodin, J. (1991). Mothers, daughters, and disordered eating. *Journal of Abnormal Psychology, 100*, 198–204.

Plener, P. L., Libal, G., Keller, F., Fegert, J. M., & Muehlenkamp, J. J. (2009). An international comparison of adolescent non-suicidal self-injury (NSSI) and suicide attempts: Germany and the USA. *Psychological Medicine, 39*, 1549–1558.

Prinstein, M. J., Boegers, J., & Spirito, A. (2001). Adolescents' and their friends' health-risk behavior: Factors that alter or add to peer influence. *Journal of Pediatric Psychology, 26*, 287–298.

Prinstein, M. J., Guerry, J. D., Browne, C. B., & Rancourt, D. (2009). Interpersonal models of nonsuicidal self-injury. In M. K. Nock (Ed.), *Understanding nonsuicidal self injury: Origins, assessment, and treatment* (pp. 79–98). Washington, DC: American Psychological Association.

Rigby, K., & Slee, P. (1999). Suicidal ideation and adolescent school children, involvement in bully-victim problems, and perceived social support. *Suicide and Life-Threatening Behavior, 29*, 119–130.

Rodham, K., & Hawton, K. (2009). Epidemiology and phenomenology of nonsuicidal self-injury. In M. K. Nock (Ed.), *Understanding nonsuicidal self-injury: Origins, assessment, and treatment* (pp. 37–62). Washington, DC: American Psychological Association.

Rodham, K., Hawton, K., & Evans, E. (2004). Reasons for deliberate self-harm: Comparison of self-poisoners and self-cutters in a community sample of adolescents. *Journal of the American Academy of Child & Adolescent Psychiatry, 43*(1), 80–87.

Rosen, P. M., & Walsh, B. W. (1989). Patterns of contagion in self-mutilation epidemics. *The American Journal of Psychiatry, 146*, 656–658.

Ross, S., & Heath, N. (2002). A study of the frequency of self-mutilation in a community sample of adolescents. *Journal of Youth and Adolescence, 31*, 67–77.

Ross, S., Heath, N., & Toste, J. (2009). Non-suicidal self-injury and eating pathology in high school students. *The American Journal of Orthopsychiatry, 79*, 83–92.

Schutz, H. K., & Paxton, S. J. (2007). Friendship quality, body dissatisfaction, dieting, and disordered eating in adolescent girls. *British Journal of Clinical Psychology, 46*, 67–83.

Siegel, J., Yancey, A., Aneshensel, C., & Schuler, R. (1999). Body image, perceived pubertal timing and adolescent mental health. *Journal of Adolescent Health, 25*, 155–165.

Silberg, J., & Bulik, C. (2005). The developmental association between eating disorders and symptoms of depression and anxiety in juvenile twin girls. *Journal of Child Psychology and Psychiatry, and Allied Disciplines, 46*, 1317–1326.

Sim, L., Adrian, M., Zeman, J., Cassano, M., & Friedrich, W. (2009). Adolescent deliberate self-harm: Linkages to emotion regulation and family emotional climate. *Journal of Research on Adolescence, 19*, 75–91.

Sroufe, L. A., & Rutter, M. (1984). The domain of developmental psychopathology. *Child Development, 17–29.*

Stein, A., Woodley, H., Cooper, S., Winterbottom, J., Fairburn, C., & Cortina-Borja, M. (2006). Eating habits and attitudes among 10 year old children of mothers with eating disorders: Longitudinal study. *The British Journal of Psychiatry, 189*, 324–329.

Stice, E., Marti, C., & Durant, S. (2011). Risk factors for onset of eating disorders: Evidence of multiple risk pathways from an 8-year prospective study. *Behaviour Research and Therapy, 49*, 622–627.

Stice, E., Marti, C. N., Shaw, H., & Jaconis, M. (2009). An 8-year longitudinal study of the natural history of threshold, subthreshold, and partial eating disorders from a community sample of adolescents. *Journal of Abnormal Psychology, 118*, 587.

Stice, E., Mazotti, L., Weibel, D., & Agras, W. S. (2000). Dissonance prevention program decreases thin-ideal internalization, body dissatisfaction, dieting, negative affect, and bulimic symptoms: A preliminary experiment. *International Journal of Eating Disorders, 27*, 206–217.

Stice, E., Presnell, K., & Bearman, S. (2001). Relation of early menarche to depression, eating disorders, substance abuse, and comorbid psychopathology among adolescent girls. *Developmental Psychology, 37*, 608–619.

Stice, E., Presnell, K., & Spangler, D. (2002). Risk factors for binge eating onset in adolescent girls: A 2-year prospective investigation. *Health Psychology, 21*, 131–138.

Strober, M., Freeman, R., Lampert, C., Diamond, J., & Kaye, W. (2001). Controlled family study of anorexia and bulimia nervosa: Evidence of shared liability and transmission of partial syndromes. *The American Journal of Psychiatry, 157*, 393–401.

Suyemoto, K., & MacDonald, M. (1995). Self-cutting in female adolescents. *Psychotherapy, 32*, 162–171.

Swanson, S. A., Crow, S. J., Le Grange, D., Swendsen, J., & Merikangas, K. R. (2011). Prevalence and correlates of eating disorders in adolescents: Results from the national comorbidity survey replication adolescent supplement. *Archives of General Psychiatry, 68*, 714.

Taliaferro, L. A., Muehlenlamp, J. J., Borowsky, I. W., McMorris, B. J., & Bugler, K. C. (2012). Factors distinguishing youth who report self-injurious behavior: A population-based sample. *The Academy of Pediatrics, 12*, 205–213.

Yates, T. (2009). Developmental pathways from child maltreatment to nonsuicidal self-injury. In M. K. Nock (Ed.), *Understanding nonsuicidal self-injury: Origins, assessment, and treatment* (pp. 79–98). Washington, DC: American Pyschological Association.

Zahn-Waxler, C. (2000). The development of empathy, guilt and internalization of distress: Implications for gender differences in internalizing and externalizing problems. In R. Davidson (Ed.), *Anxiety, depression, and emotion* (pp. 222–265). New York, NY: Oxford University Press.

Etiological Models of Non-suicidal Self-Injury and Eating Disorders

4

Kathryn H. Gordon, Mun Yee Kwan, Allison M. Minnich, and Darren L. Carter

Abstract

The high rate of non-suicidal self-injury (NSSI) among individuals with eating disorders is a well-documented and clinically significant phenomenon (Svirko and Hawton, Suicide Life Threat Behav 37:409–421, 2007). Several shared risk factors have been identified for disordered eating and NSSI. These common risk factors were examined within the context of etiological models that have the potential to explain why they so frequently co-occur. Thus, data on the relevance of the shared risk factors are reviewed within the framework of multiple conceptual models for eating disorders and/or NSSI. Moreover, empirical data and the explanatory potential for the overlapping nature of these maladaptive behaviors are evaluated for each model. A summary of the commonalities and limitations of the various etiological models is then presented. Finally, the chapter concludes by highlighting clinical implications and future directions for the advancement of knowledge regarding this pernicious problem, with a focus on the need for additional research and the development of integrative, comprehensive etiological models for non-suicidal self-injury and eating disorders.

4.1 Overview of the Problem

Non-suicidal self-injury (NSSI), defined as "the deliberate, self-inflicted destruction of body tissue without suicidal intent and for purposes not socially sanctioned" (International Society for the Study of Self-Injury, 2013), is a significant problem among individuals who suffer from eating disorders (Svirko & Hawton, 2007). Common NSSI behaviors include cutting, burning, scratching, and head banging; culturally sanctioned behaviors such as tattoos and body piercing are typically

K.H. Gordon (✉) • M.Y. Kwan • A.M. Minnich • D.L. Carter
Department of Psychology, North Dakota State University, Fargo, ND, USA
e-mail: kathryn.gordon@ndsu.edu

L. Claes and J.J. Muehlenkamp (eds.), *Non-Suicidal Self-Injury in Eating Disorders*, DOI 10.1007/978-3-642-40107-7_4,

excluded. NSSI is slated to appear in the appendix of the *Diagnostic and Statistical Manual of Mental Disorders, Fifth Edition* (*DSM-5*; APA, 2013), as a disorder in need of further study, which is a testament to growing empirical data on the clinical significance of this problem (e.g., Selby, Bender, Gordon, Nock, & Joiner, 2012). According to the *DSM-5* criteria, an individual will qualify for this diagnosis if they have engaged in self-harm without suicidal intent on 5 or more days in the past year and if it is associated with clinically significant distress or impairment. However, because this is not an official diagnosis, studies referenced in this chapter typically refer to dimensional conceptualizations of NSSI rather than NSSI as a qualitative syndrome. It is worth noting that many of the individuals in the research would likely qualify for the diagnosis, however.

For the purposes of this chapter, which provides an overview of etiological models for NSSI among individuals with eating disorders, studies on disordered eating will include those that reflect the symptoms of the main eating disorder diagnostic categories defined by the *DSM-IV-TR* (APA, 2000): anorexia nervosa (AN), bulimia nervosa (BN), eating disorder not otherwise specified (EDNOS), and binge-eating disorder (BED). Though BED is currently in the appendix of the *DSM-IV-TR*, it will be added as a formal diagnostic category in the next edition of the *DSM-5* and is therefore included in this review. AN is characterized by a refusal to maintain minimal body weight and an overwhelming fear that, despite being quite underweight, one will become fat. Meanwhile, BN is characterized by recurrent binge-eating episodes (eating substantially more in a discrete period of time than most people would in the same situation) and inappropriate compensatory behaviors (e.g., vomiting, taking laxatives, excessive exercise; APA, 2000). BED is characterized by recurrent binge-eating episodes, similar to BN, where the individual feels a loss of control while eating and eats until she/he is uncomfortably full, but, unlike an individual with BN, does not regularly engage in compensatory behaviors with the intent of preventing weight gain. Finally, an EDNOS is a clinically significant disordered eating syndrome that is diagnosed when an individual's eating problems are causing distress and impairment despite not meeting criteria for AN or BN (APA, 2000).

Following a review of studies on the co-occurrence of NSSI and disordered eating, Svirko and Hawton (2007) estimated that the prevalence of NSSI among people with eating disorders ranged from 25 to 55 %, while the rate of eating disorders among patients who engage in NSSI ranged from 54 to 61 %. These statistics indicate clear, elevated rates of NSSI among individuals with eating disorders, as estimates of NSSI in other samples are much lower (e.g., 4 % in the general population (Briere & Gil, 1998), 12–14 % in adolescent and college samples (Ross & Heath, 2002), 11 % in a psychiatric control sample (Welch & Fairburn, 1996); for a review, see Muehlenkamp, Claes, Havertape, & Plener, 2012).

Explanations for the NSSI and eating disorder overlap often highlight shared commonalities between the phenomena. For example, both NSSI and eating disorders tend to onset in adolescence or early adulthood and may be increasing in recent years (Svirko & Hawton, 2007). In addition to these commonalities,

NSSI and eating disorders also share risk factors such as impulsivity, obsessive-compulsive characteristics, affect dysregulation, self-criticism, a need for control, dissociation, trauma, and problematic family environments (Svirko & Hawton, 2007). The current chapter seeks to expand upon previous reviews on the topic by identifying and evaluating extant empirical evidence for shared risk factors within the context of theoretical or conceptual etiological models. The chapter includes a review of data relevant to models specifically designed to explain both NSSI and eating disorders, as well as models of NSSI or eating disorders that may also be pertinent to the explanation of high rates of comorbidity. The purpose of reviewing existing knowledge on this topic is to highlight directions for future work addressing this challenging clinical problem, which is associated with significant suffering, costs, and the increased risk for death by suicide (Nock, Joiner, Gordon, Lloyd-Richardson, & Prinstein, 2006).

4.2 Etiological Models of SSI and Eating Disorders

4.2.1 Emotional Cascade Model

The emotional cascade model (Selby & Joiner, 2009) was developed to explain the etiology of borderline personality disorder, but has also been tested as a general conceptual model linking emotion dysregulation and behavioral dysregulation (including maladaptive behaviors such as disordered eating and NSSI). The main premise is that distal factors such as childhood abuse (which occurs at elevated rates among individuals with eating disorders and NSSI; Svirko & Hawton, 2007) render an individual more susceptible to "emotional cascades," which purportedly precede dysfunctional coping behaviors. The model proposes that rumination, a style of responding to stress that involves focusing on the feelings of distress, as well as potential causes and consequences of the distress, in a repetitive, passive manner Nolen-Hoeksema (2003), exacerbates negative affect and leads to emotional and behavioral dysregulation. Emotional cascades are posited to occur when an event triggers a negative emotion and the individual ruminates about the event, thereby increasing the intensity of the resultant negative emotion. The amplified emotion then purportedly leads to even greater levels of rumination, which leads to yet more intense negative feelings. This emotional cascade is proposed to continue gaining strength until the negative mood state is so powerful that engaging in an equally intense coping behavior (e.g., NSSI) is viewed as the only way to sufficiently distract oneself from the aversive emotions. According to the model, less extreme coping strategies (e.g., talking to a friend) are not engaging enough to distract from and change these high-intensity negative emotions.

There is mounting evidence that rumination and negative affect interact to predict both NSSI and binge eating in cross-sectional (Selby, Anestis, & Joiner, 2008; Selby, Anestis, Bender, & Joiner, 2009) and ecological momentary assessment studies (Selby & Joiner, 2013) in samples which include participants from the community and college students. Furthermore, consistent with the model, laboratory studies have provided evidence that the experience of physical pain does decrease negative emotion in college students who engage in NSSI significantly more than non-painful, comparable stimuli (Bresin & Gordon, 2013) and that physical pain reduces negative affect for individuals with relatively high levels of emotional reactivity (Bresin, Gordon, Bender, Gordon, & Joiner, 2010).

In addition, though not designed to directly test the emotional cascade model, multiple studies have documented a link between negative affect and/or rumination with NSSI (e.g., Hoff & Muehlenkamp, 2009; Kerr & Muehlenkamp, 2010; Nock, Prinstein, & Sterba, 2009; Selby, Connell, & Joiner, 2010) and bulimic behaviors (e.g., Selby & Joiner, 2009; Gordon, Holm-Denoma, Troop-Gordon, & Sand, 2012; Holm-Denoma & Hankin, 2010; Selby, Connell et al., 2010; Smyth et al., 2007), which is consistent with the model. Important in the current context, data supports the connection of these variables with NSSI specifically occurring in the context of an eating disorder (Claes, Klonsky, Muehlenkamp, & Vandereycken, 2010; Muehlenkamp et al., 2009). Moreover, the emotional cascade model may also be relevant to individuals with AN, who also appear to have elevated levels of negative affect and ruminative tendencies in initial studies (e.g., Cowdrey & Park, 2011; Engel et al., 2005; Rawal, Park, & Williams, 2010).

Consistent with the emotional cascade model, Engel et al. (2005) proposed that negative affect may precede restrictive behaviors among individuals with AN, though this hypothesis has not yet been tested to our knowledge. Therefore, in light of existing data, it is plausible that this model may potentially explain the relatively high co-occurrence of NSSI and disordered eating even though its main intention is to explain borderline personality disorder (incidentally, borderline personality disorder symptoms are associated with NSSI among patients with eating disorders; e.g., Selby et al., 2010). Perhaps individuals who experience emotional cascades are drawn to intensely stimulating, attention-engaging, distracting behaviors such as eating disorder behaviors (binge eating, purging, excessive exercise, dietary restriction) and NSSI to cope with their very intense emotions, and this may explain the overlap. If this is the case, clinicians may be able to help their clients find more adaptive behaviors for disrupting the emotional cascades by using strategies suggested by Nolen-Hoeksema (2003) such as taking a break to engage in a distracting activity before returning to the problem (e.g., going for a walk), cognitively reappraising the situation, or utilizing thought-stopping techniques. Other potentially useful clinical interventions may include non-harmful coping behaviors that serve the function of distracting from intense emotions such as those suggested by Linehan (1993) for dialectical behavior therapy. For example, Linehan (1993) recommends a variety of distracting behaviors for tolerating intense negative emotions such as holding an ice cube tightly, completing a crossword puzzle, changing body temperature through a cold shower, or listening to loud music.

4.2.2 Four-Function Model

Nock and Prinstein (2004) proposed a contextual model for NSSI which outlines the four main functions of the behavior, as identified by individuals who engage in NSSI. They posit that NSSI has four major functions that fall along two dimensions (1) automatic (within oneself) versus social and (2) positive versus negative reinforcement. Specifically, the model uses these two dimensions to specify four main functions: intrapersonal negative reinforcement (to cease unpleasant emotions; this is the most commonly endorsed function), automatic positive reinforcement (to create an emotion that replaces numbness or dissociative experiences, which have been linked with both NSSI and disordered eating; (Svirko & Hawton, 2007), social negative reinforcement (to avoid an undesired situation), and social positive reinforcement (to gain attention or help from others). It is important to note that interpersonal/social support problems have also been linked to both NSSI and disordered eating (e.g., Adrian, Zeman, Erdley, Lisa, & Sim, 2011; Bodell, Smith, Holm-Denoma, Gordon, & Joiner, 2011; Claes et al., 2012) and that empirical support has been garnered for this model in NSSI samples (e.g., Nock et al., 2009; Nock & Prinstein, 2005).

Of particular interest, Wedig and Nock (2010) hypothesized that this four-function model could also apply binge-eating and purging behavior, given that these are also harmful behaviors that may be driven by intrapersonally and interpersonally related motives. In a sample of individuals who had engaged in binge-eating or purging behavior in the past 3 months, Wedig and Nock reported that results of a confirmatory factor analysis supported the fit of the four-function model to binge-eating and purging behaviors. This model has not yet been tested in patients with eating disorders or with regard to symptoms of AN.

However, the fit of Nock and Prinstein's (2004) functional model for both NSSI and bulimic behaviors suggests that the high rates of co-occurrence in these maladaptive behaviors may be attributable to the fact that individuals with skill deficits for achieving goals in an adaptive manner (e.g., decreasing distressing feelings through healthy means, asserting one's desires adaptively in interpersonal situations) may be drawn to NSSI and/or disordered eating behaviors as methods for achieving their goals. In line with this assertion, poor coping skills have been linked to both NSSI and disordered eating (e.g., Cawood & Huprich, 2011; Nock & Mendes, 2008; Svaldi, Dorn, & Trentowska, 2011). The identification of the automatic negative reinforcement function of NSSI and bulimic behaviors is compatible with the emotional cascade model assertion that individuals engage in these maladaptive behaviors to cope with intense negative emotions. Future research testing this model in eating disorder samples, particularly among those who also engage in NSSI, is needed before conclusions can be drawn about its explanatory value for the co-occurrence of NSSI and eating disorders. Additionally, in light of the similar motives found to drive both behaviors, it would be of theoretical and clinical interest to determine why some individuals selected disordered eating versus NSSI and how they may differ from individuals who engage in both behaviors (Muehlenkamp, Peat, Claes, & Smits, 2012).

4.2.3 Escape Theory

The escape theory of binge eating (Heatherton & Baumeister, 1991) proposes that binge eating is motivated by a desire to escape aversive self-awareness. Specifically, Heatherton and Baumeister (1991) posit that the chain of events that leads to binge eating begins with an individual failing to meet a personal standard. According to the theory, once an individual experiences this type of failure to meet a standard, they blame themselves and enter a state of aversive self-awareness about their perceived inadequacy, which leads to a negative mood. These negative mood states are theorized to drive a person to a state of cognitive deconstruction (cf. dissociation), which then leads to binge eating as a means of focusing their attention away from their painful self-awareness and toward the physical sensations of eating (e.g., chewing, tasting). Of interest in this particular context, the escape theory was initially designed as an explanation of suicide, with the same causal chain leading to a different outcome in that case (a suicide attempt; Baumeister, 1990). The escape theory and emotional cascade model are similar in that they purport that the destructive behaviors are driven by a desire to escape painful affective states. However, the pathways differ in that the escape theory focuses on behavioral dysregulation resulting from dissociation emerging from aversive self-awareness about a failure to meet a personal standard, while the emotional cascade model focuses on negative emotions building intensity through a ruminative cycle. While the escape theory hinges on these behaviors acting as an escape from the self, the emotional cascade model posits that maladaptive coping behaviors like NSSI and disordered eating act to distract from broader sources of negative affect.

While the original escape theory focuses on suicide attempts (with some intent of death as an outcome) rather than NSSI (which, by definition, cannot include the intent to die as a result), it seems logical that this theory could also explain NSSI and the overlap of NSSI and disordered eating. The escape theory's proposed pathway of psychological processes may also lead individuals to NSSI and other concrete, physical eating disorder behaviors beyond binge eating (e.g., excessive exercise, purging) to escape from aversive self-awareness. This possibility is supported by evidence that both individuals who engage in NSSI and disordered eating exhibit constructs identified in the theory's pathway. For example, Heatherton and Baumeister propose that individuals with high levels of perfectionism may be particularly susceptible to the initial step (failing to meet a standard) as they, by definition, have very high and often unattainable standards. Indeed, perfectionism is a correlate of both NSSI and disordered eating (e.g., Bardone-Cone, Wonderlich, Frost, Bulik, & Mitchell, 2007; Claes, Soenens, Vansteenkiste, & Vandereycken, 2012; Hoff & Muehlenkamp, 2009). Also consistent with the escape theory, the components of self-blame and aversive self-awareness (cf. low self-esteem and self-criticism) have been linked to both NSSI and disordered eating (e.g., Cawood & Huprich, 2011; Holm-Denoma et al., 2005; Svirko & Hawton, 2007). Moreover, both types of behaviors have an association with dissociative tendencies (Svirko & Hawton, 2007) and negative affect (e.g., Muehlenkamp et al., 2009; Smyth et al., 2007). It is also noteworthy that the escape theory of binge eating states that the failure to meet any type of personal standard (e.g., career achievement) may trigger binge eating, but there is a particular emphasis on failing to meet standards related to the body, and that negative attitudes about the body are relevant for both NSSI and disordered eating (e.g., Muehlenkamp & Brausch, 2012; Muehlenkamp, Peat et al., 2012). Altogether, a multitude of studies have supported various components of the escape theory for binge eating, and many of the components have been linked to both NSSI and eating disorders. Therefore, exploration of the escape theory's applicability to NSSI and other disordered eating behaviors, as well as its possible explanation of overlap for NSSI and disordered eating (as driven by similar pathways) is warranted.

4.2.4 Experiential Avoidance Model

The experiential avoidance model (Chapman, Gratz, & Brown, 2006) posits that individuals engage in NSSI in the pursuit of temporary relief and avoidance of undesired emotional arousal and that this becomes increasingly negatively reinforcing with repetition (Gordon et al., 2010). Furthermore, the model suggests that particular characteristics make people more susceptible to coping with undesired emotions through NSSI: poor distress tolerance, emotion regulation skill deficits, high emotional intensity, and difficulty self-regulating when aroused. This model is compatible with the emotional cascade model, and the four-function model claims that individuals engage in NSSI as a means to decrease or avoid undesired affect.

Though the experiential avoidance model has not yet been tested with regard to eating disorders, it may explain the elevated rates of NSSI among individuals with eating disorders in that many of the proposed factors are also relevant for people with eating disorders. For example, multiple studies have found that people who exhibit NSSI or eating disorders have tendencies toward experiential and emotional avoidance (e.g., Corstorphine, Mountford, Tomlinson, Waller, & Meyer, 2007; Fulton et al., 2012; Kingston, Clark, & Remington, 2010). Moreover, extant research suggesting that negative emotions precede binge eating, vomiting, and NSSI, and then decrease after engaging in the behaviors (e.g., Haines, Brain, & Wilson, 1995; Smyth et al., 2007; Claes et al., 2010), is compatible with the crucial negative reinforcement aspect of the model.

There are also empirical findings that corroborate the model's predictions about individual difference variables that render people especially susceptible to engaging NSSI. Specifically, poor distress tolerance (e.g., Anestis, Fink, Smith, Selby, & Joiner, 2011; Nock & Mendes, 2008) and emotion regulation difficulties (e.g., Burns, Fischer, Jackson, & Harding, 2012; Gratz & Roemer, 2008; Muehlenkamp, Peat et al., 2012) have been linked to NSSI as well as disordered eating. Moreover, negative urgency, which is conceptually similar to the model's construct of difficulty self-regulating when aroused, has been identified as a specific facet of impulsivity (Whiteside & Lynam, 2001). Data are accumulating which particularly link this facet of impulsivity to both eating pathology (Anestis,

Selby, & Joiner, 2007; Anestis, Smith, Fink, & Joiner, 2009; Claes, Vandereycken, & Vertommen, 2005; Peterson & Fischer, 2012) and NSSI (e.g.,Lynam, Miller, Miller, Bornovalova, & Lejuez, 2011; Peterson & Fischer, 2012). Therefore, the experiential avoidance model may not only be useful for understanding the nature of NSSI. It also has promise of explaining the co-occurrence of NSSI and disordered eating via its identification of characteristics of people who are particularly drawn toward these forms of emotionally avoidant coping (e.g., people with poorer distress tolerance).

4.2.5 Conceptual Model of Childhood Traumatic Experiences

Childhood maltreatment, including sexual, physical, and emotional abuse, has been linked to both disordered eating and NSSI (Svirko & Hawton, 2007). Muehlenkamp, Claes, Smits, Peat, and Vandereycken (2011) proposed a conceptual model that described one hypothesized pathway for NSSI among individuals with eating disorders. This model states that one major starting point for the development of these behaviors is childhood maltreatment. Specifically, Muehlenkamp et al. (2011) put forth a pathway suggesting that childhood trauma leads to low self-esteem, which leads to affective pathology (e.g., anxiety, depression), which may lead to dissociation and or/body dissatisfaction, and that all of these variables lead to NSSI. In support of this conceptual model, each of these variables is related to both NSSI and disordered eating and specifically with NSSI among individuals with eating disorders (Muehlenkamp et al., 2011; Svirko & Hawton, 2007).

This conceptual model was tested in a sample of 422 women who were admitted to an inpatient eating disorder unit, and empirical support for multiple aspects of the model emerged (Muehlenkamp et al., 2011). Specifically, structural equation modeling analyses yielded statistically significant paths from childhood abuse and low self-esteem to pathology and from pathology to dissociation to NSSI, as well as significant pathways from childhood maltreatment to body dissatisfaction and from body dissatisfaction to NSSI. However, the authors note that the connection from body dissatisfaction to NSSI was not particularly strong and that there was no evidence of a direct pathway from pathology to NSSI.

This conceptual model of childhood traumatic experiences has multiple strengths and the potential for explaining the link between NSSI and eating disorders. It was specifically designed to address the question as to why the behaviors frequently co-occur, integrates multiple shared risk factors, and specifies how each of the variables are related and may lead to one another. Currently, only one test of the model with a sample of inpatient females with eating disorders exists.

4.2.6 Emotion Dysregulation Expressed Through the Body

Difficulties regulating emotions appear to underlie both NSSI and disordered eating (e.g., Burns et al., 2012; Lavender & Anderson, 2010; Svirko & Hawton, 2007).

However, emotion dysregulation has also been associated with a host of other psychopathology-related problems such as substance abuse (e.g., Bradley et al., 2011), risky sexual behavior (e.g.,Messmann-Moore, Walsh, & DiLillo, 2010), and aggression (e.g., Herts, McLaughlin, & Hatzenbuehler, 2012). Therefore, it is possible that emotion dysregulation could simply be a general risk factor for multiple types of psychopathology and/or impulsive behaviors. Muehlenkamp, Peat, et al. (2012) thus proposed that emotion dysregulation may be a more specific and particularly potent risk factor for disordered eating and/or NSSI when paired with negative attitudes toward the body (e.g., body dissatisfaction, low investment in the body).

Specifically, Muehlenkamp, Peat, et al. (2012), referencing Orbach's (1996) hypothesis that negative experiences of the body (e.g., disconnection, negative attitudes, and feelings) facilitate self-destructive behaviors, proposed that individuals who engage in NSSI and disordered eating behaviors are utilizing their body to cope with distressing emotions. Orbach's (1996) model is supported by data demonstrating that suicidal individuals tend to harbor more negative feelings about their bodies than non-suicidal individuals (Orbach et al., 2006), which is consistent with the notion that negative bodily attitudes facilitate thoughts and behaviors affiliated with harm to one's body. Muehlenkamp et al.'s model is also consistent with previous findings that individuals with eating disorders who engage in NSSI have significantly higher levels of body dissatisfaction than those who do not engage in NSSI (Anderson, Carter, McIntosh, Joyce, & Bulik, 2002). Moreover, this is in line with research showing that negative attitudes toward the body are correlates of NSSI and disordered eating (e.g., Gordon et al., 2012; Muehlenkamp & Brausch, 2012; Nelson & Muehlenkamp, 2012).

Based upon previous empirical findings and Orbach's (1996) model, Muehlenkamp, Peat, and colleagues (2012) proposed that individuals with the highest levels of negative attitudes toward the body, depression symptoms, and emotion dysregulation would be at highest risk for exhibiting co-occurring disordered eating and NSSI in a sample of college undergraduate women. Indeed, they found that individuals who reported these co-occurring behaviors had significantly higher levels of depression symptoms and emotion dysregulation than individuals who reported either NSSI or disordered eating alone. This is further support for etiological models which propose that the presence of negative affect and emotion regulation deficits drives NSSI and/or disordered eating (e.g., the emotion cascade model, experiential avoidance model, escape theory, four-function model) and may explain why these behaviors so frequently overlap. Perhaps the behaviors are particularly likely to co-occur in individuals with the highest levels of emotion dysregulation and depression symptoms (cf. negative affect) because they are the most desperate to reduce painful emotions and are willing to try multiple types of extreme, destructive behaviors in this effort.

A second major finding by Muehlenkamp, Peat, et al. (2012) may illuminate differentiating motives for individuals to choose NSSI or disordered eating (for those who do not engage in both). In their study, women with disordered eating had greater body dissatisfaction than women who exhibited NSSI alone, and women who exhibited NSSI alone had lower levels of psychological investment in their body image than individuals who only engaged in disordered eating and not NSSI. This suggests that individuals who are dissatisfied with their bodies but who are more invested in their appearance may be more inclined to engage in disordered eating behaviors (e.g., dietary restriction, purging) in an effort to cope with their emotions in ways that are more culturally valued. Meanwhile, people with less investment in their appearance may turn to NSSI in an attempt to regulate their emotions, as they have less concern about what behaviors such as cutting and burning will do their appearance (e.g., scarring).

In conclusion, a major strength of the model of NSSI and disordered eating as expressions of emotion dysregulation through the body is that it integrates and prioritizes specific risk factors for the co-occurring phenomena and identifies emotion dysregulation deficits as underlying both NSSI and disordered eating. Moreover, it identifies that individuals with the highest levels of emotion dysregulation are most likely to exhibit both behaviors and highlights distinguishing factors between the different groups. The concept of utilizing the body to cope with emotion dysregulation may be unique to these specific maladaptive behaviors and therefore has promise for deepening the understanding of their etiology and the nature of the frequent overlap. It may be useful for future research to further break down the body experience component by examining the facets that Orbach and Mikulincer (1998) delineated in their body investment scale (i.e., body image feelings and attitudes, comfort in touch, body care, and body protection) to see if these differential components may lend even greater specificity to the model.

4.2.7 Altered Physical Pain Perception

Altered physical pain perception is a final variable that is considered with regard to potentially being related to the etiology of NSSI among individuals with eating disorders. As noted in Muehlenkamp, Peat, et al.'s (2012) model, NSSI and disordered eating appear to share the commonality of emotion dysregulation being expressed through the body. Individuals who engage in disordered eating behaviors (e.g., excessive exercise, fasting, binge eating, purging, laxative abuse) endure physical pain and discomfort as do individuals who engage in NSSI (e.g., cutting, puncturing, burning). Therefore, it is possible that one factor that leads emotionally dysregulated individuals toward the selection of physically inflicting harm on their bodies as a coping strategy may be related to a characteristic of experiencing physical pain as less aversive than the general population.

Consistent with this idea, individuals who engage in NSSI appear to be less sensitive to physical pain and can tolerate more pain in laboratory tests (e.g., thermally and pressure-induced pain) than healthy controls (Hooley, Ho, Slater, & Lockshin, 2010) and psychiatric controls who do not engage in NSSI (e.g., Hooley et al., 2010; Kemperman et al., 1997). Moreover, many individuals subjectively report that they experience little or no pain while engaging in NSSI despite the bodily damage (e.g., Claes, Vandereycken, & Vertommen, 2006; Nock &

Prinstein, 2005). Similarly, there is evidence from laboratory pain assessment tasks that individuals with eating disorders have decreased pain sensitivity compared to healthy controls (e.g., de Zwaan, Biener, Schneider, & Stacher, 1996; Raymond et al., 1995, 1999). In addition to these findings on altered physical pain perception, there is also some initial evidence of a reduced sense of fear about physical pain among individuals who engage in NSSI (Selby, Connell et al., 2010) and disordered eating behaviors (e.g., particularly among those who engage in overly vigorous exercising; Smith et al., 2013).

Therefore, a potentially fruitful area for future research on the etiology of NSSI among individuals with eating disorders could involve models which incorporate the variable of altered pain perception (including less subjectively experienced negative attitudes and fear about pain, as well as decreased physical sensitivity to pain). This variable may fit well into extant models, such as Muehlenkamp, Peat, et al.'s (2012) model of NSSI and disordered eating as emotion dysregulation expressed through the body. It stands to reason that individuals with decreased emotional and physical sensitivity to pain would also feel less investment/more disconnection from their bodies and therefore be at higher risk for damaging their bodies through disordered eating behaviors and NSSI. In addition, it may be useful to examine the possibility that altered pain perception is another facet of altered bodily experiences theorized to result from trauma or abuse (e.g., Muehlenkamp et al., 2011; Orbach, 1996).

Conclusions, Clinical Implications, and Future Directions

In summary, etiological models of NSSI (the experiential avoidance model, the four-function model), disordered eating (escape theory), and emotional and behavioral dysregulation (the emotional cascade model) and models specifically focused on explaining the etiology of NSSI in eating disorders (the conceptual model of childhood maltreatment, emotion dysregulation expressed through the body) and an additional shared risk factor (altered pain perception) have been reviewed. There is evidence that several variables in these models are linked to NSSI and disordered eating independently and that many of the variables are featured across models. For example, emotion dysregulation (the emotional cascade model, the four-function model, the experiential avoidance model), dissociation (the escape theory, the conceptual model of childhood maltreatment), negative evaluation of the self and body (the escape theory, the conceptual model of childhood maltreatment, emotion dysregulation expressed through the body), and a desire for avoidance of undesired emotional experiences (the emotional cascade model, the escape theory, the four-function model, the experiential avoidance model) are components that are featured across models. While many models feature overlapping variables, each also offers unique explanatory variables. For example, rumination is a major factor in the case of the emotional cascade model, perfectionism plays an important role in escape theory, and a tendency to act rashly/impulsively rather than tolerate distress is highlighted in the experiential avoidance model. The model focusing on emotion dysregulation expressed through the body identified specific risk factors associated with disordered eating (body dissatisfaction), NSSI (depression symptoms and decreased investment in appearance), and with those who exhibited both behaviors (greater levels of emotion dysregulation). Finally, a potential etiological variable that has not been examined as much in this context (altered pain perception) but that may contribute to the development of NSSI, disordered eating, and their frequent co-occurrence was proposed, and initial data consistent with this hypothesis was presented.

Some clinical implications may be derived from this review. Specifically, if a client with an eating disorder presents with a history of childhood trauma, depression symptoms, an insensitivity to physical pain, a tendency to act rashly in the face of distress, or other types of emotion regulation problems, it may be particularly important to regularly assess for the presence of NSSI and try to prevent it. Moreover, clinicians may directly target some of these factors with the aim of reducing NSSI behaviors in people with eating disorders. For example, coping and cognitive reappraisal methods such as those utilized in integrative cognitive affect therapy for bulimia nervosa (Wonderlich, Peterson, Mitchell, & Crow, 2000) and cognitive behavioral therapy-enhanced (Fairburn, Cooper, Shafran, & Wilson, 2008) may help to decrease negative evaluation of the self and body, perfectionism, depression symptoms, and beliefs about an inability to tolerate painful emotions. Additionally, adaptive coping strategies proposed by Linehan (1993) in dialectical behavior therapy and by Nolen-Hoeksema (2003), such as mindfulness and distraction activities to cope with intense emotions and rumination, may be healthy substitution behaviors for NSSI.

The majority of the models presented here have been developed relatively recently (with the exception of the escape theory, which has had more extensive study), and initial data appears to be in line with hypotheses derived from the models. However, with the exception of the emotion dysregulation expressed through the body and conceptual childhood traumatic experiences models, they were not specifically designed as etiological models that explain why there are high rates of NSSI among individuals with eating disorders. Therefore, some of the models may prove to be more general models of behavioral and emotional dysregulation with less ability to explain this particular phenomenon. Thus, limitations in the current literature include the fact that the majority of the models have not been tested in samples of individuals who have both eating disorders and engage in NSSI (many samples focused on only one of the behaviors) and most of them consisted of female, White, adolescent or young adult samples. Therefore, the generalizability and extent of the explanatory power for the etiological models in is currently unknown. Finally, the vast majority of the studies were cross-sectional and nonexperimental in nature, which limits knowledge on the temporal order and causal relationships between variables.

Future work is needed to expand upon existing models and to determine how applicable they may be to explaining the etiology of NSSI among individuals with eating disorders. Additional work in the area should prioritize integrating the multitude of risk factors that NSSI and eating disorders share (Svirko & Hawton, 2007), as well as identification of variables which may be uniquely associated with the co-occurrence of these behaviors and not maladaptive behaviors in general (e.g., bodily investment attitudes, altered pain perception). Theoretical development and research which seeks to refine and create parsimonious models which identify the most relevant factors for this phenomenon are greatly needed. Advancement in the ability to decrease suffering associated with these pernicious behaviors depends upon our understanding of the nature and causes of these behaviors. The development of an integrative, cohesive etiological model of co-occurring NSSI and eating disorders would pave the way for clinicians to effectively target the most potent maintenance factors for NSSI and eating disorders in treatment as well as guide the development of effective prevention efforts. Such models should stand up to longitudinal tests, which can reveal the temporal ordering and risk factors prior to the onset of the behaviors, experimental tests from which causal relationships between variables can be inferred, and generalizability as evidenced by applicability across a range of samples.

References

Adrian, M., Zeman, J., Erdley, C., Lisa, L., & Sim, L. (2011). Emotional dysregulation and interpersonal difficulties as risk factors for nonsuicidal self-injury in adolescent girls. *Journal of Abnormal Child Psychology, 39*, 389–400.

American Psychiatric Association. (2000). *Diagnostic and statistical manual of mental disorders* (4th ed.) text revision. Washington, DC: Author.

American Psychiatric Association. (2013). *Diagnostic and statistical manual of mental disorders* (5th ed.). Washington, DC: Author.

Anderson, C. B., Carter, F. A., McIntosh, V. V., Joyce, P., & Bulik, C. M. (2002). Self-harm and suicide attempts in individuals with bulimia nervosa. *Eating Disorders: The Journal of Treatment and Prevention, 10*, 227–243.

Anestis, M. D., Selby, E. A., & Joiner, T. E. (2007). The role of urgency in maladaptive behaviors. *Behaviour Research and Therapy, 45*, 3018–3029.

Anestis, M. D., Smith, A. R., Fink, E. L., & Joiner, T. E., Jr. (2009). Dysregulated eating and distress: Examining the specific role of negative urgency in a clinical sample. *Cognitive Therapy and Research, 33*, 390–397.

Anestis, M. D., Fink, E. L., Smith, A. R., Selby, E. A., & Joiner, T. E. (2011). Eating disorders. In M. J. Zvolensky, A. Bernstein, & A. A. Vujanovic (Eds.), *Distress tolerance: Theory, research, and clinical applications* (pp. 245–260). New York: Guilford Press.

Bardone-Cone, A. M., Wonderlich, S. A., Frost, R. O., Bulik, C. M., & Mitchell, J. E. (2007). Perfectionism and eating disorders: Current status and future directions. *Clinical Psychology Review, 27*, 384–405.

Baumeister, R. F. (1990). Suicide as escape from self. *Psychological Review, 97*, 90–113.

Bodell, L., Smith, A. R., Holm-Denoma, J. M., Gordon, K. H., & Joiner, T. E., Jr. (2011). Low social support and negative life events interact to predict bulimic symptoms. *Eating Behaviors, 12*, 44–48.

Bradley, B., Defife, J. A., Guarnaccia, C., Phifer, J., Fani, N., Ressler, K. J., et al. (2011). Emotion dysregulation and negative affect: Association with psychiatric symptoms. *Journal of Psychiatry, 72*, 685–691.

Bresin, K., & Gordon, K. H. (2013). Changes in negative affect following pain (vs. nonpainful) stimulation in individuals with and without a history of nonsuicidal self-injury. *Personality Disorders: Theory, Research, and Treatment, 4*, 62–66.

Bresin, K., Gordon, K. H., Bender, T. W., Gordon, L. J., & Joiner, T. E., Jr. (2010). No pain, no change: Reductions in prior negative affect following physical pain. *Motivation and Emotion, 34*, 280–287.

Briere, J., & Gil, E. (1998). Self-mutilation in clinical and general population samples: Prevalence, correlates, and functions. *American Journal of Orthopsychiatry, 68*, 609–620.

Burns, E. E., Fischer, S., Jackson, J. L., & Harding, H. G. (2012). Deficits in emotion regulation mediate the relationship between childhood abuse and later eating disorder symptoms. *Child Abuse and Neglect, 36*, 32–39.

Cawood, C., & Huprich, S. K. (2011). Late adolescent nonsuicidal self-injury: The roles of coping style, self-esteem, and personality pathology. *Journal of Personality Disorders, 25*, 765–781.

Chapman, A. L., Gratz, K. L., & Brown, M. Z. (2006). Solving the puzzle of deliberate self-harm: The experiential avoidance model. *Behaviour Research and Therapy, 44*, 371–394.

Claes, L., Vandereycken, W., & Vertommen, H. (2005). Impulsivity-related traits in eating disorder patients. *Personality and Individual Differences, 39*, 739–749.

Claes, L., Vandereycken, W., & Vertommen, H. (2006). Pain experience related to self-injury in eating disorder patients. *Eating Behaviors, 7*, 204–213.

Claes, L., Klonsky, E. D., Muehlenkamp, J. K., & Vandereycken, W. P. (2010). The affect-regulation function of nonsuicidal self-injury in eating-disordered patients: Which affect states are regulated? *Comprehensive Psychiatry, 51*, 386–392.

Claes, L., Jiménez-Murcia, S., Agüera, Z., Castro, R., Sánchez, I., Ménchon, J. M., et al. (2012). Male eating disorder patients with and without non-suicidal self-injury: A comparison of psychopathological and personality features. *European Eating Disorders Review, 20*, 335–338.

Claes, L., Soenens, B., Vansteenkiste, M., & Vandereycken, W. (2012). The scars of the inner critic: Perfectionism and nonsuicidal self-injury in eating disorders. *European Eating Disorders Review, 20*, 196–202.

Corstorphine, E., Mountford, V., Tomlinson, S., Waller, G., & Meyer, C. (2007). Distress tolerance in eating disorders. *Eating Behaviors, 8*, 91–97.

Cowdrey, F. A., & Park, R. J. (2011). Assessing rumination in eating disorders: Principal component analysis of a minimally modified ruminative response scale. *Eating Behaviors, 12*, 321–324.

de Zwaan, M., Biener, D., Schneider, C., & Stacher, G. (1996). Relationship between thresholds to thermally and to mechanically induced pain in patients with eating disorders and healthy subjects. *Pain, 67*, 511–512.

Engel, S. G., Wonderlich, S. A., Crosby, R. D., Wright, T. L., Mitchell, J. E., Crow, J. E., et al. (2005). A study of patients with anorexia nervosa using ecological momentary assessment. *International Journal of Eating Disorders, 38*, 335–339.

Fairburn, C. G., Cooper, Z., Shafran, R., & Wilson, G. T. (2008). Eating disorders: A transdiagnostic protocol. In D. Barlow (Ed.), *Clinical handbook of psychological disorders: A step-by-step treatment manual* (4th ed.). New York: Guilford Press.

Fulton, J. J., Lavender, J. M., Tull, M. T., Klein, A. S., Muehlenkamp, J. J., & Gratz, K. L. (2012). The relationship between anxiety sensitivity and disordered eating: The mediating role of experiential avoidance. *Eating Behaviors, 13*, 166–169.

Gordon, K. H., Selby, E. A., Anestis, M. D., Bender, T. W., Witte, T. K., Braithwaite, S., et al. (2010). The reinforcing properties of repeated deliberate self-harm. *Archives of Suicide Research, 14*, 329–341.

Gordon, K. H., Holm-Denoma, J. M., Troop-Gordon, W., & Sand, E. (2012). Rumination and body dissatisfaction interact to predict binge eating. *Body Image, 9*, 352–357.

Gratz, K. L., & Roemer, L. (2008). The relationship between emotion dysregulation and deliberate self-harm among female undergraduate students at an urban commuter university. *Cognitive Behaviour Therapy, 37*, 14–25.

Haines, J. W., Brain, C. L., & Wilson, G. V. (1995). The psychophysiology of self-mutilation. *Journal of Abnormal Psychology, 104*, 471–489.

Heatherton, T. F., & Baumeister, R. F. (1991). Binge eating as escape from self-awareness. *Psychological Bulletin, 110*, 86–108.

Herts, K. L., McLaughlin, K. A., & Hatzenbuehler, M. L. (2012). Emotion dysregulation as a mechanism linking stress exposure to adolescent aggressive behavior. *Journal of Abnormal Child Psychology, 40*, 1111–1122.

Hoff, E. R., & Muehlenkamp, J. R. (2009). Nonsuicidal self-injury in college students: The role of perfectionism and rumination. *Suicide and Life-Threatening Behavior, 39*, 576–587.

Holm-Denoma, J. M., & Hankin, B. L. (2010). Perceived physical appearance mediates the rumination and bulimic symptom link in adolescent girls. *Journal of the Clinical Child and Adolescent Psychology, 39*, 537–544.

Holm-Denoma, J. M., Gordon, K. H., Bardone-Cone, A. M., Vohs, K. D., Abramson, L. Y., Heatherton, T. F., et al. (2005). A test of an interactive model of bulimic symptomatology in adult women. *Behavior Therapy, 36*, 311–321.

Hooley, J. M., Ho, D. T., Slater, J., & Lockshin, A. (2010). Pain perception and nonsuicidal self-injury: A laboratory investigation. *Personality Disorders: Theory, Research, and Treatment, 1*, 170–179.

International Society for the Study of Self-Injury. (2013). *Definition of non-suicidal self-injury*. Retrieved from http://www.isssweb.org/

Kemperman, I., Russ, M. J., Clark, W. C., Kakuma, T., Zanine, E., & Harrison, K. (1997). Pain assessment in self-injurious patients with borderline personality disorder using signal detection theory. *Psychiatry Research, 70*, 175–183.

Kerr, P. L., & Muehlenkamp, J. J. (2010). Features of psychopathology in self-injuring female college students. *Journal of Mental Health Counseling, 32*, 290–308.

Kingston, J., Clark, S., & Remington, B. (2010). Experiential avoidance and problem behavior: A mediational analysis. *Behavior Modification, 34*, 145–163.

Lavender, J. M., & Anderson, D. A. (2010). Contribution of emotion regulation difficulties to disordered eating and body dissatisfaction in college men. *International Journal of Eating Disorders, 43*, 352–357.

Linehan, M. M. L. (1993). *Skills training manual for treating borderline personality disorder*. New York: Guilford Press.

Lynam, D. R., Miller, J. D., Miller, D. J., Bornovalova, M. A., & Lejuez, C. W. (2011). Testing the relations between impulsivity-related traits, suicidality, and nonsuicidal self-injury: A test of the incremental validity of the UPPS model. *Personality Disorders: Theory, Research, and Treatment, 2*, 151–160.

Messmann-Moore, T. L., Walsh, T. L., & DiLillo, D. (2010). Emotion dysregulation and risky sexual behavior in revictimization. *Child Abuse and Neglect, 34*, 967–976.

Muehlenkamp, J. J., & Brausch, A. M. (2012). Body image as a mediator of non-suicidal self-injury in adolescents. *Journal of Adolescence, 35*, 1–9.

Muehlenkamp, J. J., Engel, S. G., Wadeson, A., Crosby, R. D., Wonderlich, S. A., Simonich, H., et al. (2009). Emotional states preceding and following acts of non-suicidal self-injury in bulimia nervosa patients. *Behaviour Research and Therapy, 47*, 83–87.

Muehlenkamp, J. J., Claes, L., Smits, D., Peat, C. M., & Vandereycken, W. (2011). Non-suicidal self-injury in eating disordered patients: A test of a conceptual model. *Psychiatry Research, 188*, 102–108.

Muehlenkamp, J. J., Claes, L., Havertape, L., & Plener, P. L. (2012). International prevalence of adolescent non-suicidal self-injury and deliberate self-harm. *Child and Adolescent Psychiatry and Mental Health, 10*, 1–9.

Muehlenkamp, J. J., Peat, C. M., Claes, L., & Smits, D. (2012). Self-injury and disordered eating: Expressing emotion dysregulation through the body. *Suicide and Life-Threatening Behavior, 42*, 416–425.

Nelson, A., & Muehlenkamp, J. J. (2012). Body attitudes and objectification in non-suicidal self-injury: Comparing males and females. *Archives of Suicide Research, 16*, 1–12.

Nock, M. K., & Mendes, W. (2008). Physiological arousal, distress tolerance, and social problem-solving deficits among adolescent self-injurers. *Journal of Consulting and Clinical Psychology, 76*, 28–38.

Nock, M. K., & Prinstein, M. J. (2004). A functional approach to the assessment of self-mutilative behavior. *Journal of Consulting and Clinical Psychology, 72*, 885–890.

Nock, M. K., & Prinstein, M. J. (2005). Contextual features and behavioral functions of self-mutilation among adolescents. *Journal of Abnormal Psychology, 114*, 140–146.

Nock, M. K., Joiner, T. E., Jr., Gordon, K. H., Lloyd-Richardson, E., & Prinstein, M. J. (2006). Non-suicidal self-injury among adolescents: Diagnostic correlates and relation to suicide attempts. *Psychiatry Research, 144*, 65–72.

Nock, M. K., Prinstein, M. J., & Sterba, S. K. (2009). Revealing the form and function of self-injurious thoughts and behaviors: A real-time ecological assessment study amongst adolescents and young adults. *Journal of Abnormal Psychology, 118*, 816–827.

Nolen-Hoeksema, S. (2003). *Women who think too much*. New York: St. Martin's Press.

Orbach, I. (1996). The role of body experience in self-destruction. *Clinical Child Psychology and Psychiatry, 1*, 607–619.

Orbach, I., & Mikulincer, M. (1998). The body investment scale: Construction and validation of a body experience scale. *Psychological Assessment, 10*, 415–425.

Orbach, I., Gilboa-Schechtman, E., Sheffer, A., Meged, S., Har-Even, D., & Stein, D. (2006). Negative bodily self in suicide attempters. *Suicide and Life-Threatening Behavior, 36*, 136–153.

Peterson, C. M., & Fischer, S. (2012). A prospective study of the influence of the UPPS model of impulsivity on the co-occurrence of bulimic symptoms and non-suicidal self-injury. *Eating Behaviors, 13*, 335–341.

Rawal, A., Park, R. J., & Williams, J. M. G. (2010). Rumination, experiential avoidance, and dysfunctional thinking in eating disorders. *Behaviour Research and Therapy, 48*, 851–859.

Raymond, N. C., de Zwaan, M., Faris, P. L., Nugent, S. M., Ackard, D. M., Crosby, R. D., et al. (1995). Pain thresholds in obese binge-eating disorder subjects. *Biological Psychiatry, 37*, 202–204.

Raymond, N. C., Faris, P. L., Thuras, P. D., Eiken, B., Howard, L. A., Hofbauer, R. D., et al. (1999). Elevated pain threshold in anorexia nervosa subjects. *Biological Psychiatry, 45*, 1389–1392.

Ross, S., & Heath, N. (2002). A study of the frequency of self-mutilation in a community sample of adolescents. *Journal of Youth and Adolescence, 31*, 67–77.

Selby, E. A., & Joiner, T. E., Jr. (2009). Cascades of emotion: The emergence of borderline personality disorder from emotional and behavioral dysregulation. *Review of General Psychology, 13*, 219–229.

Selby, E. A., & Joiner, T. E., Jr. (2013). Emotional cascades as prospective predictors of dysregulated behaviors in borderline personality disorder. *Personality Disorders: Theory, Research, and Treatment, 4*, 168–174.

Selby, E. A., Anestis, M. D., & Joiner, T. E., Jr. (2008). Understanding the relationship between emotional and behavioral dysregulation: Emotional cascades. *Behaviour Research and Therapy, 46*, 593–611.

Selby, E. A., Anestis, M. D., Bender, T. W., & Joiner, T. E., Jr. (2009). An exploration of the emotional cascade model in borderline personality disorder. *Journal of Abnormal Psychology, 118*, 375–387.

Selby, E. A., Bulik, C. M., Thornton, L. B., Crawford, H. A., Fichter, S., Halmi, M. M., et al. (2010). Refining behavioral dysregulation in borderline personality disorder using a sample of women with anorexia nervosa. *Personality Disorders: Theory, Research, and Treatment, 1*, 250–257.

Selby, E. A., Connell, L. D., & Joiner, T. E., Jr. (2010). The pernicious blend of rumination and fearlessness in non-suicidal self-injury. *Cognitive and Therapy Research, 34*, 421–428.

Selby, E. A., Bender, T. W., Gordon, K. H., Nock, M. K., & Joiner, T. E. (2012). Nonsuicidal self-injury (NSSI) disorder: A preliminary study. *Personality Disorders: Theory, Research, and Treatment, 3*, 167–175.

Smith, A. R., Fink, E. L., Anestis, M. D., Ribeiro, J. D., Gordon, K. H., Davis, H., et al. (2013). Exercise caution: Over-exercise is associated with suicidality among individuals with disordered eating. *Psychiatry Research, 206*, 246–255.

Smyth, J. M., Wonderlich, S. A., Heron, K. E., Sliwinski, M. J., Crosby, R. D., Mitchell, J. E., et al. (2007). Daily and momentary mood and stress are associated with binge eating and vomiting in bulimia nervosa patients in the natural environment. *Journal of Consulting and Clinical Psychology, 75*, 629–638.

Svaldi, J., Dorn, C., & Trentowska, M. (2011). Effectiveness for interpersonal problem-solving is reduced in women with binge eating disorder. *European Eating Disorders Review, 19*, 331–341.

Svirko, E., & Hawton, K. (2007). Self-injurious behavior and eating disorders: the extent and nature of the association. *Suicide & Life-Threatening Behavior, 37*, 409–421.

Wedig, M. M., & Nock, M. K. (2010). The functional assessment of maladaptive behaviors: A preliminary evaluation of binge eating and purging among women. *Psychiatry Research, 178*, 518–524.

Welch, S. L., & Fairburn, C. G. (1996). Impulsivity or comorbidity in bulimia nervosa: A controlled study of deliberate self-harm and alcohol and drug misuse in a community sample. *British Journal of Psychiatry, 169*, 451–458.

Whiteside, S. P., & Lynam, R. D. (2001). The Five Factor Model and impulsivity: Using a structural model of personality to understand impulsivity. *Personality and Individual Differences, 30*, 669–689.

Wonderlich, S. A., Peterson, C. B., Mitchell, J. E., & Crow, S. J. (2000). Integrative cognitive therapy for bulimic behavior. In K. J. Miller & S. J. Mizes (Eds.), *Comparative treatments for eating disorders* (pp. 258–282). New York: Springer.

Psychological Meanings and Functions of Non-suicidal Self-Injury and Eating Disorders

5

Michelle M. Wedig

Abstract

Non-suicidal self-injury (NSSI) and eating disorder behaviors have many things in common, including some of the reasons why people do them. Many researchers have taken a syndromal approach, whereby such behaviors are seen as symptoms of some underlying illness, but it may be more fruitful to examine these behaviors from a functional approach, in which maladaptive behaviors are instead goal-directed behaviors performed to obtain some desired end. This chapter focuses on a functional perspective, presenting evidence for a four-factor model that might underlie both eating disorders and NSSI behavior. This model proposes two dichotomous dimensions including contingencies that are automatic versus social and reinforcement that is positive (i.e., followed by the presentation of a favorable stimulus) versus negative (i.e., followed by the removal of an aversive stimulus). Such an approach has a considerable impact on methodological considerations in research and clinical assessment and treatment. It suggests that a functional assessment might be useful in evaluating such patients and influencing treatment options, especially when these behaviors overlap.

5.1 Introduction

The reasons why some individuals intentionally harm themselves continue to puzzle scientists, clinicians, and the public. Most research over the past several decades has taken a syndromal approach to these behaviors, in which maladaptive behaviors are conceptualized as signs or symptoms of some underlying disease process, and they have been examined as independent disorders. An alternative approach is to consider the functions of these maladaptive behaviors—that is, what

M.M. Wedig (✉)
McLean Hospital and Harvard Medical School, Belmont, MA 02478, USA
e-mail: mwedig@mclean.harvard.edu

L. Claes and J.J. Muehlenkamp (eds.), *Non-Suicidal Self-Injury in Eating Disorders*, DOI 10.1007/978-3-642-40107-7_5,

purposes they serve in their immediate environment. From a functional perspective, maladaptive behaviors are not necessarily manifestations of an underlying disease, but instead are goal-directed behaviors performed to obtain some desired end (Claes & Vandereycken, 2007).

This chapter will focus on the psychological meanings and functions of NSSI and eating disorder behaviors. First, the literature surrounding the functions of NSSI and eating disorder behaviors will be reviewed individually, then the overlap of the functions of the two behaviors will be discussed as well as the differences in the functions of the two behaviors. Finally, methodological considerations and clinical implications of such an approach to these behaviors are discussed.

5.2 Functions of Non-suicidal Self-Injury

There have been a number of functions given in the literature for NSSI. The first of these and perhaps the most well known is the four-function model provided by Nock and Prinstein (2004). This model is drawn from that of experimental studies of stereotypic self-injurious behaviors in the developmentally disabled. This population has demonstrated that their self-injurious behaviors are maintained through social (i.e., interpersonal or reinforced by others) and automatic (i.e., intrapersonal or reinforced by oneself) contingencies (Iwata et al., 1994). Drawing on these findings, Nock and Prinstein (2004) proposed and evaluated four functions of NSSI that differ among two dichotomous dimensions. These two dimensions are contingencies that are automatic versus social and reinforcement that is positive (i.e., followed by the presentation of a favorable stimulus) versus negative (i.e., followed by the removal of an aversive stimulus). In this model, *automatic-negative reinforcement* (ANR) refers to a process in which behavior is maintained by the removal of a negative affective state. In contrast, *automatic-positive reinforcement* (APR) refers to a process in which behavior is maintained by the consequent occurrence of a desired internal state. Engaging in a behavior for *social-negative reinforcement* (SNR) refers to doing so to avoid interactions with others or other social tasks. In contrast, the *social-positive reinforcement* (SPR) function focuses on getting attention from others or to communicate information to another. To test their theory, Nock and Prinstein used the Functional Assessment of Self-Mutilation (FASM, Lloyd-Richardson, Kelley, & Hope, 1997) as well as a confirmatory factor analysis to confirm the factors of their model. Important to note is that these authors found that over 50 % of self-injurers in their study indicated they engage in the behavior "to stop bad feelings," an ANR function, suggesting that perhaps ANR is the most commonly used function of NSSI.

Additional authors have also examined other functions of NSSI. They have similarly found an emotion regulation function to be the most common function of NSSI. For example, Brown and colleagues (2002) reported that non-suicidal acts were intended to express anger, punish oneself, generate normal feelings, and distract oneself. These functions were differentiated from suicide attempts which were reported to function "to make others better off." But both suicidal and NSSI were reported to function to relieve negative emotions, again an ANR function.

In a review paper of the functions of NSSI, Klonsky (2007) identified seven different models of the functions of NSSI. He reported based on 18 studies that NSSI serves to alleviate acute negative affect or aversive affective arousal (*affective-regulation model*; i.e., ANR); to end the experience of depersonalization or dissociation (*anti-dissociation model*); to replace, compromise with, or avoid the impulse to commit suicide (*anti-suicide model*); to assert one's autonomy or a distinction between self and other (*interpersonal boundaries model*); to seek help from or manipulate others (*interpersonal-influence model*); to derogate or express anger toward oneself (*self-punishment model*); and to generate exhilaration or excitement (*sensation-seeking model*). Many of these functions appear to fit within the Nock and Prinstein four-function model, but additional research is required to confirm this, such that the specific functional domains fit under the two superordinate domains of interpersonally related functions and intrapersonal functions. One study by Glenn and Klonsky (2011) did confirm that the functions of NSSI fit under these two overarching functions. However, in two empirical studies, Klonsky (2009, 2011) found that self-injury related to affect regulation was the most highly endorsed function of the behavior.

Klonsky and Olino (2008) also conducted a latent class analysis of 205 young adults with a history of one or more NSSI behaviors. They found four subgroups of self-injurers; the first subgroup contained 61 % of the participants who performed relatively few NSSI behaviors and displayed the fewest clinical symptoms. This might suggest that most of those who engage in NSSI are "experimenting" with the behavior. In comparison to the first group, the second group had an earlier age of onset of NSSI and performed more NSSI behaviors. This group comprised 17 % of the sample. Therefore, this group appeared to represent more than just occasional experimentation. This second group might engage in NSSI to manage their psychiatric distress, as they had more psychiatric symptoms than the first group. The third group (11 % of the sample) utilized a variety of NSSI methods and heavily endorsed both automatic and social functions of the behavior. This group had an early age of onset of NSSI and displayed more symptoms of anxiety than any other group. The fourth group comprised of 10 % of the sample and engaged in their NSSI almost exclusively in private and reported waiting more than 1 h after the urge to engage in the behavior set in before acting, suggesting they were less impulsive in their behaviors. This group also heavily endorsed emotion regulation functions of their behaviors. These individuals were also more likely to carry a diagnosis of borderline personality disorder, have attempted suicide, and to have required medical treatment for a suicide attempt.

Similarly, Turner, Chapman, and Layden (2012) also supported the automatic and social model of Nock and Prinstein. They had 162 female participants' complete online measures of self-injury, emotion regulation strategies and abilities, trait affectivity, social problem-solving styles, and interpersonal problems. They found through an exploratory factor analysis that each of these measures was associated with functions of emotion relief (i.e., ANR), feeling generation (i.e., APR), self-punishment, interpersonal influence (i.e., SPR), and interpersonal communication (i.e., SPR). Franklin et al. (2010) also supported this model. They used 112 participants (33 controls, 39 no-pain controls, 16 NSSI individuals, and 24 controls matching the affect dysregulation levels of the NSSI group). They employed a startle task and a prepulse inhibition task (where a stimulus is presented 30–500 ms before a startle-eliciting stimulus and causes decreased startle activity to the startle stimulus relative to non-prepulse trials) (Blumenthal, 1999) and a cold pressor task as an NSSI-proxy. Their results showed not only support for an affect regulation function of NSSI but also a cognitive regulation function and an improvement in cognitive processing.

While an ANR has been shown to be the most common function of NSSI, social reinforcement functions cannot be forgotten. Evidence that NSSI is maintained by social reinforcement is suggested in at least a substantial minority of instances. NSSI may be used when more common, less intense strategies fail (e.g., speaking, yelling, crying) and may also gain attention and caregiving from others thus strengthening affiliation with others (Nock, 2008). A recent empirical article by Muehlenkamp and colleagues (2013) suggests that interpersonal reasons for NSSI were often given for initiating rather than repeating the behavior. It also suggests that approximately 59 % of participants had disclosed their NSSI, though rarely to mental health professionals, and that conversations with others about the behavior were rated as generally unhelpful. Such research suggests that addressing the interpersonal reinforcement functions along with the automatic and affective reinforcement functions of NSSI is imperative.

5.3 Functions of Eating Disorders

The functions of eating disorder behaviors are less well researched than those of NSSI. This may be partly due to the predominantly syndromal approach taken to these behaviors based on their status in the DSM-IV. Eating disorder behaviors also vary considerably from restricting food intake to binge eating and purging, suggesting that each behavior may have a separate function.

One study of anorexia nervosa surveyed 18 women ages 20–34 from three different clinical institutions in Norway. Using unstructured interviews this study found that anorectic behavior can be summarized in eight functions: *security* (feeling of stability and safety), *avoidance* (avoiding negative emotions), *mental strength* (inner sense of mastery), *self-confidence* (feeling acknowledged and worthy of compliments), *identity* (achieving a new identity), *care* (eliciting care from others), *communication* (communicating difficulties), and *death* (wishing to starve oneself to death) (Nordbo, Espeset, Gulliksen, Skarderud, & Holte, 2006).

Another study (Jackson, Cooper, Mintz, & Albino, 2003) examined "motivations to eat" in general, including restricting behaviors, binge eating, and purging. They based their model on a four-factor model of drinking alcohol proposed by Cooper (1994), and Jackson et al. found that motivations to eat fit into this same model proposed by Cooper: *coping, social, compliance, and pleasure*. Cooper's model was further supported by the fact that each eating motivation was associated with a unique pattern of eating behavior. Coping and compliance motivations both positively predicted restrictive eating, bingeing, and purging, though coping predicted bingeing more strongly and compliance predicted restricting and purging more strongly. Pleasure also positively predicted binge eating and negatively predicted restricting, but showed no relation to purging. Finally, social motivations negatively predicted restrictive eating and purging but positively predicted bingeing.

Heatherton and Baumeister (1991) have proposed that bingeing functions to escape from negative self-awareness. According to this theory, some people, especially those who maintain high standards for themselves, find it aversive to be aware of themselves and their shortcomings and thus binge to avoid the negative feelings that may arise from this awareness (Heatherton, Herman, & Polivy, 1991; Heatherton, Striepe, & Wittenber, 1998). A similar model has been proposed for NSSI where NSSI is hypothesized to be maintained by avoidance of negative experiences (Chapman, Gratz, & Brown, 2006). Several studies support this model by showing that people often report high negative mood before the occurrence of binge episodes (Agras & Telch, 1998; Davis, Freeman, & Garner, 1988; Davis, Freeman, & Solyom, 1985; Lingswiler, Crowther, & Stephens, 1989; Powell & Thelen, 1996; Telch & Agras, 1996) and decreases in negative mood following binge eating (Kaye, Gwirtsman, George, Weiss, & Jimerson, 1986). Others have suggested that negative mood may actually increase immediately following binge episodes (Hilbert & Tuschen-Caffier, 2007) but then decrease following compensatory behaviors (i.e., purging) (Lynch, Everingham, Dubitzky, Hartman, & Kasser, 2000; Smyth et al., 2007).

Additional work provides support for other functions. For instance, dissociation often precedes binge eating episodes (Engelberg, Steiger, Gauvin, & Wonderlich, 2007; Lyubomirsky, Casper, & Sousa, 2001), suggesting that binge eating may function as an attempt to ground oneself via feeling generation. However, in this case, binge eating may also occur as an attempt to relieve the distress caused by dissociation. Furthermore, although the link between bingeing and purging and social influence is less clear, research has highlighted the overlap between bulimia and social anxiety (Grabhorn, Stenner, Kaufbold, Overbeck, & Stangier, 2005; McLean, Miller, & Hope, 2007). Thus, binge eating may be used to avoid others in the context of this anxiety. Furthermore, an evolutionary perspective has suggested bulimia may be the result of competition for mates (Faer, Hendriks, Abed, & Figueredo, 2005). In this theory, high body dissatisfaction and drive for thinness contribute to bulimic symptoms which function to improve this body dissatisfaction and increase attraction from potential mates.

5.4 Overlap of Functions of Non-suicidal Self-Injury and Eating Disorders

It may be clear by now that there are many overlaps in the functions of NSSI and the various eating disorders, primarily, that a four-function model seems to fit best for both types of behaviors. That is, an automatic negative reinforcement function (ANR; emotion regulation), automatic positive reinforcement (APR; feeling generation), social negative reinforcement (SNR; to avoid others), and social positive reinforcement function (SPR; to bring others closer) fit both types of behaviors. A similar four-function model has been demonstrated as appropriate for the psychological functions of self-injury (Nock & Prinstein, 2004), alcohol use (Cooper, Frone, Russell, & Mudar, 1995; Cox & Klinger, 1988), and healthy eating patterns (Jackson et al., 2003).

Klonsky (2007) suggests a number of functions of self-injury that might fit into Nock and Prinstein's four-function model. Similarly, his latent class analysis (Klonsky & Olino, 2008) supports both intrapersonal and interpersonal functions. Turner et al. (2012) also supported the automatic and social model of Nock and Prinstein, as did Franklin et al. (2010). Thus, while there are some papers that emphasize a four-function model, others find that a two-function model fits better (i.e., automatic/intrapersonal versus social/interpersonal, Zetterqvist, Lundh, Dahlstrom, & Svedin, 2013). Furthermore, in his 2008 paper Nock emphasized the importance of not excluding the social functions of NSSI, and Muehlenkamp et al. (2013) reinforced this in her article on the importance of interpersonal reinforcement functions of NSSI.

Similarly, many eating disorder functions seem to fit into this same model. Prior theoretical models of bingeing and purging are consistent with the Nock and Prinstein four-function model of NSSI (Heatherton & Baumeister, 1991; Polivy & Herman, 1999). Heatherton and Baumeister's model is consistent with the common ANR model as it is proposed that binge eating diminishes the aversive self-awareness. As pointed out above, the Chapman et al. (2006) article also seems to fit this model. This is also true for the several studies that show negative affect prior to binge eating and a decrease in binge eating following the behavior or following purging. Binge eating secondary to dissociation (Engelberg et al., 2007; Lyubomirsky et al., 2001) may be an example of APR, as individuals may be trying to generate feelings, or it may be an attempt to reduce the aversive experience of dissociating (ANR). Binge eating to avoid social anxiety may also be ANR but might also be SNR, if it is done in the service of avoiding other people.

Claes and colleagues (2010) examined 177 female inpatients with eating disorders and investigated the affect regulation function of different types of NSSI in these patients. They found a clear pattern for the reason "to avoid or suppress negative feelings" referring to the ANR function of NSSI. However, though they looked at this in those with eating disorders, they did not look at the functions of the participants' eating disorder behaviors.

One study has explicitly examined whether binge eating and purging statistically fit this four-function model. Wedig and Nock (2010) collected 298 adult females who had engaged in binge eating or purging in the last 3 months and who provided data for an online survey. They modified the Functional Assessment of Self-Mutilation (Lloyd-Richardson et al., 1997) to be used with a wide range of maladaptive behaviors and titled it the Functional Assessment of Maladaptive Behaviors. They performed confirmatory factor analyses for binge eating and purging separately and found a good fit for both models for the four-function model. This suggests that the model found to be useful with NSSI (Nock & Prinstein, 2004) may also help to explain pathological eating behaviors, particularly binge eating and purging.

5.5 Differences in Functions of Non-suicidal Self-Injury and Eating Disorders

There are some differences in the functions of NSSI and eating disorders though they seem to be few. One of the most obvious differences is the emphasis on weight and shape in eating disorders, which is not as prevalent in NSSI. Those with eating disorders often engage in behaviors in an attempt to lose weight, which is different from those who engage in NSSI. The issue of perfectionism is often more highly cited in the eating disorder literature as well (i.e., Claes, Soenens, Vansteenkiste, & Vandereycken, 2012).

5.6 Methodological Considerations

The results reported here suggest that certain methodological considerations should be considered. First, these results show the importance of conducting a functional assessment of both NSSI and eating disorder behaviors to understand what is driving the behaviors. How this assessment is done is another question and may vary depending on one's professional setting (e.g., clinical versus academic). Most of the studies reported above have used predominantly self-report methods, but other methods might be considered, such as ecological momentary assessment (EMA, i.e., Muehlenkamp et al., 2009; Nock, Prinstein, & Sterba, 2009). One study found specifically that EMA was a better predictor of actual binge eating episodes than was retrospective self-reporting (Anestis et al., 2010). Regardless, it is important to conduct one's assessment from a theoretical model.

Additionally, one might consider other models besides the four-function model for there might be other functions of these behaviors the model does not include, such as focusing on a two-function model or some of Klonsky's (2007) functions found in his review like his anti-dissociation function, anti-suicide function, self-punishment model, and sensation-seeking model. It might be important when assessing both NSSI and eating disorders to assess for these functions as well as it is not yet clear that these functions are not part of the model. Furthermore, the focus here was on the consequences of the behaviors, and a focus on the antecedents might also be useful (e.g., sexual abuse, overevaluation of weight and shape, the breaking of dietary restraint).

5.7 Clinical Implications

The functional model supported by the research presented here has implications for understanding and treating these behaviors. This model suggests that people do not engage in NSSI or bingeing or purging for any one reason, but instead do so in the service of several different functions, and treatment may be most effective if it appropriately targets these functions in each individual case. For example, a person who engages in these behaviors to escape negative emotions (ANR) may benefit most from learning skills for better emotion regulation and distress tolerance, while an individual who does so to avoid social interactions (SNR) may benefit more from work on exposure to social situations.

Several existing treatments have components that map directly onto the four functions hypothesized in our model. For instance, dialectical behavior therapy (DBT, Linehan, 1993a, 1993b) includes modules aimed at teaching people to regulate distressing affect and to develop interpersonal effectiveness skills. These modules are designed to help individuals develop more adaptive methods of serving these functions. This treatment was initially developed to treat suicidal and non-suicidal self-injury (Linehan, 1993a, 1993b) but has been successfully adapted for those with substance use disorders (Linehan et al., 1999), as well as bulimia nervosa (Chen, Matthews, Allen, Kuo, & Linehan, 2008; Safer, Telch, & Agras, 2000, 2001) and binge eating disorder (BED, Chen et al., 2008; Telch, 1997; Telch, Agras, & Linehan, 2001, 2000). Similarly, acceptance and commitment therapy (ACT) is based on the idea that maladaptive behaviors function as a way of avoiding emotional experience (Hayes, Strosahl, & Wilson, 1999; Hayes, Wilson, Gifford, Follette, & Strosahl, 1996) and these concepts have also been applied to the treatment of eating disorders (see Wilson, 1996, 2004). The success of these treatment modules, which were designed to target specific functional areas, with the very behaviors shown to serve similar functions, provides additional support for the idea that matching treatment to functionality may be an effective form of treatment and that these functions might operate transdiagnostically.

It will be important for future treatment studies to include pretreatment measures of the functions served by the maladaptive behavior being targeted and to test the usefulness of tailoring treatment to match the identified function in each individual case. We have no knowledge yet whether such matching of treatment to function is effective, but research to date has suggested that this may be an effective way to treat both NSSI and various forms of eating disorders. Using measures such as the Functional Assessment of Maladaptive Behaviors (Wedig & Nock, 2010) may be useful in both research and clinical practice, with the caveat that this measure has only been tested on binge eating and purging and requires further validation for other behaviors. The Functional Assessment of Self-Mutilation (Lloyd-Richardson et al., 1997; Nock & Prinstein, 2004) may be useful for the assessment of NSSI, but how to translate that into effective treatment is still in question.

Oftentimes, we see "symptom substitution," where one symptom (e.g., cutting) is substituted for another (e.g., restricting). This might provide additional support for a functional approach suggesting that these behaviors might serve the same function. Hopefully future research will embrace the functional approach underlying these disorders and empirically test whether matching treatment to function is in fact the most effective way to treat these behaviors.

References

Agras, W. S., & Telch, C. F. (1998). The effects of caloric deprivation and negative affect on binge-eating in obese binge-eating disordered women. *Behavior Therapy, 29*, 491–503.

Anestis, M. D., Selby, E. A., Crosby, R. D., Wonderlich, S. A., Engel, S. G., & Joiner, T. E. (2010). A comparison of retrospective self-report versus ecological momentary assessment measures of affective lability in the examination of its relationship with bulimic symptomatology. *Behaviour Research and Therapy, 48*(7), 607–613.

Blumenthal, T. D. (1999). Short lead interval modification. In M. E. Dawson, A. M. Schell, & A. H. Bohmelt (Eds.), *Startle modification: Implications for neuroscience, cognitive science, and clinical science* (pp. 51–71). Cambridge: Cambridge University Press.

Brown, M. Z., Comtois, K. A., & Linehan, M. (2002). Reasons for suicide attempts and nonsuicidal self-injury in women with borderline personality disorder. *Journal of Abnormal Psychology, 111*(1), 198–202.

Chapman, A. L., Gratz, K. L., & Brown, M. Z. (2006). Solving the puzzle of deliberate self-harm: The experiential avoidance model. *Behaviour Research and Therapy, 44*(3), 371–394.

Chen, E. Y., Matthews, L., Allen, C., Kuo, J. R., & Linehan, M. M. (2008). Dialectical behavior therapy for clients with binge-eating disorder or bulimia nervosa and borderline personality disorder. *International Journal of Eating Disorders, 41*(6), 505–512.

Claes, L., Klonsky, E. D., Muehlenkamp, J., Kuppens, P., & Vandereycken, W. (2010). The affect-regulation function of nonsuicidal self-injury in eating-disordered patients: Which affect states are regulated? *Comprehensive Psychiatry, 51*(4), 386–392.

Claes, L., Soenens, B., Vansteenkiste, M., & Vandereycken, W. (2012). The scars of the inner critic: Perfectionism and nonsuicidal self-injury in eating disorders. *European Eating Disorder Review, 20*(3), 196–202.

Claes, L., & Vandereycken, W. (2007). Self-injurious behavior: Differential diagnosis and functional differentiation. *Comprehensive Psychiatry, 48*(2), 137–144.

Cooper, M. L. (1994). Motivations for alcohol use among adolescents: Development and validation of a four factor model. *Psychological Assessment, 6*, 117–128.

Cooper, M. L., Frone, M. R., Russell, M., & Mudar, P. (1995). Drinking to regulate positive and negative emotions: A motivational model of alcohol use. *Journal of Personality and Social Psychology, 69*(5), 990–1005.

Cox, W. M., & Klinger, E. (1988). A motivational model of alcohol use. *Journal of Abnormal Psychology, 97*(2), 168–180.

Davis, R., Freeman, R. J., & Garner, D. M. (1988). A naturalistic investigation of eating behavior in bulimia nervosa. *Journal of Consulting and Clinical Psychology, 56*(2), 273–279.

Davis, R., Freeman, R., & Solyom, L. (1985). Mood and food: An analysis of bulimic episodes. *Journal of Psychiatric Research, 19*(2/3), 331–335.

Engelberg, M. J., Steiger, H., Gauvin, L., & Wonderlich, S. A. (2007). Binge antecedents in bulimic syndromes: An examination of dissociative and negative affect. *International Journal of Eating Disorders, 40*, 531–536.

Faer, L. M., Hendriks, A., Abed, R. T., & Figueredo, A. J. (2005). The evolutionary psychology of eating disorders: Female competition for mates or for status? *Psychology and Psychotherapy: Theory, Research and Practice, 78*, 397–417.

Franklin, J. C., Hessel, E. T., Aaron, R. V., Arthur, M. S., Heilbron, N., & Prinstein, M. J. (2010). The functions of nonsuicidal self-injury: Support for cognitive-affective regulation and opponent processes from a novel psychophysiological paradigm. *Journal of Abnormal Psychology, 119*(4), 850–862.

Glenn, C. R., & Klonsky, E. D. (2011). One-year test-retest reliability of the Inventory of Statements about Self-Injury (ISAS). *Assessment, 18*(3), 375–378.

Grabhorn, R., Stenner, H., Kaufbold, J., Overbeck, G., & Stangier, U. (2005). Shame and social anxiety in anorexia and bulimia nervosa. *Zeitschrift für Psychosomatische Medizin und Psychotherapie, 51*(2), 179–193.

Hayes, S. C., Strosahl, K., & Wilson, K. G. (1999). *Acceptance and commitment therapy: An experiential approach to behavior change*. New York: The Guilford Press.

Hayes, S. C., Wilson, K. G., Gifford, E. V., Follette, V. M., & Strosahl, K. (1996). Experiential avoidance and behavioral disorders: A functional dimensional approach to diagnosis and treatment. *Journal of Consulting and Clinical Psychology, 64*(6), 1152–1168.

Heatherton, T. F., & Baumeister, R. F. (1991). Binge eating as escape from self-awareness. *Psychological Bulletin, 110*(1), 86–108.

Heatherton, T. F., Herman, C. P., & Polivy, J. (1991). The effects of physical threat and ego threat on eating. *Journal of Personality and Social Psychology, 60*, 138–143.

Heatherton, T. F., Striepe, M., & Wittenber, L. (1998). Emotional distress and disinhibited eating: The role of self. *Personality and Social Psychology Bulletin, 24*(3), 301.

Hilbert, A., & Tuschen-Caffier, B. (2007). Maintenance of binge eating through negative mood: A naturalistic comparison of binge eating disorder and bulimia nervosa. *International Journal of Eating Disorders, 40*, 521–530.

Iwata, B. A., Pace, G. M., Dorsey, M. F., Zarcone, J. R., Vollmer, T. R., Smith, R. G., et al. (1994). The functions of self-injurious behavior: An experimental-epidemiological analysis. *Journal of Applied Behavior Analysis, 27*(2), 215–240.

Jackson, B., Cooper, M. L., Mintz, L., & Albino, A. (2003). Motivations to eat: Scale development and validation. *Journal of Research in Personality, 37*, 297–318.

Kaye, W. H., Gwirtsman, H. E., George, D. T., Weiss, S. R., & Jimerson, D. C. (1986). Relationship of mood alterations to bingeing behaviour in bulimia. *British Journal of Psychiatry, 149*, 479–485.

Klonsky, E. D. (2007). The functions of deliberate self-injury: A review of the evidence. *Clinical Psychology Review, 27*, 226–239.

Klonsky, E. D. (2009). The functions of self-injury in young adults who cut themselves: Clarifying the evidence for affect-regulation. *Psychiatry Research, 166*(2–3), 260–268.

Klonsky, E. D. (2011). Non-suicidal self injury in United States adults: Prevalence, sociodemographics, topography and functions. *Psychological Medicine, 41*, 1981–1986.

Klonsky, E. D., & Olino, T. M. (2008). Identifying clinical distinct subgroups of self-injurers among young adults: A latent class analysis. *Journal of Consulting and Clinical Psychology, 76*(1), 22–27.

Linehan, M. M. (1993a). *Cognitive-behavioral treatment of borderline personality disorder*. New York: The Guilford Press.

Linehan, M. M. (1993b). *Skills training manual for treating borderline personality disorder*. New York: The Guilford Press.

Linehan, M. M., Schmidt, H., Dimeff, L. A., Craft, J. C., Kanter, J., & Comtois, K. A. (1999). Dialectical behavior therapy for patients with borderline personality disorder and drug-dependence. *American Journal on Addictions, 8*(4), 279–292.

Lingswiler, V. M., Crowther, J. H., & Stephens, M. A. P. (1989). Affective and cognitive antecedents to eating episodes in bulimia and binge eating. *International Journal of Eating Disorders, 8*(5), 533–539.

Lloyd-Richardson, E. E., Kelley, M. L., & Hope, T. (1997). *Self-mutilation in a community sample of adolescents: Descriptive characteristics and provisional prevalence rates*. Poster session presented at the annual meeting of the Society for Behavioral Medicine, New Orleans, LA.

Lynch, W. C., Everingham, A., Dubitzky, J., Hartman, M., & Kasser, T. (2000). Does binge eating play a role in the self-regulation of moods? *Integrative Physiological and Behavioral Science, 35*(4), 298–313.

Lyubomirsky, S., Casper, R. C., & Sousa, L. (2001). What triggers abnormal eating in bulimic and nonbulimic women? *Psychology of Women Quarterly, 25*(3), 223–232.

McLean, C. P., Miller, N. A., & Hope, D. A. (2007). Mediating social anxiety and disordered eating: The role of expressive suppression. *Eating Disorders, 15*(1), 41–54.

Muehlenkamp, J. J., Brausch, A., Quigley, K., & Whitlock, J. (2013). Interpersonal features and functions of nonsuicidal self-injury. *Suicide and Life Threatening Behavior, 43*, 67–80.

Muehlenkamp, J. J., Engel, S. G., Wadeson, A., Crosby, R. D., Wonderlich, S. A., Simonich, H., et al. (2009). Emotional states preceding and following acts of non-suicidal self-injury in bulimia nervosa patients. *Behaviour Research and Therapy, 47*(1), 83–87.

Nock, M. K. (2008). Actions speak louder than words: An elaborated theoretical model of the social functions of self-injury and other harmful behaviors. *Applied and Preventive Psychology, 12*(4), 159–168.

Nock, M. K., & Prinstein, M. J. (2004). A functional approach to the assessment of self-mutilative behavior. *Journal of Consulting and Clinical Psychology, 72*(5), 885–890.

Nock, M. K., Prinstein, M. J., & Sterba, S. K. (2009). Revealing the form and function of self-injurious thoughts and behaviors: A real-time ecological assessment study among adolescents and young adults. *Journal of Abnormal Psychology, 118*(4), 816–827.

Nordbo, R. H., Espeset, E. M., Gulliksen, K. S., Skarderud, F., & Holte, A. (2006). The meaning of self-starvation: Qualitative study of patients' perception of anorexia nervosa. *International Journal of Eating Disorders, 39*(7), 556–564.

Polivy, J., & Herman, C. P. (1999). Distress and eating: Why do dieters overeat? *International Journal of Eating Disorders, 26*, 153–164.

Powell, A. L., & Thelen, M. H. (1996). Emotions and cognitions associated with bingeing and weight control behavior in bulimia. *Journal of Psychosomatic Research, 40*(3), 317–328.

Safer, D. L., Telch, C. F., & Agras, W. S. (2000). Dialectical behavior therapy adapted for bulimia: A case report. *International Journal of Eating Disorders, 30*, 101–106.

Safer, D. L., Telch, C. F., & Agras, W. S. (2001). Dialectical behavior therapy for bulimia nervosa. *American Journal of Psychiatry, 158*(4), 632–634.

Smyth, J. M., Wonderlich, S. A., Heron, K. E., Sliwinski, M. J., Crosby, R. D., Mitchell, J. E., et al. (2007). Daily and momentary mood and stress are associated with binge eating and vomiting in bulimia nervosa patients in the natural environment. *Journal of Consulting and Clinical Psychology, 75*(4), 629–638.

Telch, C. F. (1997). Skills training treatment for adaptive affect regulation in a woman with binge-eating disorder. *International Journal of Eating Disorders, 22*, 77–81.

Telch, C. F., & Agras, W. S. (1996). Do emotional states influence binge eating in the obese? *International Journal of Eating Disorders, 20*(3), 271–279.

Telch, C. F., Agras, W. S., & Linehan, M. M. (2000). Group dialectical behavior therapy for binge-eating disorder: A preliminary, uncontrolled trial. *Behavior Therapy, 31*, 569–582.

Telch, C. F., Agras, W. S., & Linehan, M. (2001). Dialectical behavior therapy for binge eating disorder. *Journal of Consulting and Clinical Psychology, 69*(6), 1061–1065.

Turner, B. J., Chapman, A. L., & Layden, B. K. (2012). Intrapersonal and interpersonal functions of non-suicidal self injury: Associations with emotional and social functioning. *Suicide and Life-Threatening Behavior, 42*(1), 36–55.

Wedig, M. M., & Nock, M. K. (2010). The functional assessment of maladaptive behaviors: An evaluation of binge eating and purging. *Psychiatry Research, 178*(3), 518–524.

Wilson, G. T. (1996). Acceptance and change in the treatment of eating disorders and obesity. *Behavior Therapy, 27*(3), 417–439.

Wilson, G. T. (2004). Acceptance and change in the treatment of eating disorders. In S. C. Hayes, V. M. Follette, & M. Linehan (Eds.), *Mindfulness and acceptance*. New York: The Guilford Press.

Zetterqvist, M., Lundh, L. G., Dahlstrom, O., & Svedin, C. G. (2013). Prevalence and Function of Non-Suicidal Self-Injury (NSSI) in a Community Sample of Adolescents, Using Suggested DSM-5 Criteria for a Potential NSSI Disorder. *Journal of Abnormal Child Psychology, 41*, 759–773.

Part II

Assessment and Treatment

Functional Assessment of Non-suicidal Self-Injury and Eating Disorders

6

Margaret S. Andover, Caroline S. Holman, and Marguerite Y. Shashoua

Abstract

Non-suicidal self-injury (NSSI) and eating disorders, both important public health concerns, co-occur at a considerable rate. As many as 55–61 % of individuals with NSSI or eating disorders report engaging in the other type of self-destructive behavior. This significant overlap suggests that a common mechanism may be involved in the development and maintenance of the disorders. One potential common mechanism may be explained by principles of operant conditioning. Operant conditioning is important in understanding factors that maintain problem behaviors, such as NSSI and eating disorder behaviors, as well as in the treatment of these behaviors. The purpose of this chapter is to discuss the application of the behavioral technique of functional assessment, which is based on principles of operant conditioning, to the assessment and treatment of comorbid NSSI and eating disorders. We will first review the empirical research and theory that support behavioral models for the maintenance of NSSI and eating disorders. Second, we will demonstrate the use of functional assessment to identify the factors associated with the maintenance of these problem behaviors and discuss the implications of functional assessment to the treatment of comorbid NSSI and eating disorders.

6.1 Functional Assessment of Non-suicidal Self-Injury and Eating Disorders

By definition, non-suicidal self-injury (NSSI) involves deliberate tissue damage without suicidal intent. Common methods of NSSI include cutting, carving, scratching, interfering with wound healing, self-hitting, and burning. NSSI is not

M.S. Andover (✉) • C.S. Holman • M.Y. Shashoua
Department of Psychology, Fordham University, Bronx, New York, NY, USA
e-mail: andover@fordham.edu

L. Claes and J.J. Muehlenkamp (eds.), *Non-Suicidal Self-Injury in Eating Disorders*, DOI 10.1007/978-3-642-40107-7_6, © Springer-Verlag Berlin Heidelberg 2014

associated with any one psychiatric disorder; rather, the behavior occurs across psychiatric disorders (Nock, Joiner, Gordon, Lloyd-Richardson, & Prinstein, 2006). For example, NSSI has been associated with mood disorders such as major depressive disorder and dysthymia, anxiety disorders such as obsessive-compulsive disorder and posttraumatic stress disorder, substance abuse, and eating disorders (i.e., Claes, Vandereycken, & Vertommen, 2001; Jacobson & Gould, 2007; Klonsky & Muehlenkamp, 2007; Serras, Saules, Cranford, & Eisenberg, 2010). The co-occurrence of NSSI and eating disorders is particularly alarming. Studies have shown that among NSSI samples, as many as 61 % have a diagnosis of an eating disorder (Svirko & Hawton, 2007). Similarly, high school students with a history of NSSI are more likely than their non-injuring counterparts to report disordered eating (Ross, Heath, & Toste, 2009). Among samples of patients with eating disorders, between 19 and 55 % report a history of NSSI (Claes et al., 2013; Claes, Klonsky, Muehlenkamp, Kuppens, & Vandereycken, 2010; Claes, Soenens, Vansteenkiste, & Vandereycken, 2012; Stein, Lilenfeld, Wildman, & Marcus, 2004; Svirko & Hawton, 2007). Research suggests that NSSI is associated with specific eating disorder behaviors and diagnoses. For example, eating disorder patients with a history of NSSI were more likely than those without an NSSI history to report binging and purging behaviors. In addition, those with an NSSI history were more likely to engage in multiple methods of purging than those without NSSI (Stein et al., 2004). Claes et al. (2013) found that NSSI was significantly more likely among patients with bulimia nervosa (BN) and eating disorder not otherwise specified (EDNOS) diagnoses than with obesity. Prevalence rates in this study suggest that NSSI behaviors are less common in eating disorders characterized by extreme weight, such as the restricting subtype of anorexia nervosa (AN) and obesity. Consistent with these findings, Svirko and Hawton (2007) suggest that NSSI is more common among individuals with BN and the binge/purge subtype of AN than among those with the restricting subtype of AN.

The comorbidity between NSSI and eating disorders, especially those involving binging and purging, suggests the presence of a common mechanism underlying the disorders. Further, research on and theoretical models for both eating disorders and NSSI suggest similarities among the factors that contribute to the maintenance of the behaviors. The purpose of this chapter is to discuss the application of the behavioral technique of functional assessment to the treatment of comorbid NSSI and eating disorders. As such, we will first briefly review behavioral models of NSSI, followed by models of eating disorder, each with an emphasis on the aspects most directly relevant to functional assessment. We will then review the functional overlap between NSSI and eating disorder symptoms. Lastly, we will provide an overview on conducting and utilizing functional assessment in the treatment of comorbid NSSI and eating disorders.

6.2 Functional Models of Non-suicidal Self-Injury

The reasons for which some individuals purposely injure themselves without intent to die have long been a focus of attention and theory (Favazza, 1998; Suyemoto, 1998), and research investigating the reasons and motivations for NSSI has increased substantially in recent years. A number of reasons for NSSI have been proposed or reported (e.g., Suyemoto, 1998). For example, in a survey of households in the USA, Klonsky (2011) found that 64 % of self-injurers reported engaging in NSSI to release emotional pressure, 60 % to get rid of bad feelings, and 36 % to feel something. In addition, 32 % reported engaging in NSSI for self-punishment, and 28 % reported engaging in NSSI to communicate with others or to get attention. Engaging in NSSI for multiple reasons is common; nearly 70 % of those surveyed with a history of NSSI reported doing so for more than one reason (Klonsky, 2011). Research most strongly supports affect or emotion regulation and self-punishment as functions of NSSI (e.g., Klonsky, 2007), although a number of studies suggest the role of social factors in the behavior as well (e.g., Klonsky, 2011; Nock & Prinstein, 2004, 2005).

The role of affect regulation as a consequence of NSSI has been supported in both self-report studies and laboratory studies. Using ecological momentary assessment, Armey, Crowther, and Miller (2011) found that episodes of NSSI were preceded by an increase in *negative affect* and followed by a decrease in negative affect. In addition, decreases in negative affect have been reported following the administration of a painful stimulus as an NSSI proxy (Bresin & Gordon, 2013; Bresin, Gordon, Bender, Gordon, & Joiner, 2010; Franklin et al., 2013). The role of NSSI in affect regulation has also been reported using objective, non-self-report measures. Researchers have shown that imagining an episode of NSSI is associated with a decrease in physiological arousal among individuals with a history of NSSI (Brain, Haines, & Williams, 1998; Haines, Williams, Brain, & Wilson, 1995), supporting the function of affect regulation. The studies discussed here provide only a sample of research on the regulation of negative affect through NSSI; consistent results have been found in numerous studies.

Although research often focuses on the reduction of negative affect, recent studies suggest that *positive affect* increases following NSSI behavior (e.g., Franklin et al., 2013; Jenkins & Schmitz, 2012; Muehlenkamp et al., 2009). In fact, among individuals with greater affect dysregulation, frequency of NSSI over time was predicted by positive affect, but not negative affect (Jenkins & Schmitz, 2012). Other research, however, has not supported an increase in positive affect following NSSI (e.g., Bresin et al., 2010).

In addition to affect regulation, NSSI may serve to regulate *cognitive processing*. Franklin et al. (2010) found that following a painful stimulus, performance on a physiological measure of information processing increased among individuals with a history of NSSI, suggesting that the behavior may improve information processing and therefore provide a method of cognitive regulation. Further research on the role of NSSI in cognitive regulation and the regulation of positive affect is needed.

Although affect regulation is the most commonly reported function of NSSI, individuals also engage in NSSI for other reasons, sometimes simultaneously (e.g., Klonsky, 2011; Nock, 2009; Nock & Prinstein, 2004, 2005). It is therefore imperative that a model of NSSI function be flexible enough to accommodate the range of consequences of the behavior.

One such model is based on behavioral principles of reinforcement, which makes it ideal for application to the functional assessment of NSSI behaviors. According to Nock and Prinstein (2004, 2005), NSSI is reinforced by the consequences of the behavior; these consequences make it more likely that NSSI will be repeated. NSSI may be performed for automatic negative reinforcement (i.e., removal of an aversive stimulus), automatic positive reinforcement (i.e., generation of a favorable stimulus), social negative reinforcement (i.e., escape from interpersonal situations or demands), and social positive reinforcement (i.e., gaining attention from others or access to environmental or interpersonal resources; Nock & Prinstein, 2004, 2005). Research has provided empirical support for this functional model of NSSI. The *automatic reinforcement functions* of NSSI are consistent with research on affect regulation, self-punishment, and other models of NSSI such as the experiential avoidance model (Chapman, Gratz, & Brown, 2006). When NSSI is performed to cause a change in the environment, this would be considered *social reinforcement*. Engaging in NSSI in order to communicate distress or get attention would be considered social positive reinforcement, while performing NSSI behaviors to avoid an interpersonal situation or demand would be social negative reinforcement.

Although, historically, many reasons and motivations for NSSI behaviors have been suggested, research suggests that individuals primarily engage in NSSI for affect regulation, self-punishment, and social communication (e.g., Klonsky, 2007; Nock & Prinstein, 2004, 2005). Given the substantial research on affect regulation as a function of NSSI, researchers have suggested that interventions target this specifically (Slee, Spinhoven, Garnefski, & Arensman, 2008). However, interventions for NSSI should be flexible enough to address other functions of the behavior as well. Behavioral assessment and intervention strategies, such as functional assessment, are ideal for this task (Nock, Teper, & Hollander, 2007; Muehlenkamp, 2006), as their purpose is to identify and target the factors that reinforce and therefore maintain NSSI behaviors.

6.3 Functional Models of Eating Disorders

Various cognitive-behavioral models for bulimia nervosa (BN) have been proposed, and symptoms of BN and other eating disorders, such as binge eating (Lee & Miltenberger, 1997), can be conceptualized as a function of antecedent and consequent behaviors. Cognitive-behavioral treatments (CBT) have been found to be effective in the treatment of BN (e.g., Agras, Walsh, Fairburn, Wilson, & Kraemer, 2000; Shapiro et al., 2007; Whittal, Agras, & Gould, 1999). As cognitive-behavioral models of BN are largely concerned with factors that maintain

BN symptoms, this suggests an important role for behavioral interventions based on functional assessment. Cognitive-behavioral approaches have also been developed and are often used to treat anorexia nervosa (AN), but there is debate as to their effectiveness, especially in the outpatient treatment of adults (Bulik, Berkman, Brownley, Sedway, & Lohr, 2007; Fairburn, 2005). Some researchers suggest that function-based behavioral approaches to AN may be useful, and treatments based on a functional conceptualization of the disorder would resolve the shortcomings previously attributed to behavioral techniques (Wiese, 2009).

In order to determine the symptoms of eating disorders that would be appropriate targets of functional assessment, we turn to existing models of the disorders. Although a complete review of theoretical models is beyond the scope of this chapter, we will draw from specific pathways common to cognitive-behavioral models in our formulation of a functional assessment of these disorders.

6.3.1 Models of Bulimia Nervosa

Cognitive-behavioral models of BN overlap considerably in the *cognitive factors* theorized to contribute to the etiology of this disorder. For example, models have suggested that cognitive factors such as perfectionism, low self-esteem, inability to tolerate intense feelings or mood intolerance, interpersonal difficulties, negative self-referent beliefs, and maladaptive beliefs about eating contribute to the development and maintenance of BN (e.g., Cooper, Wells, & Todd, 2004; Fairburn, Cooper, & Shafran, 2003). Body dissatisfaction that emerges from the internalization of sociocultural standards and overvaluation of weight and shape are also cognitive factors theorized to play a direct role in BN symptomology (Fairburn, Cooper, & Cooper, 1986; Fairburn, Marcus, & Wilson, 1993; Stice, 1994). These cognitions about the body and eating lead to dietary restriction, which in turn leads to binging behaviors (Fairburn et al., 2003; Stice, 1994) either because restriction leads to disinhibited eating (Stice, 1994), a lapse in restriction leads to a loss of control (Fairburn et al., 2003), or because restriction leads to negative affect through caloric deprivation or lack of weight loss (Stice, 1994). The binge, however, further contributes to concerns about weight and shape, resulting in even more stringent dietary restriction (Fairburn et al., 2003). Although models of BN have specific implications for cognitive treatments, they also provide a theoretical framework with which to apply behavioral interventions, including functional assessment.

Most relevant to interventions based on a functional assessment of BN are the mechanisms by which symptoms of BN are maintained. Although the specific relationships between antecedents, behaviors, and consequences vary across models, research has shown that binging behaviors across eating disorders are often preceded by *negative affect* (e.g., Berg et al., 2013; Smyth et al., 2007; Stein et al., 2007). Stice and colleagues (1994) and Stice, Shaw, and Nemeroff (1998) proposed that negative affect occurs through two separate pathways in BN. First, body dissatisfaction and related cognitions are associated with negative affect. Second, negative affect may be caused by dietary restriction itself. This may be a result of repeated failures with dieting, which have been proposed to impact self-esteem and cause negative affect (Heatherton & Polivy, 1992). In addition, negative affect may be associated with mood changes related to caloric deprivation (Keys, Brozek, Henschel, Mickelsen, & Taylor, 1950). Researchers have also suggested that specific events that may or may not be related to eating and weight, but that are construed as challenges to the individual's perceived self-worth, may activate initial negative self-referential beliefs and subsequent negative thoughts. These negative beliefs and thoughts lead to an increase in negative affect, triggering a binge/purge episode (Cooper et al., 2004). The cycle of binging and purging is theorized to be maintained through specific cognitions, including thoughts about the consequences of eating on body shape and weight, thoughts that are permissive of eating, thoughts of uncontrollability, and thoughts that food will improve affect through avoidance (Cooper et al., 2004). The use of binging to improve affect suggests that this behavior may be amenable to behavioral treatment targeted at the function of the binge.

In sum, binges are largely conceptualized as functioning to reduce negative affect that may be associated with body dissatisfaction, dietary restriction itself, or an external trigger (Cooper et al., 2004; Fairburn et al., 2003; Stice, 1994; Stice et al., 1998), while purging is most often proposed as a means of mitigating the consequences of the binge. As the models discussed above and others suggest, many cognitive factors in the development and maintenance of BN must be addressed in treatment, potentially through cognitive therapy. However, the reduction of negative affect and cognitions associated with binging and purging behaviors provide negative reinforcement, increasing the likelihood that these behaviors will occur again.

6.3.2 Models of Anorexia Nervosa

Although the reinforcing properties of BN symptoms have been identified in models of the disorder and have received some empirical support, behavioral approaches for AN have been less evident. Early approaches to the treatment of AN included behavioral interventions with the specific goal of initiating weight gain (Garfinkel, Garner, & Moldofsky, 1977; Stunkard, 1972). To accomplish this goal, behavioral modification using operant conditioning principles (Agras, Barlow, Chapin, Abel, & Leitenberg, 1974), behavioral contracts (Solanto, Jacobson, Heller, Golden, & Hertz, 1994), and systematic desensitization to food and weight gain (Schnurer, Rubin, & Roy, 1973) have been used. Although these strategies may restore weight in patients with AN during hospitalization, they have been criticized as being dangerously unsustainable after hospital discharge and for ignoring the complexity of factors that underlie this disorder (Bruch, 1974). However, some researchers suggest that treatments based on a functional conceptualization of AN would resolve the shortcomings previously attributed to behavioral techniques (Wiese, 2009).

Like BN, models of AN emphasize both cognitive factors and reinforcement principles in the development and maintenance of AN symptomology. Factors implicated in the development of AN include perfectionism, low satisfaction with life, and decreased self-esteem that occur as a result of normal adolescent development, interpersonal conflict, and experiences with failure (Slade, 1982). Together, these factors lead to a perceived need for control over some aspect of the individual's life. A pervasive need for control that transitions to a focus on eating is central to several theoretical models of AN (i.e., Fairburn, Shafran, & Cooper, 1999; Garner & Bemis, 1982; Schmidt & Treasure, 2006; Slade, 1982). In addition, entrenched pro-anorexia beliefs regarding the importance of food restriction to maintaining thinness and emotional stability make the disorder more difficult to treat (Garner & Bemis, 1982; Schmidt & Treasure, 2006).

Although initial dieting may stem from common social cues, in the context of the previously mentioned intrapersonal characteristics, dieting may serve as the first step towards more pathological dietary restriction (Slade, 1982). Following early attempts at dieting where weight loss is achieved, dietary restriction is perpetuated through positive and negative reinforcement. Resulting increases in positive mood, feelings of accomplishment, increased control, and increased self-worth positively reinforce food restriction behaviors (Fairburn et al., 1999; Garner & Bemis, 1982; Schmidt & Treasure, 2006; Slade, 1982). Dietary restriction is negatively reinforced through avoidance of weight gain. Further, preoccupation with food intake provides a means of avoiding other life problems, which negatively reinforces food restriction and preoccupation (Fairburn et al., 1999; Slade, 1982). Overvaluation of thinness and distorted beliefs about food and eating may justify the avoidance of normal eating behaviors and result in constant hypervigilance for any food-related temptations, which further reinforces dietary restriction (Fairburn et al., 1999; Garner & Bemis, 1982; Schmidt & Treasure, 2006). Dietary restriction may also be reinforced by social factors; the behavior may lead to positive social reinforcement, first in the context of initial dieting and weight loss and eventually as displays of concern by others as the disease progresses (Garner & Bemis, 1982; Schmidt & Treasure, 2006). Restriction may also negatively reinforce itself, as its physiological consequences such as hunger and impaired concentration may be interpreted as threats to self-control to be avoided through further food restriction and constant monitoring (Fairburn et al., 1999).

Negative reinforcement pathways that emphasize avoidance are often included in models of AN, suggesting a role in functional assessment. Emotional avoidance has been proposed as an important element of AN and has been found to mediate the associations among depression, anxiety, and eating symptoms (Wildes, Ringham, & Marcus, 2010). Further supporting the role of emotional avoidance in AN, research has shown that AN is associated with emotion suppression (Geller, Cockell, & Goldner, 2000). In addition, AN is associated with disorder-specific rumination, which has been posited as a cognitive avoidance strategy (Cowdrey & Park, 2012). Interestingly, some researchers have shown that fewer emotional regulation difficulties were associated with lower body mass indexes among individuals with acute AN, suggesting that dietary restriction may serve an emotion regulation function (Brockmeyer et al., 2012). In fact, Haynos and Fruzzetti (2011) propose that AN is a disorder of emotional dysregulation, and difficulties in emotion regulation may be central to the maintenance of this disorder.

Although models of AN often have less emphasis on behavioral aspects of the disorder, research suggests that several symptoms of AN may be suitable for behavior therapy. Specifically, factors that reinforce food restriction and binging behaviors and AN symptoms that function to avoid emotional experiences may be addressed by functional assessment in conjunction with treatments focused on addressing the cognitive aspects of the disorder.

6.3.3 Transdiagnostic Model of Eating Disorders

With the goal of conducting functional assessment of eating disorder behaviors in mind, it is important to recognize that a considerable amount of overlap exists between symptoms of BN, AN, binge-eating disorder (BED), and eating disorders not otherwise specified (EDNOS), as each involves restricting, binging, and/or purging with relative frequency (American Psychiatric Association, 2000). Fluidity among the disorders has also been found (Agras et al., 2000; Sullivan, Bulik, Fear, & Pickering, 1998), which suggests the potential for functional commonality of these symptoms across the disorders. In an effort to address these concerns, Fairburn and colleagues (2003) developed a transdiagnostic model of eating disorders. An extension of Fairburn's updated cognitive-behavioral model of bulimia nervosa, this formulation maintains at its core the overvaluation of weight and size and specific pathways that lead to dietary restriction (Fairburn et al., 2003). In addition, low self-esteem, perfectionism, mood intolerance, and interpersonal difficulties are again hypothesized to play a role in the maintenance of eating symptoms in some individuals.

Fairburn and colleagues (2003) suggest that eating disorders can be differentiated by a relative tendency by the individual to binge or restrict. Instead of engaging in binging and compensatory behavior, restricting behaviors leading to a low weight in AN may be maintained by the physical and psychological consequences of the starvation itself (Fairburn et al., 1999). Notably, Fairburn and colleagues (2003) argue that the binge/purge subtype of AN may be particularly resistant to treatment (Steinhausen, Rauss-Mason, & Seidel, 1991), as it may be reinforced by both the consequences of binging and purging and by the physical and psychological consequences of extreme restriction.

6.4 Functional Overlap Between Non-suicidal Self-Injury and Eating Disorders

Research has demonstrated that patients with an eating disorder and NSSI behaviors are more likely to report binging and purging behaviors or have a diagnosis that includes binging and purging in its symptomology (Claes et al., 2013; Stein et al., 2004; Svirko & Hawton, 2007), suggesting an underlying commonality to the behaviors. Research suggests that negative affect is a common antecedent to binging behaviors, and individuals binge in order to reduce this negative affect (Cooper et al., 2004; Fairburn et al., 2003; Stice, 1994; Stice et al., 1998). Individuals purge in order to mitigate the binge and negative affect associated with the binge, which again reinforces the purging behavior. Although these behavioral models were developed specifically for binging and purging behaviors in BN, the transdiagnostic model (Fairburn et al., 2003) suggests that the same reinforcement principles may maintain binge/purge behaviors across eating disorders. Similar to the affect regulation function of NSSI, these maladaptive coping behaviors are automatically negatively reinforced by the reduction of negative affect and potentially automatically positively reinforced by an increase in positive affect.

Although behavioral techniques have been used to increase weight among patients with AN during hospitalization, the ability to sustain these gains after hospitalization has been questioned (Bruch, 1974). However, some researchers suggest that interventions based on individualized functional assessments may be beneficial to the treatment of AN (Wiese, 2009). Dietary restriction in AN and across eating disorders is often maintained by positive and negative reinforcement. Dietary restriction is positively reinforced by increases in positive mood, control, and accomplishment resulting from initial weight loss and negatively reinforced through the avoidance of weight gain (Fairburn et al., 1999; Garner & Bemis, 1982; Schmidt & Treasure, 2006; Slade, 1982). In addition, preoccupation with dietary restriction and food intake may provide a means of avoiding emotions and other problems (Fairburn et al., 1999; Slade, 1982); this emotional and experiential avoidance may negatively reinforce restricting behaviors. These factors provide automatic reinforcement for restricting behaviors, but the external environment may also provide social reinforcement. For example, the individual's social group may provide praise and compliments regarding initial weight loss, socially reinforcing the behavior. Social reinforcement continues as the social group expresses concern as the disease progresses (Garner & Bemis, 1982; Schmidt & Treasure, 2006). Although patients with the restricting subtype of AN may be less likely to engage in NSSI (Claes et al., 2013), dietary restriction occurs across eating disorders and in disordered eating among nonclinical samples, suggesting that it may be appropriate to target the behavior in treatment of eating disorders and comorbid NSSI.

Models of eating disorder development and maintenance are quite complex, and it is unlikely that simply addressing binge/purge and restricting behaviors would resolve the disorders. However, these behaviors are clearly maintained by reinforcement principles, the same principles that maintain NSSI behaviors. By integrating a focus on the factors reinforcing NSSI and eating disorder behavior into eating disorder treatment, the clinician and client may be better able to address some of the factors that are important in maintaining the maladaptive coping behaviors.

6.5 Functional Assessment of NSSI and Eating Disorders

A functional approach to assessment can inform our understanding of the factors that maintain maladaptive behaviors and provide opportunities for treatment based on learning principles. Functional assessment can provide the therapist and client with an understanding of the context surrounding problem behaviors, as well as identify factors that increase or decrease the likelihood of engaging in the behavior (e.g., Cipaini & Schock, 2011; Haynes & O'Brien, 1990). Functional assessment focuses on the factors that maintain behavior rather than the factors that led to the development of the behavior. It is important to keep in mind that factors associated with the development of a behavior may not be the same as the factors associated with its maintenance (e.g., Cipaini & Schock, 2011). Understanding the factors that maintain problem behaviors, such as NSSI, binging, purging, and restricting, will guide the strategies that will produce the greatest impact on intervention (Nock et al., 2007; Wiese, 2009).

The learning principle most applicable to functional assessment is operant, or instrumental, conditioning. In operant conditioning, consequences occur that are the direct result of a behavior produced by an organism. The resulting consequence can increase the likelihood that a behavior will be repeated (i.e., reinforcement) or decrease the likelihood (i.e., suppression) (e.g., Domjan, 2009; Iwata, Vollmer, & Zarcone, 1990; O'Donohue & Ferguson, 2004). These consequences either involve the production of a stimulus (i.e., positive) or the removal or avoidance of a stimulus (i.e., negative). When a behavior produces a stimulus that increases the likelihood the behavior will be repeated, the behavior is positively reinforced by the stimulus; a behavior that eliminates a stimulus or prevents a stimulus from occurring, which increases the likelihood the behavior will be repeated, is negatively reinforced. One of the benefits of behavioral assessment in general is that it allows for an individualized assessment of each client. Although research and theory may suggest specific functions for NSSI and eating disorder behavior, it is important that the functional assessment reflects the unique reinforcement and antecedent patterns of each individual.

In a functional assessment of NSSI or eating disorder behaviors, the therapist is usually initially concerned with factors that reinforce the behaviors, as the initial goal of the assessment is to determine factors that maintain the behavior. However, factors that decrease the likelihood that the behavior will be produced may also be important in treatment. Punishment, or positive punishment, occurs when a behavior produces a stimulus that decreases the likelihood that the behavior will be repeated, while omission training occurs when a behavior eliminates a stimulus or prevents a stimulus from occurring, which in turn decreases the likelihood that the behavior will be repeated (e.g., Domjan, 2009; Iwata et al., 1990; O'Donohue & Ferguson, 2004). Important for treatment of NSSI and eating disorder behaviors is a type of omission training called differential reinforcement of other behaviors (DRO). Rather than the target behavior simply eliminating or preventing a desired stimulus, thereby reducing the likelihood that the target behavior will occur, an individual is able to receive the desired stimulus by engaging in a behavior other than the targeted problem behavior. The desired stimulus would then positively reinforce the alternative behavior, increasing the likelihood that the alternative behavior will be repeated.

The first step in conducting a functional assessment is to identify the target behaviors of interest (e.g., Cipaini & Schock, 2011). It is important that the target behaviors be as specific as possible. For example, a target of "disordered eating" would be too broad; "binge eating" would be more appropriate. Similarly, "non-suicidal self-injury" would be too broad a behavior to be appropriate for a target of functional assessment, as preliminary data suggests that different methods of NSSI may perform different functions (Andover, Schatten, & Morris, 2010). Targeted NSSI behaviors for a functional assessment should include the specific NSSI methods used, such as cutting, biting, or skin picking.

Second, it is important to obtain baseline data on each of the target behaviors. Baseline data should include characteristics of the target behaviors such as frequency, duration, and location of the behavior. Although functional assessments traditionally favor direct observation, this may not be possible with the targeted behaviors associated with NSSI and eating disorders, especially with outpatient treatment. Although there are several methods of collecting data for a functional assessment, the method most commonly used in functional assessment with NSSI and eating disorder behaviors is an analysis of the antecedents and consequences of the behavior conducted through a behavioral interview.

The antecedent-behavior-consequence (A-B-C) analysis is used to collect data on the situations that lead a target behavior to occur and what happens when the individual does engage in the target behavior. The A-B-C analysis is also used to test hypotheses regarding the factors maintaining the target behavior (e.g., Cipaini & Schock, 2011). Although observable factors are traditionally focused upon in an A-B-C analysis, factors that maintain NSSI and eating disorder behaviors can be either external and observable or internal (i.e., automatic reinforcement). Given the importance of internal states and the difficulty in directly observing these behaviors, behavioral interview is an important method of obtaining information. However, one is not solely reliant on the client's level of insight into the behaviors. As discussed earlier, research suggests that NSSI and eating disorder behaviors are maintained by specific factors, including negative reinforcement (e.g., engaging in a behavior to reduce negative affect or to avoid emotional experiences) and positive reinforcement (e.g., concern from peers and family). Such a priori hypotheses based in research may be used to guide the interview.

Emotional, cognitive, and external variables should be included in an assessment of antecedents of a targeted behavior. Although the presence of an antecedent is easier to discern, a stimulus does not need to be present in order to be an antecedent. An antecedent may also consist of the lack of a stimulus (e.g., feeling lonely) or the possibility that a stimulus may occur (e.g., physiological sensations associated with anxiety or distress). Generally, an antecedent also includes two specific factors: a motivating operation and a discriminative stimulus. A motivating operation is a factor that changes the effectiveness of a reinforcer (e.g., Simó-Pinatella et al., 2013). For example, if a client cuts for social positive reinforcement, the presence of a friend who does not reinforce the behavior may serve as a motivating operation, as the potential for NSSI to lead to social positive reinforcement is reduced. A discriminative stimulus signals the availability of a behavior or outcome. For example, the presence of food may serve as a discriminative stimulus for a binge, while not having access to cutting implements (a possible discriminative stimulus for this behavior) may prevent NSSI from occurring following an antecedent.

Antecedents alone will alert one to the factors that trigger the problem behavior; investigating the effects of the behavior on the antecedents (i.e., consequences) will alert one to the behavior's function and the factors maintaining it. When assessing consequences of a targeted behavior, it is important to note that multiple consequences may exist. For example, consequences of a binge may include feeling ill, decreased self-worth, and feeling disappointed. However, these are not likely to be the consequence of the behavior desired by the client. The therapist must assess for the contingency that maintains the behavior, which, in the case of binging, may be a reduction of negative affect.

In order to determine the factors responsible for the maintenance of the problem behavior, it is imperative that multiple A-B-C analyses be reviewed for patterns in antecedents and consequences (e.g., Cipaini & Schock, 2011). For this reason, it is important to include both NSSI and eating disorder behaviors in functional assessment with eating disorder clients who engage in NSSI or with clients with comorbid NSSI and disordered eating, regardless of diagnosis. Although different behaviors may be performed for different functions (Andover et al., 2010), it is equally possible that different behaviors may be performed for the same function. For example, an individual may engage in both NSSI and binging in order to reduce negative affect; it is possible that the choice in behavior may be determined by the presence of a specific discriminative stimulus or another factor. Upon review of the A-B-C analyses, the therapist and client may determine that multiple behaviors serve the same function, that multiple behaviors serve different functions, or that a single behavior may serve multiple functions.

Following the identification of factors maintaining the behaviors, the therapist and client should experimentally evaluate them in order to ensure that they are correct. A functional analysis is performed when the antecedent variables or reinforcements are experimentally modified (e.g., Cipaini & Schock, 2011; Haynes & O'Brien, 1990; O'Donohue & Ferguson, 2004). However, this may be difficult to do when the problem behaviors provide automatic reinforcement. Additional data may be obtained through in situ hypothesis testing, such as through single-case experimental designs (e.g., Cipaini & Schock, 2011).

One of the main goals of behavioral assessment is to inform treatment. Although interventions will likely address more than the behavioral modification of specific symptoms (e.g., treatments for eating disorders will address body dissatisfaction and the overvaluation of weight and shape), directly addressing the functions of the behavior is likely to be beneficial (Muehlenkamp, 2006; Nock et al., 2007; Wiese, 2009). The results of the functional assessment may provide specific points to intervene. First, when a behavior is reinforced through environmental or social contingencies, it may be possible to directly modify these contingencies to remove the reinforcement. For example, if the functional assessment reveals that family members responding to a client's self-injury with increases in attention and concern provides positive reinforcement for the behavior, then directly intervening with the family to provide care while minimizing reinforcement may be possible. Second, the pattern of antecedents to a problem behavior may suggest a specific skills deficit or underlying problem that may be addressed through specific therapeutic techniques. For example, engaging in problem behaviors to avoid or terminate negative affect may suggest a deficit in emotion regulation. For such individuals, an intervention with a focus on emotion regulation, for example, dialectical behavior therapy (DBT; Linehan, 1993) or acceptance-based emotion regulation (e.g., Gratz & Tull, 2011), may strengthen skills so that the antecedent is no longer problematic. Similarly, if a client reports engaging in NSSI to reduce anger, then treatment might focus on alternative ways to cope with, regulate, or tolerate anger (Turner, Chapman, & Layden, 2012). Third, performing a functional assessment for the lack of behavior may be insightful. After antecedents and reinforcers have been identified, it may be informative to conduct a functional assessment of occasions where the antecedent was present, but the client did not engage in the behavior. This may provide data on other behaviors the client engages in that fill the same or a similar function, which can then be incorporated into treatment. Fourth, the majority of interventions based on functional assessment should include the differential reinforcement of other (DRO) behavior. As discussed earlier, DRO paradigms allow the client access to the reinforcing stimulus, but only when another, more appropriate behavior is performed. Inclusion of DRO is particularly important in the functional treatment of NSSI and eating disorder behavior as it provides access to the reinforcing stimulus. For example, if behaviors such as dietary restriction or NSSI are being performed to gain social positive reinforcement through displays of concern from others, elimination of the reinforcing stimulus may lead to increases in the behavior. By using DRO, the client would still be able to obtain the desired stimulus (i.e., concern from others), but only through engaging in an appropriate behavior, such as asking someone for help.

Continued assessment is an integral part of functional assessment. Baseline data that include functional assessments of multiple problem behaviors across multiple situations are important in order to identify antecedents and factors that reinforce the behaviors. Functional analysis, when possible, can confirm or refute previously identified hypotheses. Continuing functional assessment throughout treatment allows the therapist to modify the intervention if a strategy does not appear to be working, if a new or previously unidentified antecedent or reinforcing stimulus is discovered, or if the hypothesized function of the behavior was in fact incorrect. Single-case experimental designs, such as AB or ABAB designs, can be particularly useful in ongoing assessment. In addition to testing hypothesized functions of behavior and the effectiveness of interventions, single-case experimental designs have the added benefit of focusing on improving behavior in the individual and have been used in the treatment of self-injurious behaviors (e.g., Rizvi & Nock, 2008).

Conclusion

Eating disorders and NSSI involve complex behaviors that are difficult to treat. Although not the only factors involved, both research and theory suggest that NSSI and specific eating disorder behaviors such as binging, purging, and dietary restriction are maintained by reinforcement. The behavioral strategy of functional assessment allows the therapist and client to identify the emotional, cognitive, social, and environmental factors that trigger and maintain problem behaviors. This information can provide specific points for therapeutic intervention. Although functional assessment and interventions informed by it are likely to not be the sole strategies implemented in the treatment of eating disorders and NSSI, including functional assessment and function-based treatment strategies may improve the outcome of interventions for these disorders.

References

Agras, W. S., Barlow, D. H., Chapin, H. N., Abel, G. G., & Leitenberg, H. (1974). Behavior modification of anorexia nervosa. *Archives of General Psychiatry, 30*, 279–286.

Agras, W. S., Walsh, B. T., Fairburn, C. G., Wilson, G. T., & Kraemer, H. C. (2000). A multicenter comparison of cognitive-behavioral therapy and interpersonal psychotherapy for bulimia nervosa. *Archives of General Psychiatry, 57*, 459–466.

American Psychiatric Association (2000). *Diagnostic and statistical manual of mental disorders* (4th ed., text revision). Washington, DC: Author.

Andover, M. S., Schatten, H. T., & Morris, B. W. (2010). Functional differences in methods of non-suicidal self-injury. In M. F. Armey (Chair, Ed.), *Novel approaches to the identification and assessment of non-suicidal self-injury functions*. Symposium presented at the annual meeting of the Association for Behavioral and Cognitive Therapies, San Francisco, CA.

Armey, M. F., Crowther, J. H., & Miller, I. W. (2011). Changes in ecological momentary assessment reported affect associated with episodes of nonsuicidal self-injury. *Behavior Therapy, 42*, 579–588.

Berg, K. C., Crosby, R. D., Cao, L., Peterson, C. B., Engel, S. G., Mitchell, J. E., et al. (2013). Facets of negative affect prior to and following binge-only, purge-only, and binge/purge events in women with bulimia nervosa. *Journal of Abnormal Psychology, 122*, 111–118.

Brain, K. L., Haines, J., & Williams, C. L. (1998). The psychophysiology of self-mutilation: Evidence of tension reduction. *Archives of Suicide Research, 4*, 227–242.

Bresin, K., & Gordon, K. H. (2013). Changes in negative affect following pain (vs. nonpainful) stimulation in individuals with and without a history of nonsuicidal self-injury. *Personality Disorders: Theory, Research, and Treatment, 4*, 62–66.

Bresin, K., Gordon, K. H., Bender, T. W., Gordon, L. J., & Joiner, T. R. (2010). No pain, no change: Reductions in prior negative affect following physical pain. *Motivation and Emotion, 34*, 280–287.

Brockmeyer, T., Holtforth, M. G., Bents, H., Kämmerer, A., Herzog, W., & Friederich, H. C. (2012). Starvation and emotion regulation in anorexia nervosa. *Comprehensive Psychiatry, 53*, 496–501.

Bruch, H. (1974). Perils of behavior modification in treatment of anorexia nervosa. *Journal of the American Medical Association, 230*, 1419–1422.

Bulik, C. M., Berkman, N. D., Brownley, K. A., Sedway, J. A., & Lohr, K. N. (2007). Anorexia nervosa treatment: A systematic review of randomized controlled trials. *International Journal of Eating Disorders, 40*, 310–320.

Chapman, A. L., Gratz, K. L., & Brown, M. Z. (2006). Solving the puzzle of deliberate self-harm: The experiential avoidance model. *Behaviour Research and Therapy, 44*, 371–394.

Cipaini, E., & Schock, K. M. (2011). *Functional behavioral assessment, diagnosis, and treatment: A complete system for education and mental health settings*. New York: Springer.

Claes, L., Fernández-Aranda, F., Jimenez-Murcia, S., Botella, C., Casanueva, F. F., de la Torre, R., et al. (2013). Co-occurrence of non-suicidal self-injury and impulsivity in extreme weight conditions. *Personality and Individual Differences, 54*, 137–140.

Claes, L., Klonsky, E., Muehlenkamp, J., Kuppens, P., & Vandereycken, W. (2010). The affect-regulation function of nonsuicidal self-injury in eating-disordered patients: Which affect states are regulated? *Comprehensive Psychiatry, 51*, 386–392.

Claes, L., Soenens, B., Vansteenkiste, M., & Vandereycken, W. (2012). The scars of the inner critic: Perfectionism and nonsuicidal self-injury in eating disorders. *European Eating Disorders Review, 20*, 196–202.

Claes, L., Vandereycken, W., & Vertommen, H. (2001). Self-injurious behaviors in eating-disordered patients. *Eating Behaviors, 2*, 263–272.

Cooper, M. J., Wells, A., & Todd, G. (2004). A cognitive model of bulimia nervosa. *British Journal of Clinical Psychology, 43*, 1–16.

Cowdrey, F. A., & Park, R. J. (2012). The role of experiential avoidance, rumination and mindfulness in eating disorders. *Eating Behaviors, 13*, 100–105.

Domjan, M. (2009). *Principles of learning and behavior*. Belmont, CA: Wadsworth/Thomson Learning.

Fairburn, C. G. (2005). Evidence-based treatment of anorexia nervosa. *International Journal of Eating Disorders, 37*, 26–30.

Fairburn, C. G., Cooper, Z., & Cooper, P. J. (1986). The clinical features and maintenance of bulimia nervosa. In K. D. Brownell & J. P. Foreyt (Eds.), *Handbook of eating disorders: Physiology, psychology and treatment of obesity, anorexia and bulimia* (pp. 389–404). New York: Basic Books.

Fairburn, C. G., Cooper, Z., & Shafran, R. (2003). Cognitive behaviour therapy for eating disorders: A "transdiagnostic" theory and treatment. *Behaviour Research and Therapy, 41*, 509–528.

Fairburn, C. G., Marcus, M. D., & Wilson, G. T. (1993). Cognitive-behavioral therapy for binge eating and bulimia nervosa: A comprehensive treatment manual. In C. G. Fairburn & G. T. Wilson (Eds.), *Binge eating: Nature, assessment and treatment* (pp. 361–404). New York: Guilford Press.

Fairburn, C. G., Shafran, R., & Cooper, Z. (1999). A cognitive behavioural theory of anorexia nervosa. *Behaviour Research and Therapy, 37*, 1–13.

Favazza, A. R. (1998). The coming of age of self-mutilation. *Journal of Nervous and Mental Disease, 186*, 259–268.

Franklin, J. C., Hessel, E. T., Aaron, R. V., Arthur, M. S., Heilbron, N., & Prinstein, M. J. (2010). The functions of nonsuicidal self-injury: Support for cognitive–affective regulation and opponent processes from a novel psychophysiological paradigm. *Journal of Abnormal Psychology, 119*, 850–862.

Franklin, J. C., Puzia, M. E., Lee, K. M., Lee, G. E., Hanna, E. K., Spring, V. L., et al. (2013). The nature of pain offset relief in nonsuicidal self-injury: A laboratory study. *Clinical Psychological Science, 1*, 110–119.

Garfinkel, P. E., Garner, D. M., & Moldofsky, H. (1977). The role of behavior modification in the treatment of anorexia nervosa. *Journal of Pediatric Psychology, 2*, 113–121.

Garner, D. M., & Bemis, K. M. (1982). A cognitive-behavioral approach to anorexia nervosa. *Cognitive Therapy and Research, 6*, 123–150.

Geller, J., Cockell, S. J., & Goldner, E. M. (2000). Inhibited expression of negative emotions and interpersonal orientation in anorexia nervosa. *International Journal of Eating Disorders, 28*, 8–19.

Gratz, K. L., & Tull, M. T. (2011). Extending research on the utility of an adjunctive emotion regulation group therapy for deliberate self-harm among women with borderline personality pathology. *Personality Disorders: Theory, Research, and Treatment, 2*, 316–326.

Haines, J., Williams, C. L., Brain, K. L., & Wilson, G. V. (1995). The psychophysiology of self-mutilation. *Journal of Abnormal Psychology, 104*, 471–489.

Haynes, S. N., & O'Brien, W. H. (1990). Functional analysis in behavior therapy. *Clinical Psychology Review, 10*, 649–668.

Haynos, A. F., & Fruzzetti, A. E. (2011). Anorexia nervosa as a disorder of emotion dysregulation: Evidence and treatment implications. *Clinical Psychology: Science and Practice, 18*, 183–202.

Heatherton, T. F., & Polivy, J. (1992). Chronic dieting and eating disorders: A spiral model. In J. H. Crowther, D. L. Tennenbaum, S. E. Hobfoll, & M. Stephens (Eds.), *The etiology of bulimia nervosa: The individual and familial context* (pp. 133–155). Washington, DC: Hemisphere Publishing Corporation.

Iwata, B. A., Vollmer, T. R., & Zarcone, J. R. (1990). The experimental (functional) analysis of behavior disorders: Methodology, applications, and limitations. In A. C. Repp & N. N. Singh (Eds.), *Perspectives on the use of nonaversive and aversive interventions for persons with developmental disabilities* (pp. 301–330). Sycamore, IL: Sycamore Publishing Company.

Jacobson, C. M., & Gould, M. (2007). The epidemiology and phenomenology of non-suicidal self-injurious behavior among adolescents: A critical review of the literature. *Archives of Suicide Research, 11*, 129–147.

Jenkins, A. L., & Schmitz, M. F. (2012). The roles of affect dysregulation and positive affect in non-suicidal self-injury. *Archives of Suicide Research, 16*, 212–225.

Keys, A., Brozek, J., Henschel, A., Mickelsen, O., & Taylor, H. L. (1950). *The biology of human starvation*. Minneapolis, MN: University of Minnesota Press.

Klonsky, E. (2007). The functions of deliberate self-injury: A review of the evidence. *Clinical Psychology Review, 27*, 226–239.

Klonsky, E. D. (2011). Non-suicidal self-injury in United States adults: Prevalence, sociodemographics, topography and functions. *Psychological Medicine, 41*, 1981–1986.

Klonsky, E. D., & Muehlenkamp, J. J. (2007). Self-injury: A research review for the practitioner. *Journal of Clinical Psychology, 63*, 1045–1056.

Lee, M. I., & Miltenberger, R. G. (1997). Functional assessment and binge eating: A review of the literature and suggestions for future research. *Behavior Modification, 21*, 159–171.

Linehan, M. M. (1993). *Cognitive-behavioral treatment of borderline personality disorder*. New York: Guilford Press.

Muehlenkamp, J. J. (2006). Empirically supported treatments and general therapy guidelines for non-suicidal self-injury. *Journal of Mental Health Counseling, 28*, 166–185.

Muehlenkamp, J. J., Engel, S. G., Wadeson, A., Crosby, R. D., Wonderlich, S. A., Simonich, H., et al. (2009). Emotional states preceding and following acts of non-suicidal self-injury in bulimia nervosa patients. *Behaviour Research and Therapy, 47*, 83–87.

Nock, M. K. (2009). Why do people hurt themselves? New insights into the nature and functions of self-injury. *Current Directions in Psychological Science, 18*, 78–83.

Nock, M. K., Joiner, T. E., Gordon, K. H., Lloyd-Richardson, E., & Prinstein, M. J. (2006). Non-suicidal self-injury among adolescents: Diagnostic correlates and relation to suicide attempts. *Psychiatry Research, 144*, 65–72.

Nock, M. K., & Prinstein, M. J. (2004). A functional approach to the assessment of self-mutilative behavior. *Journal of Consulting and Clinical Psychology, 72*, 885–890.

Nock, M. K., & Prinstein, M. J. (2005). Contextual features and behavioral functions of self-mutilation among adolescents. *Journal of Abnormal Psychology, 114*, 140–146.

Nock, M. K., Teper, R., & Hollander, M. (2007). Psychological treatment of self-injury among adolescents. *Journal of Clinical Psychology: In Session, 63*, 1081–1089.

O'Donohue, W. T., & Ferguson, K. E. (2004). Learning and applied behavior analysis: Foundations of behavioral assessment. In S. N. Haynes & E. M. Heiby (Eds.), *Comprehensive handbook of psychological assessment: Behavioral assessment* (pp. 57–68). Hoboken, NJ: Wiley.

Rizvi, S. L., & Nock, M. K. (2008). Single-case experimental designs for the evaluation of treatments for self-injurious and suicidal behaviors. *Suicide and Life-Threatening Behavior, 38*, 498–510.

Ross, S., Heath, N. L., & Toste, J. R. (2009). Non-suicidal self-injury and eating pathology in high school students. *American Journal of Orthopsychiatry, 79*, 83–92.

Schmidt, U., & Treasure, J. (2006). Anorexia nervosa: Valued and visible. A cognitive-interpersonal maintenance model and its implications for research and practice. *British Journal of Clinical Psychology, 45*, 343–366.

Schnurer, A. T., Rubin, R. R., & Roy, A. (1973). Systematic desensitization of anorexia nervosa seen as a weight phobia. *Journal of Behavior Therapy and Experimental Psychiatry, 4*, 149–153.

Serras, A., Saules, K. K., Cranford, J. A., & Eisenberg, D. (2010). Self-injury, substance use, and associated risk factors in a multi-campus probability sample of college students. *Psychology of Addictive Behaviors, 24*, 119–128.

Shapiro, J. R., Berkman, N. D., Brownley, K. A., Sedway, J. A., Lohr, K. N., & Bulik, C. M. (2007). Bulimia nervosa treatment: A systematic review of randomized controlled trials. *International Journal of Eating Disorders, 40*, 321–336.

Simó-Pinatella, D., Font-Roura, J., Planella-Morató, J., McGill, P., Alomar-Kurz, E., & Giné, C. (2013). Types of motivating operations in interventions with problem behavior: A systematic review. *Behavior Modification, 37*, 3–38.

Slade, P. (1982). Towards a functional analysis of anorexia nervosa and bulimia nervosa. *British Journal of Clinical Psychology, 21*, 167–179.

Slee, N., Spinhoven, P., Garnefski, N., & Arensman, E. (2008). Emotion regulation as mediator of treatment outcome in therapy for deliberate self-harm. *Clinical Psychology and Psychotherapy, 15*, 205–216.

Smyth, J. M., Wonderlich, S. A., Heron, K. E., Sliwinski, M. J., Crosby, R. D., Mitchell, J. E., et al. (2007). Daily and momentary mood and stress are associated with binge eating and vomiting in bulimia nervosa patients in the natural environment. *Journal of Consulting and Clinical Psychology, 75*, 629–638.

Solanto, M. V., Jacobson, M. S., Heller, L., Golden, N. H., & Hertz, S. (1994). Rate of weight gain of inpatients with anorexia nervosa under two behavioral contracts. *Pediatrics, 93*, 989–991.

Stein, R. I., Kenardy, J., Wiseman, C. V., Dounchis, J. Z., Arnow, B. A., & Wilfley, D. E. (2007). What's driving the binge in binge eating disorder?: A prospective examination of precursors and consequences. *International Journal of Eating Disorders, 40*, 195–203.

Stein, D., Lilenfeld, L. R. R., Wildman, P. C., & Marcus, M. D. (2004). Attempted suicide and self-injury in patients diagnosed with eating disorders. *Comprehensive Psychiatry, 45*, 447–451.

Steinhausen, H. C., Rauss-Mason, C., & Seidel, R. (1991). Follow-up studies of anorexia nervosa: A review of four decades of outcome research. *Psychological Medicine, 21*, 447–454.

Stice, E. (1994). Review of the evidence for a sociocultural model of bulimia nervosa and an exploration of the mechanisms of action. *Clinical Psychology Review, 14*, 633–661.

Stice, E., Shaw, H., & Nemeroff, C. (1998). Dual pathway model of bulimia nervosa: Longitudinal support for dietary restraint and affect-regulation mechanisms. *Journal of Social and Clinical Psychology, 17*, 129–149.

Stunkard, A. (1972). New therapies for the eating disorders: Behavior modification of obesity and anorexia nervosa. *Archives of General Psychiatry, 26*, 391–398.

Sullivan, P. F., Bulik, C. M., Fear, J. L., & Pickering, A. (1998). Outcome of anorexia nervosa: A case-control study. *American Journal of Psychiatry, 155*, 939–946.

Suyemoto, K. L. (1998). The functions of self-mutilation. *Clinical Psychology Review, 18*, 531–554.

Svirko, E., & Hawton, K. (2007). Self-injurious behavior and eating disorders: The extent and nature of the association. *Suicide and Life-Threatening Behavior, 37*, 409–421.

Turner, B. J., Chapman, A. L., & Layden, B. K. (2012). Intrapersonal and interpersonal functions of non-suicidal self-injury: Associations with emotional and social functioning. *Suicide and Life-Threatening Behavior, 42*, 36–55.

Whittal, M. L., Agras, W. S., & Gould, R. A. (1999). Bulimia nervosa: A meta-analysis of psychosocial and pharmacological treatments. *Behavior Therapy, 30*, 117–135.

Wiese, J. E. (2009). Behavior therapy for anorexia nervosa: Taking a second look. *Eating Disorders, 17*, 400–408.

Wildes, J. E., Ringham, R. M., & Marcus, M. D. (2010). Emotion avoidance in patients with anorexia nervosa: Initial test of a functional model. *International Journal of Eating Disorders, 43*, 398–404.

Cognitive-Behavioral Therapy 7

Christine M. Peat

Abstract

Cognitive-behavioral therapy (CBT) has consistently been considered the gold standard for the treatment of some eating disorders and for non-suicidal self-injury (NSSI). The majority of the literature has focused on the separate treatment of these two frequently co-occurring disorders. In light of this, CBT has demonstrated efficacy in the treatment of bulimia nervosa, the newly recognized binge eating disorder, and for NSSI; however, strong evidence is lacking for anorexia nervosa. Also lacking is a well-integrated research body examining the efficacy of CBT in treating eating disorders and NSSI concurrently. The basic structure of CBT for each of the eating disorders and for NSSI is outlined in the current chapter. The general approach focuses on identifying and modifying negative, automatic thoughts in an effort to influence behavior change and the development of healthier, more adaptive coping strategies. More specific suggestions are provided with regard to the concurrent treatment of eating disorders and NSSI using a CBT approach. Future directions for both research and practice are also discussed.

7.1 Introduction

As a therapeutic approach that focuses on modifying maladaptive thoughts and behaviors, cognitive-behavioral therapy (CBT) lends itself well to the treatment of both eating disorders and non-suicidal self-injury (NSSI). The general principles of CBT posit that changes in cognitions and thought processes can alter emotions and influence behavior change. Current conceptualizations of the core

C.M. Peat (✉)
University of North Carolina, Center of Excellence for Eating Disorders, Department of Psychiatry, Chapel Hill, NC, USA
e-mail: christine_peat@med.unc.edu

L. Claes and J.J. Muehlenkamp (eds.), *Non-Suicidal Self-Injury in Eating Disorders*, DOI 10.1007/978-3-642-40107-7_7, © Springer-Verlag Berlin Heidelberg 2014

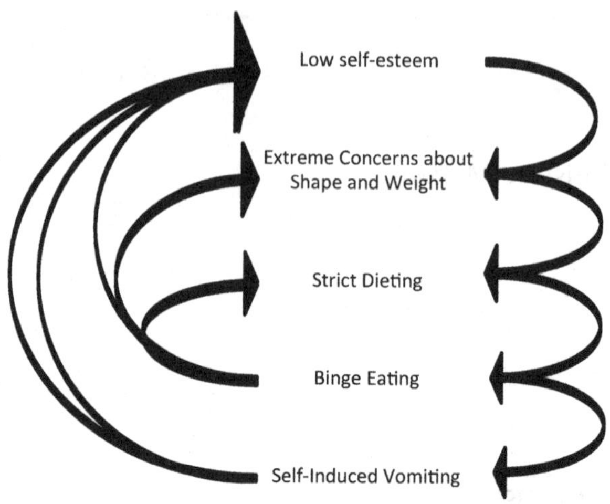

Fig. 7.1 Cognitive-behavioral model of bulimia nervosa maintenance

psychopathological features of both eating disorders and NSSI also concentrate on maladaptive thoughts and behaviors, thus fitting well within a CBT framework.

The CBT approach to eating disorder treatment generally focuses on core maladaptive beliefs about food, weight, and shape that are thought to drive eating disorder behaviors (e.g., food restriction, self-induced vomiting, compulsive exercise). In anorexia nervosa (AN) and bulimia nervosa (BN), distorted cognitions about weight and shape and a self-evaluation unduly influenced by shape and weight are common. The cognitive-behavioral conceptualization of these disorders suggests that these persistent cognitions can lead individuals to engage in eating disorder behaviors in an effort to alter their shape and weight including self-induced vomiting, extreme dietary restriction, or the use of compulsive exercise to compensate for calories consumed. Figures 7.1 and 7.2 illustrate the cognitive-behavioral model for the maintenance of both BN and AN, respectively. Similarly, the CBT model for binge eating disorder (BED) suggests that a persistent overvaluation of shape and weight can lead to dietary restriction and subsequent binge eating (without compensatory strategies). The CBT model for BED posits that binge eating becomes recurrent as dietary restriction increases and leaves a person vulnerable to binge episodes. While there are substantive differences between the eating disorders in terms of behaviors and core cognitions, all can be conceptualized within the cognitive-behavioral model of the complex interplay between negative/maladaptive thoughts, their influence on emotions, and subsequent impact on behaviors.

In a similar vein, the CBT model of NSSI focuses primarily on modifying core beliefs, attitudes, and behaviors that are central to the maintenance of NSSI (Berk, Henriques, Warman, Brown, & Beck, 2004; Slee, Arensman, Garnefski, & Spinhoven, 2007). As with many CBT models of psychopathology, the model for NSSI is grounded in the notion that core beliefs are instrumental in the development of certain attitudes and assumptions that can contribute to the use of NSSI to cope with negative, maladaptive beliefs. For example, those who struggle with NSSI may adopt the faulty belief that they are unlovable or incompetent. These faulty

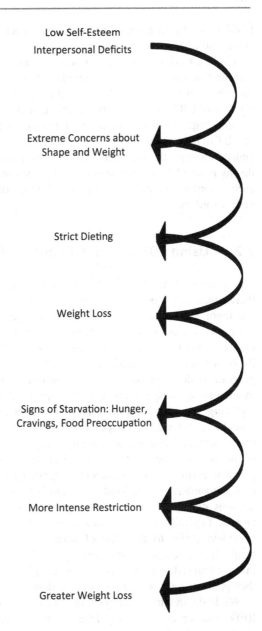

Fig. 7.2 Cognitive-behavioral model of anorexia nervosa maintenance

beliefs might then translate into assumptions that self-injury is the only way to cope with the subsequent negative affect that results from such core beliefs, thus increasing the likelihood of engaging in NSSI. In fact, the literature would suggest that a common function for NSSI is to relieve emotional/affective pain (Nock, 2009), as well as self-punishment. Thus, a central component of CBT for the treatment of

NSSI is identifying, challenging, and restructuring core beliefs so as to effect emotional and behavioral change.

While a CBT conceptualization is common to both eating disorders and NSSI and their co-occurrence is common [see Svirko and Hawton (2007) for a review], there has yet to be established a well-integrated body of literature examining the efficacy of CBT in the concurrent treatment of eating disorders and NSSI. Thus, the current chapter will provide a brief overview of the empirical evidence for the use of CBT in the treatment of eating disorders and NSSI separately. Then, based on the general therapeutic approach and the core psychopathological features of eating disorders and NSSI, more specific guidelines are detailed on CBT techniques for each disorder separately and how CBT might be adapted to concurrently address both disorders.

7.2 Using CBT for the Treatment of Eating Disorders

The general structure of CBT for AN, BN, and BED overlaps considerably; therefore, all will be presented in one overview. A more detailed version of the treatment structure can be found in any of several texts (Cooper & Fairburn, 2010; Fairburn, Marcus, & Wilson, 1993; Garner, Vitousek, & Pike, 1997; Pike, Carter, & Olmsted, 2010; Wilson, Fairburn, & Agras, 1997); thus, the following will primarily be a brief overview. In parallel with a CBT conceptualization, the treatment program is designed to focus specifically on eating disorder psychopathology to extinguish any binge eating, dietary restriction, and/or compensatory behaviors by replacing them with regular eating habits while also addressing dysfunctional thoughts about weight, shape, and dietary restraint. The primary components of this treatment focus on establishing a regular eating pattern, restructuring faulty cognitions, and preventing relapse (and weight gain in the case of AN). Thus, the primary focuses of CBT treatment center on the cornerstones of the CBT theory for eating disorders. Manualized treatment is typically comprised of 20 weekly, 1 h sessions during which there is a specific focus on the cognitive and behavioral targets. Typically, these sessions are conducted on an individual basis. The initial interview (prior to the start of formal treatment) is generally geared toward conducting a comprehensive assessment during which the nature and severity of the problem is determined and a treatment plan is formulated. Treatment options are then presented and a treatment plan is developed.

While the treatment approach in CBT for AN is quite similar to that for BN and BED (Garner et al., 1997; Pike et al., 2010), several differences should be highlighted. First, treatment motivation can be more of a pronounced obstacle in patients with AN than those with BN or BED. The, at times, ego-syntonic nature of AN symptomatology and the extreme, persistent fear of weight gain (a major aim of treatment) can interfere with a patient's willingness to engage in treatment. In contrast, patients with BN or BED are generally willing to accept the elimination of binge eating (and compensatory behaviors in the case of BN) as primary goals for recovery. In light of this, a typical component of the initial phase of treatment in

CBT for AN is a discussion and cultivation of motivation for change. Second, the issue of weight gain is unique to this patient population and therefore merits direct discussion throughout treatment. Unlike in patients with BN or BED, weight gain is a specific aim of treatment in those with AN, thus regular weekly weighing is monitored by the therapist or by another reliable source (e.g., primary care provider). Often a lack of progress in terms of weight gain (coupled with other markers of medical instability) can prompt a discussion about the medical severity of AN and the possibility of hospitalization. In addition to these features, the effects of starvation seen in patients with AN can be a further complication in the course of treatment. The "starvation state" is typically associated with food preoccupations, urges to binge eat, cognitive impairments, and emotional distress, and while some of these features are also common to patients with BN (and more rarely BED), they are particularly pronounced in AN and can impact treatment motivation and progress. Despite these sometimes significant differences, the core components and interventions used in CBT are similar across the eating disorders. Thus, the following provides a general overview of each phase of treatment and its specific goals.

7.2.1 Phase I

Typically this stage of treatment lasts approximately eight sessions and focuses on behavioral change. The initial phase of treatment is particularly important in terms of founding the rationale for treatment and establishing a sound therapeutic relationship. Oftentimes, patients with eating disorders have been referred by their primary care doctors or perhaps by a loved one; therefore, there is a certain amount of trepidation that may be apparent at the beginning of treatment. Given the nature of the discussions and the challenging behavioral tasks that will be required, establishing a solid therapeutic relationship with the patient is essential for the initial phase of treatment. Other primary focuses of treatment in Phase I include the following: psycho-education regarding the cognitive view of eating disorder maintenance and the need for both cognitive and behavioral change; regular weekly weighing (conducted with the therapist for patients with AN or either with the therapist or independently for patients with BN or BED); education about the adverse effects of dieting; the physical consequences of binge eating, dietary restriction, and/or compensatory behaviors; the introduction of a regular pattern of eating; and weight restoration (in the case of AN). Crucial in these goals is the faithful and regular practice of self-monitoring which serves to both provide the therapist with a detailed account of problematic eating behaviors and cognitions and increase the patient's awareness of his/her own eating patterns and potentially triggering situations.

7.2.2 Phase II

The second phase of treatment typically spans from sessions 9 to 16. The techniques and principles developed in Phase I are reinforced and supplemented with additional behavioral and cognitive interventions. Whereas Phase I entailed a more behavioral focus, Phase II concentrates on the cognitive aspects of an eating disorder. The primary cognitive targets of this phase include eliminating dieting and dietary restriction, cognitive restructuring, and addressing shape and weight concerns. At this point in treatment, patients have learned the cognitive view of how the eating disorder is maintained, including rigid dieting strategies and reliance on faulty cognitions regarding eating, shape, and weight. Thus, a primary goal in this phase of treatment is to introduce cognitive restructuring as to decrease reliance on thinking errors that reinforce eating disorder behaviors. The cognitive restructuring techniques involved in Phase II are adapted from Beck's original cognitive therapy for depression (Beck, Rush, Shaw, & Emery, 1979) and involve identifying a problematic thought, evaluating evidence for or against that thought, and developing a more balanced and typically less rigid thought. These cognitive restructuring techniques are used throughout treatment in an effort to address faulty cognitions about dieting, weight, and shape. When used in conjunction with behavioral interventions [e.g., problem-solving skills, eating previously avoided foods, using adaptive behaviors as an alternative to purging (BN), and/or increasing or decreasing weighing], the cognitive principles in Phase II are designed to result in changes in mood and a decreased reliance on previously entrenched behaviors.

7.2.3 Phase III

The third and final phase of treatment is aimed at relapse prevention strategies and typically encompasses sessions 17 to 20 on a biweekly basis. The longer duration of time between each session in Phase III allows patients to thoroughly practice the skills they have developed in Phases I and II and to address any remaining problem areas. The primary goal in Phase III is for patients to identify and anticipate potential difficulties they might encounter in the future. In these final sessions, patients are encouraged to discuss potentially triggering situations and how they might utilize the skills they have developed in specific and concrete terms. The rationale is that the better prepared the patient is, the more likely s/he will be able to successfully navigate the triggering situation without engaging in binge eating or compensatory behaviors (in the case of BN) or dietary restriction (as in AN). In an effort to maintain the newly developed changes accomplished in therapy, patients are encouraged to develop a maintenance plan to follow after therapy has completed. Typically these plans are tailored to the specific needs and individual styles of the patient and include written steps of how to handle triggering situations and/or relapses. While each plan is different, there are components that are generally represented including being able to identify the trigger or problem situation, using self-monitoring to "get back on track," actively using both the behavioral (e.g., regular meal plans, problem-solving skills, alternative behaviors) and the cognitive (e.g., cognitive restructuring) techniques that have been effective in the past, and setting short-term, realistic goals in order to facilitate success. Patients are also reminded that a "refresher course" of therapy is not uncommon on the road to recovery.

7.3 Evidence for the Use of CBT in the Treatment of Eating Disorders

CBT is the most frequently studied psychotherapeutic approach in the treatment of eating disorders. Typically, CBT is evaluated in isolation for each eating disorder (e.g., AN, BN, binge eating disorder) as reflective of the Diagnostic and Statistical Manual nosology (APA, 2000), and, at present, there is substantial evidence to suggest that CBT is particularly effective in the treatment BN (NICE, 2004; Shapiro et al., 2007; Wilson, Grilo, & Vitousek, 2007). In fact, the National Institute for Health and Clinical Excellence (NICE, 2004) guidelines identify manualized CBT (Fairburn et al., 1993) as the treatment of choice for adults with BN. This recommendation marked the first time NICE had endorsed a psychological intervention as frontline treatment for a psychiatric disorder (Wilson & Shafran, 2005).

7.3.1 CBT for Bulimia Nervosa

The effectiveness of CBT for BN has been assessed in several ways including examination of rates and measuring reductions in core symptoms of BN such as binge eating and purging. Estimates for overall remission rates have been calculated; however, given that estimates such as these include several studies with varying methodologies and statistical approaches, the information can overgeneralize and be misleading (Wilson et al., 1997). The more typical approach has been to evaluate CBT in terms of reducing core features of BN including binge eating, compensatory behaviors, and various cognitive features such as the overvaluation of shape and weight. In this regard, CBT has been associated with binge eating remission rates ranging from 51 to 71 % and with purging remission rates ranging from 36 to 56 % (Agras, Schneider, Arnow, Raeburn, & Telch, 1989; Agras et al., 1992; Fairburn et al., 1991; Garner et al., 1993). In addition to these core features, studies have also suggested that CBT is effective in improving attitudes toward shape and weight (Fairburn et al., 1991; Garner et al., 1993; Wilson, Eldredge, Smith, & Niles, 1991) and in reducing dietary restraint (Fairburn et al., 1991; Garner et al., 1993; Wilson et al., 1991).

CBT has also been shown to be associated with greater probability of remission and reduction in BN symptoms in comparison to several other conditions including wait-list control (Hay, Bacaltchuk, Stefano, & Kashyap, 2009; Shapiro et al., 2007) and interpersonal therapy (IPT; Hay et al., 2009; Shapiro et al., 2007). CBT was also shown to be more effective than nutritional therapy alone in reducing core BN symptoms (e.g., binge eating and purging) and body dissatisfaction (Wolk & Devlin, 2001). In addition, CBT was associated with greater reductions in food preoccupation and eating concerns when compared to supportive-expressive therapy (a nondirective psychodynamically oriented therapy) (Garner et al., 1993). The effects associated with CBT also appear to be relatively well maintained with good long-term effects at 1-year follow-up (Agras et al., 1994; Fairburn et al., 1993; Shapiro et al., 2007; Wilson et al., 1991). There is some suggestion that the benefits of CBT may not be significantly different from those of IPT at 1-year follow-up (Fairburn et al., 1991); however, CBT appears to be associated with a more rapid reduction of symptoms.

Several studies have attempted to identify the "active ingredients" in CBT, which is an inherently multimodal treatment. Studies suggest that the cognitive component is the crucial feature critical to the therapeutic outcome (Agras et al., 1989; Bulik, Sullivan, Carter, McIntosh, & Joyce, 1998; Cooper & Steere, 1995; Fairburn et al., 1991). Fairburn et al. (1991) reported that the combination of cognitive and behavioral interventions produced better eating-related outcomes when compared to behavioral interventions alone. In addition, complete CBT was associated with lower relapse rates when compared to exposure with response prevention (Cooper & Steere, 1995) and with higher abstinence rates compared to self-monitoring alone (Agras et al., 1989). Two studies evaluated the effect of adding an exposure with response prevention component to traditional CBT (Agras et al., 1989; Bulik et al., 1998) and neither reported any additive efficacy with this combination. Thus, it seems that the cognitive interventions in CBT are crucial to the success of the treatment in reducing core BN symptoms.

7.3.2 CBT for Binge Eating Disorder

In December 2012, the American Psychiatric Association made a landmark decision to recognize binge eating disorder (BED) as a formal eating disorder diagnosis in DSM-5 (APA, 2012). Previously diagnosed as "eating disorder not otherwise specified" according to DSM-IV nosology (APA, 2000), the newly recognized BED is thought to be the most prevalent eating disorder with prevalence estimates at 3.5 % in women and 2 % in men in the United States (Hudson, Hiripi, Pope, & Kessler, 2007). The formal recognition of this disorder and its relatively high prevalence estimates highlight the importance of identifying efficacious treatments for BED, and many studies have focused on CBT given the symptom overlap with BN (e.g., recurrent binge eating episodes). In fact, two recent reviews showed CBT was effective in reducing the frequency of binge episodes and binge days (Brownley, Berkman, Sedway, Lohr, & Bulik, 2007; Peat, Brownley, Berkman, & Bulik, 2012). CBT-based interventions also resulted in significant recovery rates (e.g., no longer meeting threshold or subthreshold criteria for BED) in individuals with subthreshold BED (Ricca et al., 2010) and increased abstinence rates in individuals with threshold diagnoses of BED (Dingemans, Spinhoven, & van Furth, 2007; Schlup, Munsch, Meyer, Margraf, & Wilhelm, 2009). In addition to addressing binge eating behaviors, CBT also improved the eating-related psychopathological aspects of BED [see Brownley et al. (2007) and Peat et al. (2012) for a review]. While both individually and group-administered CBT demonstrated significant overall improvements, patients who received individually administered CBT demonstrated higher recovery rates and decreases in total eating disorder concerns, as well as concerns about weight and shape as compared with patients who received group CBT (Ricca et al., 2010). Other existing studies (Grilo & Masheb, 2005; Shapiro et al., 2007; Wilson, Wilfley, Agras, & Bryson, 2010) would suggest that CBT, even when not delivered in a traditional individual or group format, is efficacious in reducing binge eating frequency and related psychopathological features. These treatment formats may be of particular interest given that not all individuals who struggle with BED have convenient access to specialty eating disorder treatment. Self-guided approaches would allow providers to disseminate empirically supported interventions to a wider range of patients who might not otherwise receive treatment.

7.3.3 CBT for Anorexia Nervosa

In contrast to the literature on BN, empirical support for the use of CBT in the treatment of AN is limited. There have been conducted a handful of trials of CBT for patients with AN [see Berkman et al. (2006) for a review]; however, currently the only empirically supported treatment for AN is the Maudsley method of family therapy for adolescents and children (Lock, Le Grange, Agras, & Dare, 2001). While features of both BN and AN can certainly overlap, there are distinct differences between the two that can make it a difficult phenomenon to study. First, the prevalence of AN is lower than that of other eating disorders (Hudson et al., 2007) which makes identifying and recruiting participants more challenging. Second, the clinical characteristics of patients with AN can hamper acceptability of treatment. Patients with AN often require inpatient hospitalization for the purposes of weight restoration, and this medically severe complication is not typically seen in patients with BN. In addition, the issue of low body weight itself further complicates both treatment and recovery. The cognitive limitations associated with low body weight can make it difficult for an individual to engage in abstract thinking as is required in CBT. Furthermore, the rigid and persistent fear of weight gain and the ego-syntonic nature of the disordered eating cognitions and behaviors can interfere with progress throughout treatment, and thus, many trials involving AN patients are plagued by significant dropout (Berkman et al., 2006). Collectively, these factors make evaluating the efficacy of CBT for AN a more challenging task.

Of the existing controlled trials that have been conducted in underweight adults with AN, a modified version of CBT is often the treatment of choice. When CBT was compared to IPT and nonspecific supportive clinical management (NCSM) in a group of underweight patients with AN, NCSM evidenced the best global outcomes as compared to IPT, and the outcomes for CBT fell somewhere in between (McIntosh et al., 2005). Another study suggested that CBT and behavioral therapy failed to show any significant differences at 1-year follow-up with regard to control over eating and weight outcomes in a group of underweight patients with AN (Channon, de Silva, Hemsley, & Perkins, 1989). Still another study reported that outpatient therapy (which comprised elements of CBT) was associated with higher weight and BMI and improvements in global eating pathology, menstruation, associated nutrition, and mental state (Crisp et al., 1991; Gowers, Norton, Halek, & Crisp, 1994). Improvements in global eating pathology, menstruation, nutrition, and mental state were relatively well maintained at 1- and 2-year follow-up (Crisp et al., 1991; Gowers et al., 1994).

Two studies have evaluated the efficacy of CBT in weight-restored patients with AN (Carter et al., 2009; Pike, Walsh, Vitousek, Wilson, & Bauer, 2003). Pike et al. (2003) reported that 77 % of the CBT group reported intermediate or better outcomes with regard to overall clinical psychopathology (including eating disorder symptoms) as compared to supportive nutritional counseling. In addition, 17 % of those receiving CBT met criteria for "full recovery" at the end of treatment which these authors defined as (a) reporting "good" outcomes according to the Morgan–Russell criteria (Morgan & Russell, 1975), (b) eating attitudes and weight concerns less than one standard deviation above the mean for a comparison group without eating disorders according to the Eating Disorders Examination (EDE; Cooper & Fairburn, 1987), and (c) absent binge eating and purging (Pike et al., 2003). In a nonrandomized trial, Carter et al. (2009) compared CBT to maintenance treatment as usual (MTAU) which was designed to be reflective of typical follow-up care in the community. These authors reported significant longer times to relapse in the CBT condition versus the MTAU condition with only 45 % of the CBT condition relapsing at 1-year follow-up as compared to 66 % in the MTAU condition at the same time point (Carter et al., 2009). Thus, it would seem that there is generally some support for the use of CBT in patients with both acute (e.g., non-weight restored) AN and also for those patients who are weight recovered. Additional well-controlled studies are needed to more firmly establish an evidence base for the use of CBT in AN.

7.4 Using CBT for the Treatment of NSSI

7.4.1 Cognitive Strategies

Similar to the treatment for eating disorders, CBT in the treatment of NSSI blends both core cognitive interventions and skills with behavioral interventions, namely, replacement behaviors. This treatment can conceptualized in a stepped-care model (Walsh, 2012a) wherein the core cognitions that support NSSI are addressed with cognitive restructuring techniques and then replacement skills are taught and practiced. Thus, the initial sessions are characterized with presenting the cognitive rationale for treatment and developing a sound therapeutic relationship. During the early sessions, the therapist will explain how automatic thoughts can lead to specific emotional states and physiological responses that support NSSI. Automatic thoughts that are common to the patient are elicited, and any apparent thinking errors are identified. Throughout this process, therapist and patient will discuss how thoughts are alterable, and the two will thus employ "collaborative empiricism" in an effort to proceed in treatment (Beck et al., 1979). Walsh (2012a) has previously outlined the five-step process utilized in targeting dysfunctional thoughts, and what is presented here is a brief overview of that approach. First, patients are asked to identify a situation that recently led to NSSI. Second, they are asked to identify the emotions or feelings that were triggered from this situation. Third, patients ascertain any thinking errors and/or automatic thoughts that might have led to the identified emotion. (A thorough review and discussion of common cognitive distortions in the initial sessions helps facilitate this process.) In this third step, patients are also asked to rate the accuracy of their belief in this situation and the intensity of the feeling associated with that belief or thought (typically on a 0–100 scale). The fourth step involves evaluating the evidence for and against the thought, and in the fifth step, patients weigh the evidence just presented and re-rate their belief in and distress associated with the original belief. Patients are then encouraged to develop alternative (and more balanced) cognitions in light of the evidence. Initially, patients may require coaching or facilitation of this process with the therapist until they become more familiar with the language and the method of restructuring cognitions. As therapy progresses, however, they should come to develop this as a core skill to utilize independently during triggering situations or urges to engage in NSSI.

7.4.2 Behavioral Strategies

The second step in this treatment approach involves teaching replacement skills to use as alternatives to NSSI. These skills should be taught during the early stages of treatment when patients are relatively calm and focused. Rehearsal of these skills during periods of non-distress will help enable patients to utilize these skills when they are in acute distress. The overarching goal is to enable patients to use replacement skills (coupled with cognitive strategies) to mitigate an episode of NSSI. However, patients can also be taught to use these replacement skills as a means of delaying the onset of an NSSI episode. This can be particularly helpful in the early stages of treatment when the ability to completely abstain from NSSI may be challenging. Thus, while completely preventing an episode of NSSI may be difficult during the initial stages of treatment, practice using multiple replacement skills increases proficiency at using the skills and can perhaps delay an episode until the most intense emotions have subsided. Again, Walsh (2012b) has previously outlined nine different skills that can be effective in extinguishing NSSI. They include:

- Negative replacement behaviors (marking the body with a red-colored marker, applying ice to the body, using a temporary tattoo and scratching it off with a fingernail, dictating a self-injury sequence into an audio recorder)

- Mindful breathing skills ("I am here…I am calm," "1 through 10 exhale" breathing, "Letting go of…" breathing)
- Visualization techniques (vividly retrieving pleasant, relaxing scenes)
- Physical exercise
- Writing (about the self-injury, about the emotions surrounding the self-injury, about important people in one's life)
- Artistic expression (painting, drawing, sculpting)
- Playing or listening to music
- Communication with others (utilizing social supports)
- Diversion techniques (play with pets, clean the house, read a book)

It should be noted that not all of these techniques will be effective for every patient but that they represent skills that have demonstrated efficacy. Thus, clinicians should work collaboratively with patients to develop replacement behaviors that are both appealing and potentially effective for each individual they work with.

7.5 Evidence for the Use of CBT in the Treatment of NSSI

Unlike the existing literature on CBT for the treatment of eating disorders, two recent reviews suggest that the number of studies providing empirical support for CBT interventions in NSSI is limited (Brausch & Girresch, 2012; Muehlenkamp, 2006). Muehlenkamp (2006) suggests that the limited empirical data available is due at least in part to ethical and legal risks inherent in studying NSSI in addition to few studies identifying these behaviors as the primary focus (many identify suicidality or suicide attempts as the primary focus). While the limited number of well-controlled trials makes it difficult to draw any firm conclusions regarding the overall efficacy of CBT for NSSI, the existing studies seem to suggest that using a CBT framework to address NSSI can be a useful therapeutic approach.

Crowe and Bunclark (2000) describe a multidisciplinary therapeutic approach that included cognitive restructuring techniques, problem-solving skills training, dynamic processing, and psychotropic medications (when necessary). The authors treated 58 patients who endorsed NSSI and reported that this multidisciplinary approach resulted in significantly decreased acts of NSSI in 38 of their patients. It is difficult to fully ascertain the effect of this intervention as there was no comparison group; however, the results suggest that a comprehensive treatment approach that included components of CBT produced modest effects. In a similar vein, Slee, Garnefski, van der Leeden, Arensman, and Spinhoven (2008) randomized 90 individuals who had recently reported NSSI to either a CBT condition or a treatment as usual condition, which involved either psychotropic medication, psychotherapy, or psychiatric hospitalizations in the community. Results of this study indicated that CBT was associated with a significant decrease in NSSI in addition to greater reductions in depression, anxiety, and suicidal cognitions as compared to treatment as usual (Slee et al., 2008). Lastly, Wood, Trainor, Rothwell, Moore, and Harrington (2001) randomized 63 patients who reported NSSI to either group therapy plus routine care or routine care alone. The group therapy intervention combined CBT, problem-solving, dialectical behavioral therapy, and psychodynamic group therapy techniques, while routine care consisted of family sessions and nonspecific counseling. Group therapy was associated with a longer time to first repetition of NSSI and fewer incidents of NSSI than routine care alone (Wood et al., 2001).

There have also been a handful of studies conducted that evaluated the potential efficacy for manual-assisted cognitive-behavioral therapy (MACT; Tyrer et al., 2003, 2004; Weinberg, Gunderson, Hennen, & Cutter, 2006). The typical treatment for MACT involves a 70-page document that combines CBT techniques and dialectical behavioral therapy (DBT; Linehan, 1993) interventions into a comprehensive manual which patients can utilize independently both in place and in support of other psychotherapeutic interventions (typically psychotherapy). While initial studies of MACT failed to demonstrate any significant differences in self-injury rates when compared to treatment as usual (Tyrer et al., 2003, 2004), these studies may have potentially obscured the effect MACT could have on NSSI as their definition of self-injury included active suicide attempts. A subsequent study by Weinberg et al. (2006) investigated the use of MACT to treat NSSI specifically (excluding active suicide attempts) in a group of patients diagnosed with borderline personality disorder. These authors reported that MACT was associated with a significant decrease in NSSI both immediately after treatment and that this effect was maintained at 6 months posttreatment as well (Weinberg et al., 2006). In addition, MACT was associated with significantly decreased NSSI severity at 6 months posttreatment. Although the sample size was small in this study ($N = 30$), the results provide some initial support for the use of MACT in treating NSSI. Further studies are needed to establish empirical support for MACT, particularly in patients who are not concurrently diagnosed with a personality disorder.

Although the literature is limited in number and in consistent methodology, the available evidence would suggest that CBT may be of some benefit in reducing the frequency of NSSI (Slee et al., 2008; Weinberg et al., 2006). Future studies are needed to more fully determine the efficacy of CBT in treating NSSI. It will be particularly important for future studies to focus specifically on NSSI (as opposed to suicidal acts) as the two are considered distinct phenomena. Also important is a focus on the use of purely CBT techniques and interventions. As it stands, many of the available studies use a blend of CBT techniques and other behavioral approaches (Crowe & Bunclark, 2000; Raj, Kumaraiah, & Bhide, 2001; Wood et al., 2001). While it is certainly beneficial to have a variety of techniques available to aid patients, it is of critical importance that CBT be studied in isolation so as to more comprehensively ascertain its potential efficacy for NSSI. In addition to these studies, it is also crucial that future studies the potential efficacy of CBT in the treatment of concurrent eating disorders and NSSI. The co-occurrence of these behaviors has been documented throughout the literature [see Svirko and Hawton (2007) for a review] and is commonly seen in clinical practice. However, there is a significant gap in the literature in that there are no currently published studies examining CBT as a treatment intervention for the comorbidity of these problems.

The addition of such studies would provide both researchers and clinicians with important insights with regard to etiology, maintenance, and effective treatment of these two disorders.

7.6 Putting it All Together: CBT for an Eating Disorder and Concurrent NSSI

Given the considerable overlap in CBT treatment for eating disorders and NSSI, it seems prudent to discuss a potential treatment structure that could simultaneously address both. While the exact structure and nature of the treatment would vary based on an individual's presentation, the general principles encompassed in CBT could be extended to restructure cognitions common to both eating disorder and NSSI pathology and to develop alternative behaviors in replacement of less adaptive responses. This would require that the therapist take a more broad view of the presenting problems and conceptualize them as connected or interrelated in some way (versus conceptualizing them as distinct presenting problems). In fact, some have conceptualized eating disorder behavior as forms of NSSI, suggesting that both lie on a continuum of self-harm (Svirko & Hawton, 2007). Thus, utilizing broad cognitive techniques and specific behavioral interventions could potentially reduce simultaneous reliance on disordered eating and NSSI. Conducting a functional assessment (see Chap. 6, Andover, Holman, and Shashoua (2013)) that evaluates the antecedents, consequences, and cognitive and emotional factors involved in concurrent episodes of NSSI and ED behavior is recommended to guide the therapy. The following represents an overview of a blended CBT approach for both BN and cutting as an illustrative example. The length of treatment is not specified given the varying nature and extent of the presenting problems; however, general guidelines regarding treatment progression are provided.

7.6.1 Case History

Catherine is a 21-year-old university student who reports having experimented with binge eating and purging since the age of 15. Over time, her binge eating and purging increased in frequency and severity, until her mother discovered her purging and enrolled her in outpatient therapy at age 16. She attended therapy for a period of 3 months but made little progress in terms of recovery. Instead she became more secretive with her eating disorder behaviors, particularly with her mother, and she would resort to binge eating in her bedroom or in the car while driving herself home from school each day.

Catherine was raised in a single parent household where her mother was responsible for raising both the patient and her younger brother after their biological father left when she was 7. Throughout much of her adolescence, Catherine and her mother emphasized the importance of education and academic achievement. In addition, Catherine was on the varsity swim team and served as the team captain her senior year. It was during her senior year that she began cutting (age of 17). Catherine reported that the onset of her NSSI occurred after her mother remarried that year. She reports she has never had a particularly close relationship with her (now) stepfather and that his arrival put considerable strain on her previously close relationship with her mother. Despite these difficulties, Catherine excelled in school and earned an athletic scholarship to a local university.

At present, Catherine just completed her first semester of college. She has continued to experience significant academic pressure, and, as a result of carrying an 18-course credit load in her first semester, she ended up failing two of her classes. This resulted in academic probation and a formal review of her scholarship eligibility. Catherine's primary source of social support throughout this ordeal has been her boyfriend Tom. He recently learned about her eating disorder, and while overall he is quite supportive of her efforts at recovery, Catherine reports finding that his frequent "checking in" can contribute to some degree of stress and that she feels pressure to demonstrate improvement even when she is struggling. Currently she is binging and purging five times per week and cutting once per week. During one recent binge/purge episode, she vomited blood and became concerned about her physical health. She thus was self-referred for outpatient treatment at a local eating disorders center and presents for her initial assessment.

7.6.2 Assessment

Before treatment had formally been initiated, the therapist would conduct a thorough assessment of the nature and extent of Catherine's chief complaints. Frequency of both binge eating and purging behaviors in addition to frequency of cutting would be determined in an effort to prioritize a focus in therapy. Standard assessments such as the EDE (Cooper & Fairburn, 1987) and the Self-Injurious Behavior Questionnaire (Schroeder, Rojahn, & Reese, 1997) could be used in addition to a clinical interview to elicit information about specific eating disorder/NSSI thoughts and behaviors. The cognitive rationale for treatment and the expected treatment trajectory would be discussed with the patient while working to establish therapeutic rapport.

7.6.3 Initial Sessions

The initial sessions of treatment would focus on psycho-education and the cognitive model of maintenance for both BN and NSSI. Throughout the initial psycho-educational sessions, the therapist would work with Catherine to solidify her understanding of how thoughts and feelings have supported her use of eating disorder and/or self-injurious behaviors in the past. Eliciting concrete examples of how this process has unfolded in Catherine's own life would vividly illustrate these principles and serve to bolster treatment motivation. The physical consequences of both BN and cutting would be discussed, and the need for both behavioral and cognitive change would be reinforced. During this phase of treatment, Catherine would start self-monitoring both her food intake (and any binge eating and purging episodes) in addition to any episodes of NSSI. A regular eating plan (e.g., three meals, two snacks) would be established, and Catherine would work with her therapist to identify any potential obstacles that might hinder progress with regular eating. She and her therapist would also work together to identify triggering situations that are common to both sets of behaviors. For example, by reviewing each week's self-monitoring, they might identify that Tom's questions about her "progress" and the upcoming review of her scholarship eligibility are triggering events that generate automatic thoughts of "I'm not good enough" which leads to anxiety, frustration, and an urge to binge and/or cut. This process of reviewing self-monitoring would take place on a weekly basis so as to develop this as a foundational skill.

7.6.4 Intermediate Sessions

The more challenging cognitive and behavioral interventions would be implemented after the initial foundation of self-monitoring, and regular eating had been established. During this phase of treatment, Catherine would be walked through the five-step process of cognitive restructuring for both her eating disorder and NSSI behaviors. For example, Catherine might recall that having found out that she was on academic probation led to a binge eating and purging cycle that lasted for 2 h. Throughout the process of cognitive restructuring, Catherine identified that her initial emotional reaction was one of extreme anxiety and the automatic thought of "I've always been a failure and I always will be." At the time, she rated her belief in that thought as 70 and the intensity of the associated anxiety as 80 (on a 100 point scale). At this point, Catherine and her therapist would work together to weigh evidence for and against this automatic thought. Her past successes in academics, athletics, and her interpersonal life could be reviewed, and she could re-rate her belief in her automatic thought and the intensity of her associated emotion. This same sequence could be implemented after an episode of NSSI.

In addition to the cognitive skills, behavioral interventions would also be crucial in this phase of treatment. Catherine would be encouraged to develop a list of "feared" or "avoided" foods with which to begin challenging herself by incorporating them into her diet. She would also be encouraged to identify replacement behaviors for cutting and alternative behaviors to binge eating/purging so that in times of distress, she would have other coping behaviors available to her. For example, Catherine might identify that dictating a self-injury sequence into an audio recorder would be a viable replacement behavior and that calling a trusted friend might be an alternative to binge eating when feeling overwhelmed by stress or anxiety. Given the underlying interpersonal difficulties Catherine has identified with her mother (after her remarriage) and more recently with her boyfriend, she and her therapist would also work on developing adaptive problem-solving skills to more effectively manage these situations. It would be crucial for the therapist to support Catherine's effective use of these behavioral skills by first introducing challenges in therapy sessions. Using "collaborative empiricism," the two would explore options for behavioral challenges and start with a minimally challenging exercise. After some degree of confidence (and competence) using alternative coping skills had been developed, the more challenging activities could then be broached.

7.6.5 Final Sessions

The final sessions of treatment would involve a summarization of the progress made throughout treatment and reinforcement of the newly developed coping skills. Catherine would be encouraged to develop a written list of alternative behaviors that she has found useful throughout the course of treatment. She would work with her therapist to develop a written plan of what to do should she experience any "slip ups" with regard to either binge eating/purging or cutting. For example, Catherine would first need to identify the problematic behavior and then resume self-monitoring. She would work to effectively use her adaptive coping skills (e.g., cognitive restructuring, alternative behaviors, using social supports) and set short-term, realistic goals for herself in terms of "getting back on track." Catherine and her therapist would also discuss the option of reentering therapy should those skills be insufficient to address a recurrence of eating disorder or self-injurious thoughts and behaviors. This process of developing a maintenance and "slip up" plan could occur in the last few sessions of treatment with the final session focusing on reinforcing Catherine's treatment progress and her confidence in maintaining the skill set she has learned.

Conclusion

While there exists considerable evidence that the co-occurrence of eating disorders and NSSI is common, the current understanding of the nature of this association is limited. Both have been conceptualized from a cognitive framework and emphasize the critical role of automatic thoughts in influencing negative affect and subsequent maladaptive behaviors (e.g., binge eating and purging and/or cutting or burning). The existing evidence on these separate clinical syndromes would suggest that using a CBT-based approach to the treatment of both eating disorders and NSSI is potentially efficacious; however, the evidence for the use of CBT in dual treatment has yet to be established. Blending the CBT approach for both separate syndromes would suggest that establishing a sound therapeutic relationship is of primary importance given the challenging nature of restructuring automatic thoughts and reducing reliance on sometimes deeply ingrained behaviors. A comprehensive CBT approach to the simultaneous treatment of these problems requires that the therapist is well grounded in cognitive techniques and behavioral interventions and is able to draw parallels in cognitions, emotions, and urges between both eating disorders and NSSI. Future studies are needed to determine the potential efficacy of standard CBT techniques in addressing these often comorbid conditions in both outpatient and inpatient settings.

References

Agras, W. S., Rossiter, E. M., Arnow, B., Schneider, J. A., Telch, C. F., Raeburn, S. D., et al. (1992). Pharmacologic and cognitive-behavioral treatment for bulimia nervosa: A controlled comparison. *American Journal of Psychiatry, 149*(1), 82–87.

Agras, W. S., Rossiter, E. M., Arnow, B., Telch, C. F., Raeburn, S. D., Bruce, B., et al. (1994). One-year follow-up of psychosocial and pharmacologic treatments for bulimia nervosa. *Journal of Clinical Psychiatry, 55*(5), 179–183.

Agras, W. S., Schneider, J. A., Arnow, B., Raeburn, S. D., & Telch, C. F. (1989). Cognitive-behavioral and response-prevention treatments for bulimia nervosa. *Journal of Consulting and Clinical Psychology, 57*(2), 215.

American Psychiatric Association (2012). American psychiatric association board of trustees approves DSM-5 [Press release]. Retrieved from http://www.psychiatry.org/advocacy–news room/news-releases.

American Psychiatric Association. (2000). *Diagnostic and statistical manual of mental disorders* (4th ed.). Washington, DC: American Psychiatric Association.

Andover, M. S., Holman, C. S., & Shashoua, M. Y. (2013). Functional assessment of non-suicidal self-injury and eating disorders. In L. Claes & J. J. Muehlenkamp (Eds.), *Non-suicidal self-injury in eating disorders*. Heidelberg: Springer.

Beck, A. T., Rush, A. J., Shaw, B. F., & Emery, G. (1979). *Cognitive therapy of depression*. New York: Guilford Press.

Berk, M. S., Henriques, G. R., Warman, D. M., Brown, G. K., & Beck, A. T. (2004). A cognitive therapy intervention for suicide attempters: An overview of the treatment and case examples. *Cognitive and Behavioral Practice, 11*, 265–277.

Berkman, N. D., Bulik, C. M., Brownley, K. A., Lohr, K. N., Sedway, J. A., Rooks, A., & Gartlehner, G. (2006). Management of eating disorders. Evidence Report/Technology Assessment No. 135. (Prepared by the RTI International-University of North Carolina Evidence-Based Practice Center under Contract No. 290-02-0016.) *AHRQ Publication No. 06-E010*. Rockville, MD: Agency for Healthcare Research and Quality.

Brausch, A. M., & Girresch, S. K. (2012). A review of empirical treatment studies for adolescent nonsuicidal self-injury. *Journal of Cognitive Psychotherapy, 26*(1), 3–18.

Brownley, K. A., Berkman, N. D., Sedway, J. A., Lohr, K. N., & Bulik, C. M. (2007). Binge eating disorder treatment: A systematic review of randomized controlled trials. *International Journal of Eating Disorders, 40*(4), 337–348.

Bulik, C. M., Sullivan, P. F., Carter, F. A., McIntosh, V. V., & Joyce, P. R. (1998). The role of exposure with response prevention in the cognitive-behavioural therapy for bulimia nervosa. *Psychological Medicine, 28*(3), 611–623.

Carter, J. C., McFarlane, T. L., Bewell, C., Olmsted, M. P., Woodside, D. B., Kaplan, A. S., et al. (2009). Maintenance treatment for anorexia nervosa: A comparison of cognitive behavior therapy and treatment as usual. *International Journal of Eating Disorders, 42*(3), 202–207.

Channon, S., de Silva, P., Hemsley, D., & Perkins, R. (1989). A controlled trial of cognitive-behavioural and behavioural treatment of anorexia nervosa. *Behaviour Research and Therapy, 27*(5), 529–535.

Cooper, Z., & Fairburn, C. G. (1987). The eating disorder examination: A semi-structured interview for the assessment of the specific psychopathology of eating disorders. *International Journal of Eating Disorders, 6*(1), 1–8.

Cooper, Z., & Fairburn, C. G. (2010). Cognitive behavior therapy for bulimia nervosa. In C. M. Grilo & J. E. Mitchell (Eds.), *The treatment of eating disorders: A clinical handbook* (pp. 243–270). New York: Guilford Press.

Cooper, P. J., & Steere, J. (1995). A comparison of two psychological treatments for bulimia nervosa: Implications for models of maintenance. *Behaviour Research and Therapy, 33*(8), 875–885.

Crisp, A. H., Norton, K., Gowers, S., Halek, C., Bowyer, C., Yeldham, D., et al. (1991). A controlled study of the effect of therapies aimed at adolescent and family psychopathology in anorexia nervosa. *British Journal of Psychiatry, 159*, 325–333.

Crowe, M., & Bunclark, J. (2000). Repeated self-injury and its management. *International Review of Psychiatry, 12*, 48–53.

Dingemans, A. E., Spinhoven, P., & van Furth, E. F. (2007). Predictors and mediators of treatment outcome in patients with binge eating disorder. *Behaviour Research and Therapy, 45*(11), 2551–2562.

Fairburn, C. G., Jones, R., Peveler, R. C., Carr, S. J., Solomon, R. A., O'Connor, M. E., et al. (1991). Three psychological treatments for bulimia nervosa. A comparative trial. *Archives of General Psychiatry, 48*(5), 463–469.

Fairburn, C. G., Marcus, M. D., & Wilson, G. T. (1993). Cognitive behaviour therapy for binge eating and bulimia nervosa: A comprehensive treatment manual. In C. G. Fairburn & G. T. Wilson (Eds.), *Binge eating: Nature, assessment, and treatment* (pp. 361–404). New York: Guilford Press.

Garner, D. M., Rockert, W., Davis, R., Garner, M. V., Olmsted, M. P., & Eagle, M. (1993). Comparison of cognitive-behavioral and supportive-expressive therapy for bulimia nervosa. *American Journal of Psychiatry, 150*(1), 37–46.

Garner, D. M., Vitousek, K. M., & Pike, K. M. (1997). Cognitive-behavioral therapy for anorexia nervosa. In D. M. Garner & P. E. Garfinkel (Eds.), *Handbook of treatment for eating disorders* (2nd ed., pp. 94–144). New York: Guilford.

Gowers, S., Norton, K., Halek, C., & Crisp, A. H. (1994). Outcome of outpatient psychotherapy in a random allocation treatment study of anorexia nervosa. *International Journal of Eating Disorders, 15*(2), 165–177.

Grilo, C. M., & Masheb, R. M. (2005). A randomized controlled comparison of guided self-help cognitive behavioral therapy and behavioral weight loss for binge eating disorder. *Behaviour Research and Therapy, 43*(11), 1509–1525.

Hay, P., Bacaltchuk, J., Stefano, S., & Kashyap, P. (2009). Psychological treatments for bulimia nervosa and binging. *Cochrane Database Systematic Reviews, 4.*

Hudson, J. I., Hiripi, E., Pope, H. G., Jr., & Kessler, R. C. (2007). The prevalence and correlates of eating disorders in the National Comorbidity Survey Replication. *Biological Psychiatry, 61*(3), 348–358.

Linehan, M. M. (1993). *Cognitive behavioral treatment of borderline personality disorder.* New York: Guilford Press.

Lock, J., Le Grange, D., Agras, W. S., & Dare, C. (2001). *Treatment manual for anorexia nervosa: A family-based approach.* New York: Guilford.

McIntosh, V. V., Jordan, J., Carter, F. A., Luty, S. E., McKenzie, J. M., Bulik, C. M., et al. (2005). Three psychotherapies for anorexia nervosa: A randomized, controlled trial. *American Journal of Psychiatry, 162*(4), 741–747.

Morgan, H., & Russell, G. (1975). Value of family background and clinical features as predictors of long-term outcome in anorexia nervosa: Four-year follow-up study of 41 patients. *Psychological Medicine, 5*(4), 355–371.

Muehlenkamp, J. (2006). Empirically supported treatments and general guidelines for non-suicidal self-injury. *Journal of Mental Health Counseling, 28*(2), 166–185.

National Institute for Health and Clinical Excellence (2004). Eating disorders – Core interventions in the treatment and management of anorexia nervosa, bulimia nervosa, and relation eating disorders. *NICE Clinical Guidance No. 9.*

Nock, M. K. (2009). Why do people hurt themselves? New insights into the nature and functions of self-injury. *Current Directions in Psychological Science, 18*(2), 78–83.

Peat, C. M., Brownley, K. A., Berkman, N. D., & Bulik, C. M. (2012). Binge eating disorder: Evidence-based treatments. *Current Psychiatry, 11*(5), 33–39.

Pike, K. M., Carter, J. C., & Olmsted, M. P. (2010). Cognitive-behavioral therapy for anorexia nervosa. In C. M. Grilo & J. E. Mitchell (Eds.), *The treatment of eating disorders: A clinical handbook* (pp. 83–107). New York: Guilford.

Pike, K. M., Walsh, B. T., Vitousek, K., Wilson, G. T., & Bauer, J. (2003). Cognitive behavior therapy in the posthospitalization treatment of anorexia nervosa. *American Journal of Psychiatry, 160*(11), 2046–2049.

Raj, M. A., Kumaraiah, V., & Bhide, A. (2001). Cognitive-behavioral intervention in deliberate self-harm. *Acta Psychiatrica Scandinavica, 104*, 340–345.

Ricca, V., Castellini, G., Mannucci, E., Lo Sauro, C., Ravaldi, C., Rotella, C. M., et al. (2010). Comparison of individual and group cognitive behavioral therapy for binge eating disorder. A randomized, three-year follow-up study. *Appetite, 55*(3), 656–665.

Schlup, B., Munsch, S., Meyer, A. H., Margraf, J., & Wilhelm, F. H. (2009). The efficacy of a short version of a cognitive-behavioral treatment followed by booster sessions for binge eating disorder. *Behaviour Research and Therapy, 47*(7), 628–635.

Schroeder, S. R., Rojahn, J., & Reese, R. M. (1997). Brief report: Reliability and validity of instruments for assessing psychotropic medication effects on self-injurious behavior in mental retardation. *Journal of Autism and Developmental Disorders, 27*(1), 89–102.

Shapiro, J. R., Berkman, N. D., Brownley, K. A., Sedway, J. A., Lohr, K. N., & Bulik, C. M. (2007). Bulimia nervosa treatment: A systematic review of randomized controlled trials. *International Journal of Eating Disorders, 40*(4), 321–336.

Slee, N., Arensman, E., Garnefski, N., & Spinhoven, P. (2007). Cognitive-behavioral therapy for deliberate self-harm. *Crisis, 28*(4), 175–182.

Slee, N., Garnefski, N., van der Leeden, R., Arensman, E., & Spinhoven, P. (2008). Cognitive-behavioural intervention for self-harm: Randomised controlled trial. *The British Journal of Psychiatry, 192*(3), 202–211.

Svirko, E., & Hawton, K. (2007). Self-injurious behavior and eating disorders: The extent and nature of the association. *Suicide and Life-Threatening Behavior, 37*(4), 409–421.

Tyrer, P., Thompson, S., Schmidt, U., Jones, V., Knapp, M., Davidson, K., et al. (2003). Randomized controlled trial of brief cognitive behaviour therapy versus treatment as usual in recurrent deliberate self-harm: The POPMACT study. *Psychological Medicine, 33*(6), 969–976.

Tyrer, P., Tom, B., Byford, S., Schmidt, U., Jones, V., Davidson, K., et al. (2004). Differential effects of manual assisted cognitive behavior therapy in the treatment of recurrent deliberate self-harm and personality disturbance: The POPMACT study. *Journal of Personality Disorders, 18*(1), 102–116.

Walsh, B. W. (2012a). Cognitive treatment. In B. W. Walsh (Ed.), *Treating self-injury: A practical guide* (2nd ed., pp. 171–185). New York: Guilford Press.

Walsh, B. W. (2012b). Replacement skills training. In B. W. Walsh (Ed.), *Treating self-injury: A practical guide* (2nd ed., pp. 147–170). New York: Guilford.

Weinberg, I., Gunderson, J. G., Hennen, J., & Cutter, C. J. (2006). Manual assisted cognitive treatment for deliberate self-harm in borderline personality disorder patients. *Journal of Personality Disorders, 20*(5), 482–492.

Wilson, G. T., Eldredge, K. L., Smith, D., & Niles, B. (1991). Cognitive-behavioral treatment with and without response prevention for bulimia. *Behaviour Research Therapy, 29*(6), 575–583.

Wilson, G. T., Fairburn, C. G., & Agras, W. S. (1997). Cognitive-behavioral therapy for bulimia nervosa. In D. M. Garner & P. E. Garfinkel (Eds.), *Handbook of treatment for eating disorders* (2nd ed., pp. 67–93). New York: Guilford Press.

Wilson, G. T., Grilo, C. M., & Vitousek, K. M. (2007). Psychological treatment of eating disorders. *American Psychologist, 62*(3), 199–216.

Wilson, G. T., & Shafran, R. (2005). Eating disorders guidelines from NICE. *The Lancet, 365* (9453), 79–81.

Wilson, G. T., Wilfley, D. E., Agras, W. S., & Bryson, S. W. (2010). Psychological treatments of binge eating disorder. *Archives of General Psychiatry, 67*(1), 94–101.

Wolk, S. L., & Devlin, M. J. (2001). Stage of change as a predictor of response to psychotherapy for bulimia nervosa. *International Journal of Eating Disorders, 30*(1), 96–100.

Wood, A., Trainor, G., Rothwell, J., Moore, A., & Harrington, R. (2001). Randomized trial of group therapy for repeated deliberate self-harm in adolescents. *Journal of the American Academy of Child and Adolescent Psychiatry, 40*(11), 1246–1253.

Dialectical Behavior Therapy

8

Barent W. Walsh and Jennifer E. Eaton

Abstract

This chapter reviews the basics of Dialectical Behavior Therapy (DBT) as applied in the treatment of co-occurring non-suicidal self-injury (NSSI) and eating disorders (ED). The four major components of DBT are discussed including individual treatment, group skills training, skills coaching between sessions, and the consultation team for treaters. Modifications to the original form of DBT are reviewed including an outpatient application for adolescents who present with suicidality and NSSI and another outpatient version for adults who present with bulimia and binge eating. A detailed case example is employed demonstrating the specific interventions of DBT for the interrelated problems of NSSI and ED.

8.1 Introduction

Dialectical Behavior Therapy (DBT) is an especially relevant treatment for non-suicidal self-injury (NSSI) and eating disorders (ED) for at least three reasons: (1) the problems of NSSI and ED frequently co-occur (Muehlenkamp, Claes, Smits, Peat, & Vandereycken, 2011; Svirko & Hawton, 2007; Chap. 1 Claes & Muehlenkamp, 2013); (2) the behaviors share the common characteristic of recurrent, painful, pervasive emotion dysregulation (Claes, Klonsky, Muehlenkamp, Kuppens, & Vandereycken, 2010; Linehan, 1993a; Muehlenkamp, Peat, Claes, & Smits, 2012); and (3) DBT has been shown to be an effective, empirically based treatment for NSSI (e.g., Miller, Rathaus, & Linehan, 2007; van den Bosch, Koeter, Stijnen, Verheul, & van den Brink, 2005; Walsh, Doerfler, & Millner-Hanley, 2012) and some eating disorders, most notably binge eating and bulimia nervosa (Safer, Robinson, & Jo, 2010; Safer, Telch, & Chen, 2009; Telch, Agras, &

B.W. Walsh (✉) • J.E. Eaton
The Bridge of Central Massachusetts, Worcester, MA, USA
e-mail: barryw@thebridgecm.org

L. Claes and J.J. Muehlenkamp (eds.), *Non-Suicidal Self-Injury in Eating Disorders*, DOI 10.1007/978-3-642-40107-7_8, © Springer-Verlag Berlin Heidelberg 2014

Linehan, 2001). To date, most evaluations of DBT have focused either on NSSI or eating disorders, rather than both in combination. Such is the contribution of this volume that the two problems are discussed at length in combination with an emphasis on successful treatment recommendations.

8.2 What Is Dialectical Behavior Therapy?

DBT is an empirically validated, cognitive-behavioral treatment, informed by the mindfulness practices of Zen Buddhism. It has four major components: (1) weekly, highly structured individual therapy (using a hierarchy of behavioral targets and diary cards), (2) weekly group skills training that focuses on four major skill areas (mindfulness, distress tolerance, emotion regulation, and interpersonal effectiveness), (3) coaching by the therapist or other treaters between sessions to assist clients with skill acquisition and generalization to the environment, and (4) a weekly consultation meeting for the treatment team, designed to enhance learning of DBT and to provide peer support and supervision. These modes of treatment are designed to teach self-destructive and self-defeating clients to employ healthier emotion regulation and interpersonal skills and thereby achieve a new, improved, "life worth living" (Linehan, 1993a, 1993b). Via the consultation team, the treatment is also designed to "treat the treaters," a phenomenon that may be unique to DBT. The team is designed to reduce caregiver burnout and enhance therapists' skills.

As suggested by the above list of core components, DBT is a complex, intensive, and comprehensive treatment that is not meant for everybody. People with minor, short-lived histories of NSSI and ED may not require a treatment as complex and multimodal as DBT. However, for those with persistent, serious NSSI and ED, DBT may well be a treatment of choice.

DBT was originally developed as a treatment for adult women with borderline personality disorder who presented with pervasive emotion dysregulation, suicidal behavior, non-suicidal self-injury, and other problems such as frequent psychiatric hospitalizations (Linehan, 1993a, 1993b). In its original form, DBT was delivered on an outpatient basis via weekly individual therapy sessions in combination with weekly group skills trainings. Completing the treatment generally took about one year.

8.3 Modifications to the Original DBT

In the 20 years since the publication of Linehan's seminal work (1993a, 1993b), DBT has been repeatedly modified in terms of number of sessions provided, specific skills taught, client populations served, and clinical problems addressed. For example, Miller et al. (2007) developed an empirically validated version of DBT for suicidal and self-injuring adolescents that (1) reduced the length of the treatment from one year to 16 weeks (with the possibility of 16-week "graduate group" extensions); (2) incorporated at least one family member, most often a parent, into group skills training; (3) introduced a fifth skills training module, named "Walking the Middle Path"; and (4) modified skills training lectures, handouts, and diary cards, based on the developmental characteristics and learning styles of adolescent clients.

In a similar vein, Safer et al. (2009) have described in book-length detail a modification of DBT for individuals with binge eating and bulimia nervosa. Their version of DBT has been endorsed by Linehan and is delivered in 20 weekly sessions including a 2-h group format for binge-eating disorder clients or a 1-h individual format for those with bulimia (Safer et al., 2009). In addition, their modified versions include three of the original four skills training modules (mindfulness, emotion regulation, distress tolerance). Their rationale for excluding DBT's interpersonal effectiveness module is "based on clinical trial design concerns regarding potential overlap with other treatments developed for binge-eating disorder or bulimia nervosa that specifically focus upon treating interpersonal problems" (Safer et al., 2009, p. 2). Worth noting is that the authors recommend utilizing standard, comprehensive DBT (i.e., Linehan, 1993a, 1993b) if additional target behaviors need to be addressed including suicidal behavior, NSSI, and substance abuse or if the client has a comorbid mood disorder or personality disorder (Safer et al., 2009, p. 2–3). Since this chapter is targeting NSSI in conjunction with eating disorders, the standard, comprehensive version of DBT will be utilized for discussion purposes.

To date the large majority of studies evaluating DBT interventions for eating disorders have focused on binge eating and bulimia (e.g., Robinson & Safer, 2012; Safer et al., 2009, Safer, Lively, Telch, & Agras, 2002, 2009) and not on anorexia nervosa. Only recently have DBT researchers turned their attention to evaluating interventions with anorexia nervosa (e.g., Safer, 2011; Safer, Darcy, & Lock, 2011). As an indication of the dearth of studies pertaining to the treatment of anorexia, Safer noted, "At present no evidence-based treatments are available for adults with anorexia nervosa" (Safer, 2011, p. 203). Fortunately, DBT can be said to be an evidence-based treatment for NSSI and for binge-eating disorder and bulimia nervosa.

8.4 Treating NSSI and Eating Disorders with DBT

As noted above, DBT has four components: (1) individual therapy, (2) group skills training, (3) skills coaching between sessions, and (4) a consultation team for treaters. The remainder of the chapter will review these components with attention to how the DBT can treat NSSI and ED simultaneously in an interrelated fashion.

8.4.1 Individual Treatment with DBT

Individual treatment in DBT is the core modality, the anchor for the treatment. The philosophy central to DBT is that the therapist must strategically balance validation with change. The importance of validation in working with clients with the combined problems of NSSI and ED cannot be overstated. As noted by Muehlenkamp et al. (2011), variables with empirical links to the relationship between NSSI and ED include childhood trauma, dissociation, affective disorders, body dissatisfaction, self-criticism and self-derogation, and especially problems with affect dysregulation. Individuals who struggle with both NSSI and ED are generally exceptionally vulnerable individuals who need a great deal of support to initiate and remain in treatment. Many have endured mistreatment in family relationships and are distrustful and wary. Facilitating behavioral change in a therapeutic environment requires a finely tuned and sensitive ability to validate. DBT places so much emphasis on validation that it articulates six different levels. These range from the simplest form of paying attention (while using basic verbal and nonverbal cues) to normalizing self-destructive behaviors (as understandable attempts to regulate emotion distress) to its most advanced form of treating clients with genuine respect as coequals in a shared project (Linehan, 1993a). With this dialectic of balancing validation and change as the bedrock for the treatment, three additional core components of individual therapy are the use of (1) the DBT hierarchy of targets, (2) diary cards, and (3) chain and solution analyses.

8.4.1.1 DBT Hierarchy of Targets

The DBT targets provide a hierarchy with which to address problems within the treatment. The DBT targets in order of importance are (1) decreasing life-threatening behaviors, (2) decreasing therapy-interfering behaviors, (3) decreasing quality of life-interfering behaviors, and (4) increasing the use of new behavioral skills. The DBT hierarchy provides a way to prioritize target behaviors within the treatment. Individuals with NSSI and ED often have multiple problems they need to address. For example, an individual may complain about having suicidal urges several times a month, cutting herself several times per week, binge eating followed by inducing vomiting several times per week, having frequent conflicts with significant others and work colleagues, and finding it difficult to attend therapy twice a week (individual and group). The DBT targets provide a way to organize and prioritize these diverse problems into a manageable list. More specifically, using the list of problems just reviewed, the therapy might identify the following targets:

- Decreasing life-threatening behaviors
  - Priority # 1: Suicidal urges (due to potential lethality)
  - Priority # 2: Cutting (due to empirical link with suicide attempts long term)
- Decreasing therapy-interfering behaviors
  - Priority # 3: Finding it difficult to get to therapy appointments (without treatment, positive change is unlikely)
- Decreasing quality of life-interfering behaviors

  - Priority # 4: Binge eating and purging (due to health concerns, risk of unstable vitals, damage to esophagus, tooth enamel, etc.)
  - Priority # 5: Frequent conflicts with significant others and colleagues (important but neither is life threatening nor health compromising)
- Increasing the use of new behavioral skills
  - Increasing use of skills learned in individual therapy and group skills training (ongoing)

In addition to prioritizing targets, the DBT hierarchy provides a basic structure to the treatment. Each session begins with a review of the targets and related homework. This structure provides predictability and containment. It also establishes some order in what might otherwise be experienced as chaotic and overwhelming. The message is: "First we'll work together on this primary target and when that has been neutralized, we'll move on to the next, and then the next. All of this will occur as you acquire, practice, and use many new helpful skills."

8.4.1.2 Diary Cards

Diary cards are reviewed at the beginning of every individual therapy session. Diary cards are self-monitoring tools to track the individual DBT targets and emotions daily, set the agenda for the individual therapy sessions, monitor skills practiced over the past week, and assess changes/trends over time (Linehan, 1993a; Miller et al., 2007; Safer et al., 2009). If a client fails to bring his or her diary card to session, the client is asked to complete it at the beginning of the session. Diary cards are emphasized as a key part of homework, and failure to complete them is deemed a "therapy-interfering behavior." The therapist addresses any non-completion quite directly in an assertive, yet validating way. The justification is that "the clients who do the most homework are likely to get the most benefit." Consistent with this principle, the therapist routinely will conduct a chain analysis (see below) to explore obstacles interfering with diary card completion and to identify potential solutions moving forward.

Figure 8.1 presents a sample diary card for Sharon, a 32-year-old mother of three who has the following DBT targets:

1. Decreasing life-threatening behaviors

   Priority #1: Sharon experiences occasional suicidal urges but has never attempted or had a specific plan. She is especially triggered after binge-eating episodes due to related self-loathing.

   Priority # 2: Sharon presents with cutting behavior 2–3 times per month. The cutting involves tissue damage to her arms and legs, but it has never required medical attention.

2. Decreasing therapy-interfering behaviors

   These are not a problem for this client. She consistently attends individual therapy and skills group and completes homework.

3. Decreasing quality of life-interfering behaviors

   Priority # 3: Sharon has been diagnosed with eating disorder, NOS due to her binge eating. Her primary care MD is concerned about her weight gain of 50 lb, elevated blood pressure, and borderline risk for diabetes. She reports

DIARY CARD **Initials: SB** **Date:** __________ Filled out in session? Yes / **No** / Maybe Went to Group? **Yes** / No How often did you complete? **Daily** / 2-3 times per week / Once / Other :______

	Suicidal Behavior		Self-Injury		Binge Eating			Meals				Emotions									Skills used, or lack thereof	
	Urges/ Thoughts	Actions	Urges/ Thoughts	Actions	Urges	Actions	Binge encour-aging behaviors	Breakfast	Lunch	Dinner	Snacks	Bored	Anger	Fear/ Anxiety	Joy	Misery	Physical pain	Sad	Shame	Guilt		
Date	*0-5*	*Yes/no*	*0-5*	*Yes/No*	*0-5*	*Yes/no*	*Describe*	*Detail food items and amounts*				*0-5*									*0-5*	*What Skills?*
Th	1	n	0	n	3	n	Walked down cookie aisle	2 eggs, toast (2), coffee	Turkey sandwich, baked potato chips-indiv bag	6 oz Chicken, rice pilaf-1c, broccoli, 1.5 cups	Apple, banana w/ PB	2	1	0	1	2	0	0	2	2	4	Scrap-booking, park w/kids
F	2	n	5	Cut 3 x on arm	3	n	n	Cereal, coffee	Tuna sandwich, small bag of chips	6 oz broiled fish, 1.5 cup beans	Tangerine, PB crackers	0	2	5	0	4	0	3	4 after ward s	4	1	Failed to use skills
Sa	1	n	1	n	5	y	Went to McDonalds for lunch	3 Scrambled eggs with coffee	5 big macs 2 large fries	Nothing	Apple in morning, nothing afterwards	0	1	3	0	4	0	5	5 after	5 after	3	Used breathing in morning and evening but not around lunch time
Su																						
Mo																						
Tu																						
W																						

Target Behaviors:
0=not at all
1=a bit
2=somewhat strong
3=rather strong
4=strong
5=very strong

Notes:

Used Skills Key:
0= didn't use skills, didn't even consider
1= thought about, didn't use skills
2= used skills, didn't work
3= used skills, partly worked
4= used skills, didn't work then did work
5= used skills, worked, success!

Fig. 8.1 Diary card

binge eating 2–4 times per week. While her binge eating is certainly concerning, it does not meet DBT criteria for "life threatening." At present her eating disorder does not pose risk to life and she has no suicidal intent in relation to it.

Priority # 4: She identifies that she is less sexually active with her husband due to self-consciousness regarding weight. She is also sexually avoidant when her wounds from cutting are fresh.

Priority # 5: She at times feels frustrated being a stay-at-home mom with little contact with fellow adults.

4. Increasing the use of new behavioral skills

   Sharon has begun actively working on skills including scrapbooking (which she finds calming); breathing mindfully; attending a gym—where she has a personal trainer; and walking which she finds relaxing and mood enhancing. Sharon has also started practicing mindful eating.

   Sharon comes from a family that she describes as large and chaotic. She is 1 of 7 siblings, the oldest of whom molested her from the ages of 9–12. She says that her childhood was massively invalidating in that her mother was often depressed and unavailable and Sharon was forced to be a primary caregiver for younger siblings. In addition, the greatest invalidation occurred when she disclosed her brother's molestation to her mother and the mother's response was to call her "a liar" and "ground" her as punishment.

The client identifies her greatest problem as her binge eating. She is self-loathing regarding her weight gain and notes that she feels suicidal primarily after binge-eating episodes due to her self-disgust. She is also concerned about her cutting behavior and is especially worried her children may notice her wounds and scars. She believes that her self-injury is usually an attempt to avoid binge eating in that both provide a self-soothing effect. However, she concedes she finds binge eating much more "gratifying" than cutting. She also concedes, "With me, it seems to be one or the other. I can never get a handle on both."

As shown in Fig. 8.1, the sample (partially completed) diary card provides a great deal of information about Sharon's DBT targets, eating plan, emotions, and skills practice in a concise format. The top panel indicates that Sharon completed her diary card daily and attended group. The information contained on the row labeled "Thursday" shows that she had a successful day in avoiding suicidal urges, self-injury, binge eating, and following her meal plan. Her emotions were at a rather low level of 2 out of 5 (see key at the bottom of the diary card), and her skills practice was effective (4 out of 5) including scrapbooking and going for a walk to the park with her children. The day labeled Friday was less successful. She cut herself three times apparently related to emotions of fear/anxiety (rating of 5) and misery (4). In addition, she reported feeling shame (4) and guilt (4) after her cutting. Not surprisingly, she reported that she failed to use her skills on the day she cut herself.

A similar pattern emerged on Saturday, when Sharon left the children in the care of their father while she went to "do some errands." This led to a binge-eating episode at McDonald's which was linked to overwhelming feelings of sadness (5) and misery (4). Moreover, after the episode she felt intense guilt (5) and shame (5). And again not surprisingly, Sharon's skills practice was rather weak on Saturday. She had attempted to do some mindful breathing in the morning but failed to use other skills as the binge-eating episode unfolded.

8.4.1.3 Chain Analysis

The next step in the DBT individual therapy process is to conduct a chain analysis of the target behavior with the client. A chain analysis provides a very detailed snapshot of a specific incident such as Sharon's binge eating at McDonald's. This careful, meticulous behavioral analysis enables the client to understand why the behavior occurred. In addition, multiple chains over time uncover recurrent patterns of behavior that can be targeted, moving towards what DBT calls "solution analysis" (Linehan, 1993a). The basic components of a chain analysis in DBT are (1) exploring vulnerabilities, (2) identifying prompting event(s), (3) exploring thoughts and feelings (links), (4) identifying the problem behavior(s), (5) exploring more thoughts and feelings (links), (6) identifying consequences (both pro and con), and (7) performing a solution analysis (i.e., identifying alternative solutions (new links)) (Linehan, 1993a). It should be noted that more elaborate versions of chain analysis have recently been articulated (see Safer et al., 2009, p. 78).

Using Sharon as an ongoing example, we will describe a chain analysis regarding her binge-eating episode (in Sharon's own words) that she completed with her therapist in session:

1. Exploring vulnerabilities: I was feeling tired after two nights of poor sleep. The cutting was a sure sign I was in trouble. I have an 8-year history of binge eating. It's my toughest problem.
2. Identifying prompting event(s): It's springtime and the weather is warming. I had taken out some summer clothes and found they did not fit.
3. Exploring thoughts and feelings (links): Thoughts were, "It's hopeless; I'll never lose weight; Age is working against me; I'm a fat cow." Feelings were hopeless, sadness, and shame.
4. Identifying the problem behavior(s): Telling my family I was going to do errands and then going to McDonald's, buying lots of food, and binge eating in my car.
5. Exploring more thoughts and feelings (links): More thoughts: "If it's hopeless, I might as well do what I do best, eat like a pig." "I'm such a loser, I even cut myself yesterday." Feelings: Even more intense sadness, shame, and hopelessness.
6. Identify consequences (both pro and con): Short-term pro: I felt some satisfaction from the good taste and being really full. Short-term con: Almost immediately afterwards, I felt nauseous plus shame and revulsion. Long-term con: continued weight gain, hatred for my body, risks to health, and less sex with my husband. And I had suicidal urges after bingeing.
7. Solution analysis: Identify alternative solutions (new links); I could have called my therapist for skills coaching. I could have used my breathing and walking skills to calm down after trying on clothes. I could have identified my thoughts

about the hopelessness of losing weight as negative and pessimistic. I could have taken my family with me to "do errands" which would have prevented the binge eating at McDonald's.

8.5 Group Skills Training

Group skills training is the other weekly modality in DBT. The expectation is that DBT groups have a leader and a coleader intensively trained in DBT. Ideally, the group leaders are not the individual therapist for any of the clients within the group; however, in practice this is not always possible. Many skills group operate with a structure like the following:

- The group begins with a brief mindfulness exercise such as relaxing breathing or a visualization.
- Members present a review of their skills practice during the past week (hopefully daily).
- Members describe the use of skills that proved successful.
- Members describe any difficulty in practicing a skill and the leaders and group members provide assistance and problem solving.
- The new skill of the week from the DBT manual (Linehan, 1993b) is then taught, modeled, and practiced. Activities and role plays are often used to enhance learning.
- Homework regarding the new skill is agreed on for the coming week.
- A concluding mindfulness activity brings the session to a close.

One caveat that is important to emphasize in delivering group treatment is that social contagion can be a major risk with individuals who present with NSSI (Linehan, 1993a; Walsh, 2012) and/or ED (Becker, Smith, & Ciao, 2005; Crandall, 1988). More specifically, when group members with NSSI and ED are exposed to detailed discussions of self-injury and/or eating disorder behaviors, they can often be triggered into relapse or exacerbation of symptoms. As a result, a key rule in providing DBT skills training groups is that clients commit not to talk in detail about NSSI or ED within the group. The explanation to group members is that discussing NSSI and ED behaviors in groups has been shown empirically to trigger the behaviors in others (Becker et al., 2005; Crandall, 1988; Walsh, 2012). Groups therefore are for teaching and practicing skills rather than discussing NSSI or ED. Individual therapy is where clients should discuss their NSSI and ED in great detail using their diary cards and chain analyses. Walsh and colleagues (2012) have shown that sticking to this principle in providing skills training groups can successfully avoid self-injury contagion in a group home for adolescents. Similar beneficial effects can be expected regarding the management of eating disorders. However, worth noting is that Safer and colleagues (2009) recommend conducting chain analyses in group when treating binge eating and bulimia. Skillful group leaders may well be able to handle such activities, but they should also be alert that the risks of social contagion are considerable.

As noted above, DBT teaches four skill modules in weekly group sessions: (1) core mindfulness, (2) distress tolerance, (3) emotion regulation, and (4) interpersonal effectiveness. These are taught step by step using the DBT skills manual (Linehan, 1993b) or other modified versions (e.g., Miller et al., 2007; Safer et al., 2009). The four skills will be discussed in order with reference to their utility with NSSI and ED problems.

8.5.1 Core Mindfulness

Mindfulness has been defined as "full awareness in the present moment without judgment" (Germer, Siegel, & Fulton, 2005). Mindfulness has the potential to offer considerable solace to those who present with NSSI and ED because it offers a specific antidote to suffering. To explain this potential for relief, it is necessary to "unpack" the definition from Germer and colleagues. Let's take "full awareness" first. Full awareness is the opposite of multitasking, distractibility, or chaos. Full awareness is focusing on only one activity at a time with full attention. This can involve pretty much any activity such as doing the dishes, or completing one's diary card, or talking with a colleague, or listening to the music, or meditating. Moreover, full awareness is grounded in the present moment. This is often a significant narrowing of focus for clients; it means they are not consumed with the past (and what frequently involves many defeats or traumas), nor are they anticipating the future (and what may be perceived as daunting, insurmountable challenges). In focusing on the present moment, mindfulness takes a break, a vacation, from past and present. In addition, this focused attention proceeds without judgment. This means the individual suspends judgment of both self and others. Suspending judgment can be no small liberation for those with NSSI and ED as they are prone to self-denigration (Muehlenkamp et al., 2011) and may be similarly critical of caregivers and significant others.

There are six mindfulness skills taught in DBT: the "what" skills of observe, describe, and participate and "how" skills of nonjudgmentally, one-mindfully, and effectively. A goal is for clients to learn that negative emotions are not steady states or permanent realities. Rather, they learn that emotions come and go and can be markedly influenced. Clients learn to step back, observe, discuss, and manage their emotions effectively, while keeping their focus on their goals. DBT uses a host of metaphors to teach new ways to manage pervasive emotion dysregulation, such as moving from "Velcro mind" where every negative emotion "sticks" and "clings" to "Teflon mind" where problems are acknowledged but allowed to "slip and slide away."

Put another way, DBT mindfulness skills emphasize clients moving away from being dominated by emotion mind (e.g., intense anxiety, shame, rage, depression) into wise mind which is a centered synthesis of reasonable mind and emotion mind (Linehan, 1993a, 1993b). All of us are in wise mind some of the time; these are the moments when we are fully in touch with our emotions but are also grounded in making wise, focused decisions in our best interest. A goal is to cultivate wise mind through practice, practice, practice. A favorite method for practicing mindfulness is through guided breathing exercises which have been shown to reduce heart and respiration rate and blood pressure (Walsh, 2012). These can be especially useful in fending off urges to self-injury.

Another form of mindfulness that can be a great match for ED problems includes mindful eating. This skill applies full awareness in the present moment without judgment to eating. It serves to counteract automatic, mindless, or rushed ingestion that often characterizes binge eating. It involves slowing down and applying full attention to the appearance, texture, smell, and taste of food.

"Alternate rebellion" is an addition to the original mindfulness module (McMain, Sayrs, Dimeff, & Linehan, 2007). It acknowledges that some NSSI or ED may be intended to "take revenge" on others who have mistreated them or judged their self-injury, appearance, weight, or eating. This skill recommends "rebelling" in a safer, more effective way such as using verbal assertiveness rather than cutting or binge eating.

In returning to the discussion of Sharon, she found it helpful to apply mindful eating to her daily life. At mealtime, especially when alone, she began eating "one-mindfully" at the dining room table rather than in front of the television or when driving. She also served herself measureable portions rather than bringing an entire large bag of chips to the table. Sharon found it helpful to become less judgmental regarding her eating and body image.

8.5.2 Distress Tolerance Skills

Distress tolerance skills help clients endure uncomfortable emotions without resorting automatically to NSSI and ED behaviors or other self-defeating acts. One of the metaphors used in DBT to teach distress tolerance skills is learning to "sit with the pain." This involves watching emotional pain ebb and flow, rather than grasping on to it which results in sustained suffering. Another metaphor is learning to "surf the urge" to self-injure or binge eat or purge or restrict. In DBT, clients learn that these urges are not irresistible, all-powerful, or permanent; rather, they are time limited and vacillating and will dissipate if one learns to "tolerate the distress."

Particularly important for Sharon was to combine her mindful breathing skills with urge surfing—which is an addition to the original distress tolerance module (McMain et al., 2007). Sharon found "breathing through her urges" particularly helpful in not submitting to intense food cravings or thoughts of cutting. A special benefit was that she was able to use this skill anywhere while "on the go."

Distress tolerance skills include both crisis survival skills and acceptance skills. Crisis survival skills help clients learn to manage crises and interrupt automatic patterns of NSSI and/or ED. Specific skills include learning to distract oneself by focusing on another activity (such as watching a movie, or shopping, or doing a crossword), self-soothe (using one's senses in a calming way such as taking a bath, listening to peaceful music), IMPROVE the moment, (an acronym for seven self-management skills including calming imagery and relaxation strategies), and conducting a pros and cons (i.e., a thorough, honest analysis of the advantages and disadvantages of proceeding with NSSI or ED behaviors).

The pros and cons skill helps clients to manage emotion mind by stepping back and using observe and describe skills in considering potential outcomes before engaging in a behavior. The act of thinking about pros and cons can interrupt the link between experiencing an urge and acting on that urge. When pros and cons seem too difficult to employ, the urge surfing skill or a mindful breathing exercise can be helpful.

A brief example of a pros and cons exercise was provided above in Sharon's chain analysis of her binge-eating episode. However, had she conducted the pros and cons exercise before her binge eating, she might have been able to avoid it. Her analysis clearly showed that the cons for binge eating much outweighed the pros. Clients often carry their pros and cons lists with them to remind them of the negative consequences of a self-harm behavior. In Sharon's case, she could have retrieved her list from her purse and reviewed it to assist in her goal not to binge.

Acceptance skills within distress tolerance include radical acceptance, turning the mind and learning the distinction between willingness and willfulness. Radical acceptance is often an especially important skill for those with NSSI and ED as it enables them to cease railing against adversity and being preoccupied with (and stuck on) past negative experiences. Radical acceptance involves the following principles presented in slogan form:

- Freedom from suffering requires acceptance from deep within.
- Letting go of fighting reality is a path to reduced distress.
- Acceptance is the only way out of hell.
- Pain creates long-term suffering when you refuse to accept and let go.
- Tolerating the moment is accepting as it is rather than trying to change the moment.

Such slogans are designed to enhance motivation and sustain hope. However, radical acceptance does not mean learning to "agree with" or "excuse" past abuse or trauma. There is no submission in radical acceptance. Rather DBT states, "A lot of your problems may not be your fault, but you have to solve them anyway" (Linehan, 1993a).

Sharon found using the distract skill helpful. She explored new hobbies outside the home that provided structure and increased her contact with fellow adults. She found a gym with a day care center and began work with a personal trainer. Walking to the park with her children was relaxing and she practiced playing with them mindfully rather than sitting and watching. Sharon also carried in her wallet lists of pros and cons regarding cutting or binge eating. She reviewed her list of "cons" when urges arose.

Sharon reported that the self-soothe skill was the most challenging as it was difficult for her to feel comfortable with her body. This discomfort was trauma derived. As a corrective response, she and her therapist negotiated that she practice self-soothe daily. With enough repetition, she came to look forward to painting her nails, brushing her hair, getting a haircut, or bathing.

8.5.3 Emotion Regulation

The emotion regulation module teaches clients to identify, name, reduce, and accept intense negative emotions. An educational component provides a definition of emotions, explains how they are experienced in the body, teaches how to differentiate emotions, and practices how to step back and observe and describe emotions. Clients are taught to reduce vulnerability to negative emotions via good nutrition, regular sleep habits, and avoiding mind-altering substances. This module also fosters experiencing positive events and emotions as an antidote to pervasive emotion dysregulation. The skill of "opposite action" involves behaving counter to what an emotion is signaling. Thus, a person who experiences avoidant anxiety regarding an activity (such as applying for a job or going to a therapy appointment) deliberately forces himself and herself to engage in it with a calm confidence. Or a person experiencing anger (and a desire to attack) deliberately behaves in a civil, considerate manner. These emotion regulation skills help individuals feel more in control of their affective lives: they learn to step off the roller coaster of emotional distress onto the firm ground of modulated affective experience.

In returning to Sharon, she found "opposite action" to be an especially helpful skill. She employed it to push herself to become active when depressed about weight or isolation. With repeated practice of this skill, she reported feeling more productive and energetic. She also used opposite action to counter feelings of loneliness by reaching out to other mothers at the gym and connecting using social media. Building on these activities, she surprised herself by reconnecting with old friends from high school.

8.5.4 Interpersonal Effectiveness

The goals of this module are to learn how to initiate, manage, and maintain relationships with others, and retain a sense of self and self-respect within those relationships. This module is the generally the last of the four taught in standard DBT. It is not intended to be a comprehensive social skills training package, but rather a targeted set of skills especially relevant for people with pervasive emotion dysregulation. It certainly is a good match for most individuals with NSSI and ED, who may be prone to stormy and/or inconsistent relationships. Recovering from NSSI in combination with ED requires a lot of social support. Therefore, interpersonal effectiveness skills can be especially important in helping maintain relationships during the taxing process of dual recovery.

The three main skills in the interpersonal effectiveness module bear the acronyms of DEARMAN, GIVE, and FAST. Each capital letter in the acronym refers to a specific skill. While it is beyond the scope of this chapter to review all these skills, the major components are important to mention. DEARMAN provides techniques for meeting one's needs in relationships, asking for help, and saying no to unwanted requests. The GIVE skills emphasize four ways to maintain relationships. For this acronym, G stands for be "Gentle," I for act "Interested,"

DBT Skills Card		*Check* **the days you practiced**							**Name: __Sharon________ Date: (month 7 in treatment)**
Module	**Skill**	**M**	**T**	**W**	**T**	**F**	**S**	**S**	**Comments about Skill Usage/Practice:** (write a note to remind yourself how you practiced the skill)
Core Mindfulness	Mindful Breathing	x	x	x		x			Practiced breathing in morning during kids' morning nap to deal with urges to cut
	Wise Mind			x			x		Used wise mind before reacting to husband to avoid argument
	Observe & Describe		x						Used when in park with urges to binge (saw ice cream truck), focused on new flowers
	Participate		x						Chased kids around park (couldn't believe how long I could do this for!...15 min straight)
	One-mindfully								
	Non-judgmentally			x			x		Tried to be non-judgmental about the scars on my legs
	Effectively								
	Mindful eating	x	x	x	x	x	x	x	Each formal meal (B,L,D) eat at dining room table. Snacks are harder—on the go.
	Urge Surfing		x				x		Went out to eat with family, urge surfed to get through desire for fish & chips. Enjoyed grilled fish and salad instead and ate only 1 French fry from husband's plate!
	Alternate Rebellion								I addressed my frustration with my husband rather than cutting to "show him"
Distress Tolerance	Distract (ACCEPTS)	x	x	x		x	x		Find myself using these skills to stay out of kitchen and avoid boredom which leads to bingeing
	Self-Soothe	x	x	x	x	x	x	x	Every day! Painted nails, put on make-up even though wasn't going anywhere, treated self to a pedicure at a spa
	IMPROVE		x					x	Encouraged myself to stay strong and not buy ice cream. Even distracted my kids from it.
	PROS & CONS								
	TIP								
	Half-smile								
	Radical Acceptance						x		Certain details of my past
	Turning the mind						x		Had to use while looking at menu to make healthy choice
	Willingness (vs. willfulness)								
Emotion Regulation	Observe Describe Emotions								
	Accumulate Positive activity								
	Build MASTERY					x			Working hard on some gym exercises and getting better at them.
	PLEASE	x	x	x	x	x	x	x	I'm getting quite good at doing this daily tool. I'm proud of the meals I ate and exercise I did.
	Opposite Action			x		x			Used skill to push myself to go to the gym.
Interpersonal Effectiveness	Balance priorities with other's demands		x		x		x		Had to juggle my needs to attend to kids' appointments and husbands late work night. Felt satisfied with outcome
	Balance wants with needs								
	DEARMAN			x					Used skill to negotiate with husband scheduling issues
	GIVE						x		Attentively listened to husband talk about work. Could tell he was happy to be attended to.
	FAST				x				Stuck to my guns with my husband so we could both get our needs met versus me giving in to him like in the past.

Fig. 8.2 Skills card

V for "Validate," and E for using an "Easy" manner. These strategies are designed to assist people prone to explosive, conflictual interactions or sullen withdrawals. The FAST skills teach individuals how to maintain self-respect and remain true to one's values in relation to others. The acronym refers to: be Fair, don't over-Apologize, Stick to your values, and be Truthful.

In Sharon's case, she found the FAST skills to be most beneficial. She emphasized the S skill (i.e., Stick to your values). Sharon was absolutely committed to presenting as a good role model for her children. She was especially dedicated to this principle because positive mentoring was so absent in her childhood. She decided that cutting herself and binge eating—both of which hurt her body—were not effective modeling for her beloved offspring (even if they weren't specifically aware of the behavior). She said, "I think my kids pick up on my self-harm in subtle ways." To counteract the NSSI and ED, she made a list of her values and carried it in her purse with her other skills prompts. Even when her judgments and feelings about herself became pessimistic and negative, she was able to redirect herself as she strove to be an ideal role model. A core value for her became extinguishing NSSI and ED "for the sake of my children."

In concluding this discussion of group skills training, it is important to show how the groups link to individual treatment and the use of diary cards. Many diary cards have a list of the DBT skills on the reverse side (see Fig. 8.2 for an example). This is commonly referred to as the "skills card." This card provides a concise list of all the skills covered in DBT and facilitates tracking (with related comments). Skills taught in group are monitored as to use in the real world both in the individual therapy and group sessions via the use of the skills card.

As shown in Fig. 8.2, Sharon found that completing her skills card kept her focused in treatment. The tracking was also useful when she experienced urges to self-injure or binge eat; it helped interrupt automatic responses. Sharon also enjoyed her therapist praising her skills practice in therapy; she was an individual who had received very little validation from women. Sharon and her therapist also identified which techniques were most helpful by reviewing the skills cards across sessions. They collaboratively created a "cheat sheet" of her favorite skills for easy reference when urges spiked. Figure 8.2 demonstrates Sharon's extensive use of skills during a single week, after she had completed a full round of skills training groups. That is to say, she had already been trained in the full roster of DBT skills.

8.6 Coaching

Coaching is included as part of standard DBT because it is common for clients to have trouble applying skills in their daily lives. Coaching typically involves phone contact and is conducted by the individual therapist. The protocol is that the client calls the therapist prior to engaging in any problematic behaviors. Coaching calls are unscheduled, brief, and problem specific. They are in-the-moment interventions, not phone therapy. Such calls help clients strategize which skills to use and how to apply them in the natural environment. Coaching also allows clients to have contact with their treaters without having to escalate to crisis level behavior.

Sharon utilized coaching on several occasions. For Sharon, long days of isolation at home were difficult. After a few upsetting relapses of NSSI and binge eating, she agreed to utilize coaching calls. One day when her children were ill, she experienced increasing urges to binge eat to bring temporary comfort. As is common with clients who have multiple target behaviors, she also considered cutting to help avoid binge eating. Motivated to avoid relapse, she called her therapist. The clinician briefly validated and then directed her—while they were on the phone together—to review her pros and cons lists for binge eating and cutting. Through this process, Sharon identified several "distract" skills she could use. These included finishing a scrapbook, connecting with friends via social media, and mindfully reorganizing her bedroom closet. In addition, her therapist reminded her to "surf the urges" and engage in some breathing exercises. Sharon agreed to call her therapist back if urges worsened. She was able not to relapse.

Although initially hesitant to utilize coaching in the treatment, Sharon found these calls especially helpful when emotions were high and self-deprecating thoughts were persistent. Coaching calls naturally tapered as she reached the end of treatment.

8.7 DBT Consultation Team

As the above description of DBT individual therapy, group skills training, and coaching has indicated, DBT is an exceptionally complicated treatment. The weekly consultation team is designed to assist DBT practitioners in learning the complexities of the treatment while delivering it according to protocol (Linehan, 1993a). A standard approach in consultation team is to review treatment strategies and listen to recordings of sessions (with consent having been obtained). Such peer consultation provides direct, validating, nonjudgmental feedback and guidance. Linehan's standard outpatient model (1993a) typically includes both the individual therapists and group skills trainers. However, anyone involved in the treatment can be part of the consultation team, including milieu counselors in a group home or inpatient unit, nutritionists, nurses, and physicians.

A second major agenda for DBT consultation teams is addressing caregiver burnout. Working with self-destructive clients can be confusing, frightening, and draining. Professionals need the opportunity to debrief their own emotional distress so that they can maintain a therapeutic frame. This support also helps professionals maintain adherence when they might be tempted to drift from protocol. Consultation team is best conceived as a "team of therapists treating a team of clients" (Linehan, 1993a). The team helps practitioners not feel alone in treating challenging individuals.

During Sharon's treatment, she alternated early on between NSSI and binge eating. The consultation team "treating Sharon" included her individual therapist and group skills trainer and other experienced DBT clinicians. The team offered her two treaters opportunity to collectively strategize on a weekly basis about how to help with her interwoven self-harm behaviors. Sharon appreciated her therapist bringing new ideas from the team to help address her DBT targets. Even though she never met the team members, Sharon perceived them to be an extra source of support, an anonymous group of cheerleaders.

8.8 Concluding Comment on the Case Example

Sharon completed standard DBT in one year. She engaged in weekly individual therapy and two rounds of skills training, where she learned each skill twice. The purpose of this repetition was to increase consolidation of skills. She was a highly motivated client who had strong attendance in the treatment modalities. She used coaching with her therapist occasionally and strategically. By the end of treatment, Sharon had ceased both binge eating and cutting. She had lost 42 of her 50 lb weight gain and was feeling much better about her body image. She attributed her success primarily to her mindfulness, distress tolerance, and "sticking to her values" skills and the restorative relationship with her consistently validating therapist. Sharon was also able to do some productive work about her trauma at the hands of her brother, which provided her profound relief.

Nine months after the treatment ended, Sharon called the therapist to refer a friend for treatment. In the course of that conversation, she confirmed that she was still free of cutting and binge eating. She reported, "I rarely think about doing those things anymore."

8.9 A Note on More Challenging Clients

The case description in this chapter involved an individual who was moderately challenged, worked hard in treatment, and responded with extinction of her problem behaviors. It should be noted that DBT has been employed successfully with far more challenging individuals than Sharon. For example, the senior author of this chapter described an application of DBT in a residential treatment program for severely disturbed adolescents (Walsh et al., 2012). The program serves youth who present with recurrent suicidality, high rates of NSSI, serious eating disorders, substance abuse, and risk-taking behaviors. Their complex problems have led to high rates of psychiatric hospitalizations and removal from their family homes.

As Walsh et al. (2012) reported in their outcome study of the adolescent program ($N = 66$), DBT has been shown to be effective in largely extinguishing suicide attempts and NSSI in the clients served (6 months post-discharge). They also found a "dosage effect" in that clients who received two rounds of DBT did better than those who received less than one. Those who received more treatment had significantly lower rates of subsequent psychiatric hospitalizations and were significantly more likely to return home to family of origin.

Conclusion

A distinct advantage of DBT is that it places great emphasis on motivational strategies to assist clients in entering into treatment. In addition, it has been shown to be successful in keeping them in treatment once involved (i.e., DBT has been shown to have lower rates of dropout than treatment as usual; Linehan, 1993a; Miller et al., 2007). Such ability to engage and retain is especially important with seriously challenged individuals who may have experienced multiple previous treatment failures. The concluding point to be emphasized is that DBT has been used successfully with persons with very severe dysfunction and should be seriously considered as a treatment option when such problems are encountered clinically. This would appear to be especially true for individuals who present with the double trouble of non-suicidal self-injury and eating disorders.

References

Becker, C. B., Smith, L. M., & Ciao, A. C. (2005). Reducing eating disorder risk factors in sorority members: A randomized trial. *Behavior Therapy, 36*(3), 245–253.

Claes, L., Klonsky, E. D., Muehlenkamp, J. J., Kuppens, P., & Vandereycken, W. (2010). The affect-regulation function of non-suicidal self-injury in eating-disordered patients: Which affect states are regulated? *Comprehensive Psychiatry, 51*, 386–392.

Claes, L., & Muehlenkamp, J. J. (2013). Non-suicidal self-injury and eating disorders: Dimensions of self-harm. In L. Claes & J. J. Muehlenkamp (Eds.), *Non-suicidal self-injury in eating disorders*. Heidelberg: Springer.

Crandall, C. S. (1988). Social contagion of binge eating. *Journal of Personality and Social Psychology, 55*(4), 588–598.

Germer, C. K., Siegel, R. D., & Fulton, P. R. (Eds.). (2005). *Mindfulness and psychotherapy*. New York, NY: Guilford.

Linehan, M. M. (1993a). *Cognitive-behavioral treatment of borderline personality disorder*. NewYork, NY: Guilford.

Linehan, M. M. (1993b). *Skills training manual for treating borderline personality disorder*. New York, NY: Guilford.

McMain, S., Sayrs, J. H. R., Dimeff, L. A., & Linehan, M. M. (2007). Dialectical behavior therapy for individuals with borderline personality disorder and substance dependence. In L. A. Dimeff, K. Koerner, & M. M. Linehan (Eds.), *Dialectical behavior therapy in clinical settings: Applications across disorders and settings*. New York, NY: Guilford.

Miller, A. L., Rathaus, J. H., & Linehan, M. M. (2007). *Dialectical behavior therapy with suicidal adolescents*. New York, NY: Guilford.

Muehlenkamp, J. J., Claes, L., Smits, D., Peat, C. M., & Vandereycken, W. (2011). Non-suicidal self-injury in eating disordered patients: A test of a conceptual model. *Psychiatry Research, 188*, 102–108.

Muehlenkamp, J. J., Peat, C. M., Claes, L., & Smits, D. (2012). Self-injury and disordered eating: Expressing emotion dysregulation through the body. *Suicide and Life-Threatening Behavior, 42*, 416–425.

Robinson, A. H., & Safer, D. L. (2012). Moderators of dialectical behavior therapy for binge eating disorder: Results from a randomized clinical trial. *International Journal of Eating Disorders, 45*(4), 597–602.

Safer, D. L. (2011). Anorexia Nervosa as a disorder of emotion dysregulation: Theory, evidence, and treatment implications. *Clinical Psychology, 18*(3), 203–207.

Safer, D. L., Darcy, A. M., & Lock, J. (2011). Use of mirtazapine in an adult with refractory anorexia nervosa and comorbid depression: A case report. *International Journal of Eating Disorders, 44*(2), 178–181.

Safer, D. L., Lively, T. J., Telch, C. F., & Agras, W. S. (2002). Predictors of relapse following successful dialectical behavior therapy for binge eating disorder. *International Journal of Eating Disorders, 32*, 155–163.

Safer, D. L., Robinson, A. H., & Jo, B. (2010). Outcome from a randomized controlled trial of group therapy for binge eating disorder: Comparing dialectical behavior therapy adapted for binge eating to an active comparison group therapy. *Behavior Therapy, 41*, 106–120.

Safer, D. L., Telch, C. F., & Chen, E. Y. (2009). *Dialectical behavior therapy for binge eating and bulimia*. New York, NY: Guilford.

Svirko, E., & Hawton, K. (2007). Self-injurious behavior and eating disorders: The extent and nature of the association. *Suicide and Life-Threatening Behavior, 37*, 409–421.

Telch, C. F., Agras, W. S., & Linehan, M. M. (2001). Dialectical behavior therapy for binge eating disorder. *Journal of Consulting and Clinical Psychology, 69*, 1061–1065.

van den Bosch, L. M., Koeter, M. W., Stijnen, T., Verheul, R., & van den Brink, W. (2005). Sustained efficacy for dialectical behavior therapy for borderline personality disorder. *Behaviour Research and Therapy, 43*(9), 1231–1241.

Walsh, B. W. (2012). *Treating self-injury: A practical guide* (2nd ed.). New York, NY: Guilford.

Walsh, B. W., Doerfler, L., & Millner-Hanley, A. (2012). Residential treatment for adolescents targeting self-injury and suicidal behavior. In B. W. Walsh (Ed.), *Treating self-injury: A practical guide* (2nd ed.). New York, NY: Guilford.

Family Therapy for Eating Disorders and Non-suicidal Self-Injury

9

Elizabeth K. Hughes, Erica Allan, and Daniel Le Grange

Abstract

Non-suicidal self-injury (NSSI) and eating disorders frequently co-occur, especially during adolescence. Several family factors have been associated with risk for NSSI and eating disorders including lack of cohesion and communication, greater conflict and criticism and physical or sexual abuse. Few studies have examined protective factors within the family, and this is an area in need of greater research investment. Overall, research on relationships between family characteristics and NSSI and eating disorders is limited. Currently, family factors are thought to be better understood as risk factors for psychopathology generally, rather than NSSI and eating disorders specifically, and to interact with other biological, psychological and environmental factors. Moreover, family dysfunction may be a consequence of disruption caused by illness behaviours, rather than a cause of the illness itself. Family-based treatment (FBT) for eating disorders does not attribute blame to the family but instead focuses on the family, especially parents, as a resource for recovery. FBT has the strongest evidence base for treatment of eating disorders in adolescents; however, NSSI can make the treatment process challenging for the family and treating team. In this chapter, we describe how NSSI and suicidal behaviour should be addressed in the context of FBT and provide case examples to illustrate three types of

E.K. Hughes (✉)
University of Melbourne, Melbourne, Australia

Murdoch Childrens Research Institute, Melbourne, Australia

Royal Children's Hospital, Melbourne, Australia
e-mail: Libby.Hughes@rch.org.au

E. Allan
Murdoch Childrens Research Institute, Melbourne, Australia

Royal Children's Hospital, Melbourne, Australia

D. Le Grange
University of Chicago, Chicago, USA

L. Claes and J.J. Muehlenkamp (eds.), *Non-Suicidal Self-Injury in Eating Disorders*,
DOI 10.1007/978-3-642-40107-7_9,

situations that may arise (i.e. suicidal patients, patients who engage in low-level NSSI and patients who engage in severe or high-risk NSSI) and how these can be managed while working towards the goals of recovery.

9.1 Non-suicidal Self-Injury and Eating Disorders in Adolescents

Non-suicidal self-injury (NSSI) and eating disorders both emerge during adolescence (American Psychiatric Association, 2000) and can frequently co-occur. A recent study of 1,432 adolescents with eating disorders revealed that 40.8 % engaged in NSSI (Peebles, Wilson, & Lock, 2011), a rate similar to that reported for adults with eating disorders (Ahren-Moonga, Holmgren, von Knorring, & Af Klinteberg, 2008; Claes, Soenens, Vansteenkiste, & Vandereycken, 2012; Paul, Schroeter, Dahme, & Nutzinger, 2002). Conversely, adolescents who engage in NSSI have been reported to have elevated levels of eating disorder symptoms. For example, a study of high school students found that adolescents who reported engaging in NSSI (13.9 %) also reported experiencing greater eating disorder pathology, including greater body dissatisfaction and bulimic tendencies, compared to those who did not report NSSI (Ross, Heath, & Toste, 2009). Of concern, Wright, Bewick, Barkham, House, and Hill (2009) reported that of the 1 in 20 university students in their study who reported both NSSI and eating disorder symptoms, very few sought help, suggesting that in many instances co-occurring disordered eating and NSSI go undetected and untreated.

In women with eating disorders, NSSI more commonly onsets after the eating disorder. For example, in one study, 49 % of women reported NSSI to have onset subsequent to eating disorder, while 25 % reported concurrent onset and 26 % reported antecedent onset (Paul et al., 2002). No studies have examined the temporal sequencing of disordered eating and NSSI in adolescents; however, in university students, NSSI has been associated with earlier age of onset of disordered eating (Wright et al., 2009). In addition, earlier age of onset of comorbid depression or anxiety and pre-existing depressive disorder have also been associated with NSSI in women with eating disorders (Wildman, Lilenfeld, & Marcus, 2004). These findings highlight the potential for psychological disturbance in childhood and adolescence to be associated with development of NSSI and the need for early intervention.

Further resembling their adult counterparts, adolescents with eating disorders and NSSI use cutting as the most common form of self-injury (Claes, Vandereycken, & Vertommen, 2003; Paul et al., 2002; Peebles et al., 2011) and are more likely to have a binge-/purge-type presentation (Ahren-Moonga et al., 2008; Paul et al., 2002; Peebles et al., 2011; Stein, Lilenfeld, Wildman, & Marcus, 2004). Peebles and colleagues (Peebles et al., 2011) reported that adolescents with eating disorders and NSSI were more likely to have a history of bingeing and purging and to be diagnosed with bulimia nervosa than those without NSSI. They were also more likely to have a comorbid mood disorder and engage in substance abuse (Peebles et al., 2011).

9.2 Family-Related Risk and Protective Factors for NSSI and Eating Disorders

9.2.1 Risk Factors

NSSI and eating disorders share several common risk factors including impulsivity, compulsivity, emotion dysregulation, dissociative tendencies and a self-criticising cognitive style (Svirko & Hawton, 2007). However, it is difficult to explicate factors which pose risk for general psychopathology from those that are specific to NSSI and eating disorders and which potentially play shared causative roles. Here we focus on family factors which have been reported to be associated with NSSI and eating disorders.

Several studies have examined the role of family environment in the development of eating disorders and NSSI by asking individuals with eating disorders to describe their families' characteristics. For example, in one study using the Family Environment Scale (FES; Moos & Moos, 1986), female eating disorder patients who reported NSSI (47 % of 131) perceived their families to be less cohesive, expressive and socially oriented and more conflictual and disorganised compared to eating disorder patients who did not engage in NSSI (Claes, Vandereycken, & Vertommen, 2004). A similar study using the Parental Bonding Instrument (PBI; Parker, Tupling, & Brown, 1979) with 80 female eating disorder patients reported that those with NSSI (31 %) perceived their fathers to be less caring and to use a more "affectionless control" style of parenting, compared to those who did not engage in NSSI (Fujimori et al., 2011). This style of parenting is characterised by high level of control together with low levels of warmth. Finally, a study of 95 females with eating disorders found that those engaging in NSSI (39 %) reported higher levels of parental criticism on the Multidimensional Perfectionism Scale (Frost, Marten, Lahart, & Rosenblate, 1990) than those without NSSI (Claes et al., 2012). This latter finding is particularly noteworthy given that parental criticism has been associated with treatment response (Eisler et al., 2000; Eisler, Simic, Russell, & Dare, 2007; Le Grange, Eisler, Dare, & Russell, 1992).

Although these findings suggest that dysfunctional family environments predispose eating disorder patients to NSSI, there are obvious methodological limitations in these studies such as self-report bias and recall bias. Importantly, it is not possible to draw conclusions regarding the direction of causation from cross-sectional and retrospective studies. It is conceivable that previously well-functioning families in which a member becomes psychologically unwell may subsequently experience a breakdown in communication, reduced warmth and increased conflict. For example, adolescent externalising behaviours have been found to predict an increase in maternal criticism over time (Frye & Garber, 2005). A further limitation of studies of associations between family factors, eating disorders and NSSI is that the dysfunctional characteristics identified in these studies are not specific to eating disorders and NSSI. Indeed, dysfunctional family profiles on the FES and PBI have been associated with various forms of psychopathology including depression, anxiety and psychosis (Canavera, Ollendick, May, & Pincus, 2010;

Gonzalez-Pinto et al., 2011; Helgeland & Torgersen, 1997; Meites, Ingram, & Siegle, 2012) and so too has parental criticism (Burkhouse, Uhrlass, Stone, Knopik, & Gibb, 2012; Frye & Garber, 2005; Lopez et al., 2004). In sum, viable explanations for existing research findings in this area include that family dysfunction poses risk for psychopathology in general and that psychopathology affects family functioning in a cumulative fashion (i.e. disordered eating and NSSI contribute to greater family dysfunction than disordered eating alone).

An additional area that has received much attention with regard to eating disorders and NSSI is trauma, especially experiences of physical and sexual abuse in childhood which often occur in the family context. Overall, females with eating disorders who engage in NSSI have been found to be more likely to have experienced a traumatic event, including physical and sexual abuse, than those who do not engage in NSSI (Claes & Vandereycken, 2007; Paul et al., 2002). Interpersonal abuse before the age of 15 years, in particular, has been associated with greater risk for developing NSSI (Claes & Vandereycken, 2007). Similar to family factors described above, trauma is likely to be a risk factor for the development of psychopathology in general, rather than eating disorders and NSSI specifically. In an extensive review of risk factor research, Jacobi, Hayward, de Zwaan, Kraemer, and Agras (2004) concluded that, while there was consistency in findings relating sexual abuse to eating disorders, it posed nonspecific risk for psychopathology. A similar conclusion was drawn by Klonsky and Moyer (2008) in their meta-analysis of sexual abuse in relation to NSSI. Thus, some researchers have examined how childhood trauma may combine with other factors to impact on the development of eating disorders and NSSI more specifically. Muehlenkamp, Claes, Smits, Peat, and Vandereycken (2011) found that, in a sample of 422 females with eating disorders, the relationship between childhood trauma and NSSI was mediated by low self-esteem, psychopathology, dissociation and body dissatisfaction. Further supporting these links, Murray, Macdonald, and Fox (2008) reported that in a sample of 14- to 41-year-olds who engaged in NSSI, those who had experienced childhood sexual abuse reported higher body dissatisfaction, eating disorders and suicidal ideation, compared to those who had not been sexually abused.

Although research has been unable to identify specific causal pathways between family factors and the development of eating disorders and NSSI, risk factor models which incorporate these factors are beginning to be developed to integrate existing research and generate new testable hypotheses. For example, in a review of the literature, Svirko and Hawton (2007) identified four potential precursors to eating disorders and self-injurious behaviour: traumatic events, personality, family environment and culture. They proposed a model suggesting that when these precursors are combined with psychopathological processes including impulsivity, affect dysregulation, dissociation, self-criticism, need for control and obsessive-compulsive tendencies, individuals are at high risk for developing co-occurring disordered eating and self-injurious behaviour. Further research is needed to test this model and, in particular, differentiate these processes from other forms of psychopathology.

9.2.2 Protective Factors

The study of protective family factors in relation to eating disorders and NSSI has been largely neglected. Although recent literature has focused less on the causative role of the family in eating disorders, there has been few converse developments in the identification of positive aspects of family life that may protect individuals from developing eating disorders (Konstantellou, Campbell, & Eisler, 2012). There is some evidence that positive parent–child interactions may protect against the development of eating disorders. For example, one study reported that positive conflict resolution and open communication between fathers and daughters were associated with lower risk for eating disorder symptoms in university students (Botta & Dumlao, 2002). Families' approach to food may also play a role, with a large study of 1,664 individuals over 16 years of age reporting that healthy family eating patterns during childhood (e.g. eating breakfast regularly, less frequent eating of fatty/sugary/salty snacks and parents paying attention to healthy eating) were associated with lowered risk for eating disorders (Krug et al., 2009). It should be noted that both these studies relied on retrospective self-reports.

With regard to NSSI, parenting style may protect adolescents at risk of engaging in self-injury. For example, Hay and Meldrum (2010) reported that the effect of bullying and victimisation on NSSI and suicidal ideation was diminished in adolescents whose parents used an authoritative parenting style. The authors suggested that these parents may help adolescents to cope effectively with bullying and, in turn, reduce risk for NSSI and suicidal ideation. A similar moderating effect may be observable in the development of eating disorders whereby potential risk factors (e.g. genetics, temperament, sociocultural pressures) are counteracted by the presence of positive parenting and other family factors. Such hypotheses, however, require testing in the large, prospective studies.

9.3 Family-Based Treatment for Eating Disorders

Within the field of eating disorders, there has been a move away from looking to the family as a causative factor in the development of eating disorders. Indeed, despite much research and theoretical musings, there is little evidence that any particular type of family or parenting style causes eating disorders (Konstantellou et al., 2012). Instead, the family is now perceived as a resource for recovery, family dysfunction is perceived as a reciprocal process in which the illness and family processes interact to maintain dysfunction, and problematic family relationships are treated without blame and typically only when they present barriers to recovery (Lock & Le Grange, 2013).

Currently, family-based treatment (FBT) has the strongest evidence base for effective treatment of adolescents with AN (Treasure, Claudino, & Zucker, 2010). Its effectiveness has been demonstrated in six randomised controlled trials (Eisler et al., 2000; Le Grange et al., 1992; Lock, Agras, Bryson, & Kraemer, 2005; Lock et al., 2010; Robin, Siegel, Koepke, Moye, & Tice, 1994; Russell, Szmukler, Dare,

& Eisler, 1987), and research supporting FBT in the successful treatment of adolescents with BN is also emerging (Le Grange, Crosby, Rathouz, & Leventhal, 2007; Le Grange & Lock, 2010). FBT is a manualised outpatient intervention in which parents are assisted by a mental health clinician to become actively involved in supporting the adolescent to gain weight, normalise eating patterns and prevent binge eating and purging behaviours (Le Grange & Lock, 2007; Lock & Le Grange, 2012). It is typically delivered over 6 months and comprises 20 treatment sessions which the whole family attends together (i.e. parents, adolescent, siblings).

The treatment progresses through three phases:

Phase I. In the first phase, the parents are empowered to take control of the adolescent's eating by monitoring all meals, supporting them to eat a sufficient amount and preventing them from engaging in subsequent purging behaviour. Each session begins with the adolescent being weighed and the parents reflecting on where they have been successful or unsuccessful in refeeding their child. The therapist encourages the parents to devise strategies for achieving the goals of treatment and overcoming any barriers. Phase I includes a family meal at session two in which the family brings along a meal to eat together. This session provides the therapist with an opportunity to observe family interactions during meal times and assist the parents in uniting to support the adolescent to eat.

Phase II. Once weight has improved and the adolescent's resistance has deceased, the family moves into Phase II in which the adolescent gradually regains independence around mealtimes. Sessions remain centred around symptoms and continued weight gain is encouraged. Family issues which may be preventing steady weight gain may also be raised and addressed in this phase.

Phase III. Once weight is restored and eating disorder behaviours have remitted, the family moves into Phase III in which the therapist ensures the adolescent has returned to a normal developmental trajectory with regard to psychosocial functioning and terminates treatment.

For a more thorough description of FBT, readers should consult the treatment manual (Lock & Le Grange, 2013). In addition to reading and following the manual guidelines, clinicians wanting to provide FBT to eating disorder patients should seek formal training (http://www.train2treat4ed.com in the USA and Canada).

9.4 Managing Suicide and NSSI in Family-Based Treatment for Eating Disorders

As described earlier, suicidal and self-injurious behaviours are common in individuals with eating disorders. Although NSSI is destructive, distressing and risky, eating disorders are life-threatening illnesses which require immediate treatment. In particular, the starvation associated with AN places individuals at risk of numerous medical complications including cardiac, electrolyte, reproductive and endocrine abnormalities, stunted growth and long-term issues with bone strength and reproductive health (Robinson & Serfaty, 2008). It is associated with the highest mortality rate of all mental illnesses, with AN patients having a tenfold increased risk of premature death (Button, Chadalavada, & Palmer, 2010). Binge eating and purging behaviours, whether a feature of AN or BN, are also associated with significant medical complications across the renal, oral, gastrointestinal, cardiovascular and endocrine systems (Mehler, 2011; Mehler, Crews, & Weiner, 2004).

Clearly, eating disorders must be treated with urgency; however, NSSI and suicidal behaviours pose significant challenges in treatment for all involved and can impede ED recovery. Both the manuals for FBT for AN (Lock & Le Grange, 2013) and FBT for BN (Le Grange & Lock, 2007) provide guidance for clinicians who are confronted with patients engaging in NSSI and suicidal behaviours. These guidelines, as describe further in this chapter, highlight the need to balance the emergency of suicidal behaviours and NSSI with the emergency of ED behaviours and ensure that attention is paid to both. Although it is difficult to capture the complexity of situations that may arise, three main categories and preferred courses of action can be described: (1) suicidal patients, (2) patients who engage in low-level NSSI and (3) patients who engage in severe or high-risk NSSI. We will address each of these situations in turn and provide a case example for each.

9.4.1 Suicidal Risk

Suicidal eating disorder patients pose a situation in which other treatment priorities must be placed on hold. Suicide is a major cause of death in young people (Viner et al., 2011) and is the cause of approximately half the deaths associated with AN (Herzog et al., 2000). It must be taken seriously and addressed as an emergency. FBT must be put on hold until such time as the acute situation has resolved. During this time it is helpful to involve the parents as much as possible in addressing suicidal ideation. This might involve having them come up with ideas and strategies for keeping their child safe, ensuring they are involved as key decision makers (e.g. deciding whether inpatient treatment is necessary or whether to commence psychotropic medication) and keeping them well informed throughout the process. In this way, the importance of parents in supporting their child and their central role in their child's treatment and recovery is reinforced.

Case Example 1. *Sarah was a 15-year-old girl who presented to the eating disorder clinic having lost 15 kg over 5 months. Her parents reported she was currently eating very small amounts of low-calorie food, and they suspected she was vomiting. Sarah reported she had started restricting her intake to lose a small amount weight, but despite her now malnourished appearance, she continued to feel fat and wanted to lose further weight. She also reported a history of fluctuating depressive symptoms over the past 2 years during which time she had regularly engaged in cutting her arms and legs and had attempted to overdose on paracetamol a year ago following a breakdown in her friendship group. She had been prescribed antidepressant medication after this episode which she continued to take until presenting to the eating disorders clinic. At the time of presentation to the* *clinic, she reported no active suicidal ideation and was diagnosed with anorexia nervosa with comorbid depression. FBT was recommended with concomitant monitoring of her depression and medical status.*

Sarah's family made good progress during the first few weeks of treatment, with her parents successfully taking control of eating, supervising all of her meals and ensuring someone sat with her after meals to provide support and prevent purging. After 1 month of treatment, Sarah had gained nearly 3 kg; however, she was becoming increasingly distressed at mealtimes, lashing out at her parents and threatening to kill herself if she put on more weight. Sarah's parents were concerned that she had become more withdrawn between meals and they could not get her involved in any of the activities she used to enjoy. On further probing by the therapist, Sarah revealed that she had been frequently cutting herself and having constant thoughts about killing herself. She felt that she was causing her family a great deal of pain and that life was not worth living. She confessed that she had stopped taking her antidepressant medication and planned to overdose on the unused tablets. When her parents were advised to remove the tablets and any other means of self-injury in the house, Sarah became increasingly distressed, sobbing and screaming that she would run in front of a car or train the first chance she had. Sarah was subsequently admitted to an adolescent psychiatric unit for observation and further assessment.

After 72 hours in the inpatient unit, Sarah's mental status was deemed to be stable, and she was no longer considered at imminent risk for suicide. That said, given her premorbid history of depression, past suicide attempt and self-injurious behaviour, managing her eating disorder meant that her mood disorder and impulsive behaviours needed to be managed concomitantly via regular reviews with the team psychiatrist. The team members involved in Sarah's care met frequently to review her progress and coordinate her care. The FBT therapist remained focused on supporting Sarah's parents with weight restoration, while team psychiatrist closely monitored and managed Sarah's mood symptoms and ensured her parents felt able to keep her safe. Over the next 2 months, Sarah's weight was restored to a healthy status, her mood improved, and she reported only occasional urges to harm herself. Although Sarah's eating disorder symptoms had remitted after 6 months in FBT, she continued to report urges to injure herself and was referred to a psychologist for individual therapy to address the impulses.

While FBT is primarily focused on weight restoration, suicide is the only behaviour that trumps self-starvation. In other words, the FBT therapist strives to remain focused on supporting the parents in their efforts at weight restoration and must postpone other issues until the self-starvation has been resolved. However, suicide and other self-injurious behaviours are the exception. The FBT therapist is not solely responsible for managing all these behaviours. In fact, FBT is ultimately a team effort and, in addition to the parents, therapist and paediatrician, in this instance the child and adolescent psychiatrist plays a pivotal role in providing the adolescent and her family with critical support.

9.4.2 Low-Level NSSI

When self-injurious behaviours are not clearly suicidal, the decision to suspend FBT can be complicated. NSSI may have always been a part of the patient's presentation or may emerge during treatment in response to parents' and professionals' attempts to challenge the ED. NSSI can also be multifunctioning in the eating disorders and its treatment. It can be self-punishing, anxiety relieving, dissociative or ritualistic. It can serve as punishment for breaking dietary rules, for increasing weight or for feelings of fatness. It can also be used by the eating disorder to heighten parents' anxiety in order to get them to back down. When NSSI remains at a low level, treatment can continue with the focus on eating disorder behaviours as the source of greatest harm. If they persist into Phase III, in which wider developmental and family issues are explored, they can be addressed at this time.

Case Example 2. *Jessica was a 16-year-old girl who was referred to the eating disorder clinic for assessment following a long history of weight and eating problems. Jessica had been overweight for most of her childhood, but lost a significant amount of weight a year ago by implementing a strict diet and exercise programme she had found on the Internet. Over the previous 6 months, however, Jessica had been overwhelmed by the need to binge eat and reported getting up most nights to secretly eat large amounts of food. She described feeling incredibly guilty and disgusted with herself after these episodes and would subsequently self-induce vomiting. Her weight had gradually increased and she had found herself cycling between periods of fasting and episodes of bingeing and purging. Her weight was currently in the expected range for her age and height, but she reported feeling fat and terrified of gaining weight. Jessica was diagnosed with bulimia nervosa and referred for family-based treatment.*

In the first week of treatment, Jessica's parents struggled to enforce a routine around mealtimes and supervision post meals. They easily backed down when Jessica protested about their choice of foods and serving sizes, and they found it difficult to stop Jessica from locking herself in the bathroom after meals to vomit. Food continued to go missing from the kitchen, and they had found a box of laxatives in Jessica's school bag. With some guidance by their therapist, Jessica's parents decided together on their expectations for meals and agreed to support each other better and not negotiate with the eating disorder. They arranged to put a lock on the pantry and removed the lock from the bathroom door. They also stopped giving Jessica her pocket money so she could not buy laxatives, and instead they put this money in a savings account and bought her what she needed directly. Over the next few weeks, these strategies worked successfully to improve Jessica's eating and prevented her from bingeing and purging. Jessica became increasingly distraught at mealtimes, however, yelling at her parents and accusing them of trying to make her fat. After meals she was so wracked by guilt for having eaten that she would punch and scratch herself until her parents allowed her to go to the bathroom unsupervised. Jessica soon began punching and scratching herself during mealtimes and would tell her parents that if she was made to eat she would "do worse".

When Jessica's parents described this in session, the therapist first reminded them that the eating disorder was separate or distinct from Jessica and explained that her eating disorder would get her to engage in behaviours she would not otherwise engage in. In other words, the parents were reminded that these behaviours, or eating disorder symptoms, were not necessarily within Jessica's control, even if sometimes it might seem that way to them. The therapist sympathised with Jessica about her awful predicament, one that gets her to be so desperate and even out of control when she is made to believe that she has eaten 'too much' when, by most people's standards, she is consuming a perfectly healthy food intake. Jessica and her parents were reminded that sometimes the eating disorder would have the sufferer feel so desperate that it would use threats of self-injury to get those who care about them (in this instance the parents) to back off from their task of supporting their daughter. When asked what she thought, Jessica acknowledge that she felt guilty for making her parents worry so much, but that threatening to hurting herself was the only thing she had been able to do to get out of eating. Once the therapist felt Jessica and her parents understood the situation better, they were able to discuss together healthier ways to deal with Jessica's distress.

In this type of situation, self-injury and threats of self-injury are the patient's way of dealing with their distress. The therapist and family must work together to help teach the adolescent healthier ways to manage this very real distress. For example, the therapist will aim to help the patient distinguish between threats to self-injury when someone is depressed (as in a mood disorder) and threats of self-injury when one is upset or distressed because of the anxiety and fear induced by the idea of eating more than what the eating disorder would 'allow'. The therapist will also aim to help the parents understand this difference. However, because it is not always possible to distinguish between suicidal threats versus managing distress around eating, the adolescent and his/her parents are coached that when they are unable to make this distinction, they should act to secure their child's safety. That means to take their child to the nearest emergency room, or to call the emergency hotline, e.g. 911 in the United States. At the same time though, the patient is supported to find more appropriate or healthier ways to deal with or express her eating-related distress. The patient is encouraged, with the help of the therapist and the parents, to find to right words that capture her distress and to figure out ways to let her/his parents know about this distress. Also, the family is encouraged to be understanding of this distress and help the adolescent with healthy ways to then explore or deal with this distress, for example, have a conversation with parents or a parent, or just go for a quiet walk around the block with a parent, journal ones thoughts and so on. The central message of the therapist is that the parents cannot back down from attending to the eating disorder, but that everyone should acknowledge that the adolescent's anxiety is real and that together they can learn different skills to deal with this anxiety in healthier ways.

9.4.3 Severe and High-Risk NSSI

Although NSSI is not intended to be life-threatening, it may escalate to the point that it becomes life endangering and cause serious and lifelong damage. In this situation, NSSI may need to be attended to in the same way as suicidal behaviour. In addition, severe NSSI is likely to significantly disrupt the treatment process and will need to be addressed as a priority.

Case Example 3. *Katie was a 14-year-old girl who was brought to the emergency department by her mother who was concerned about her lack of eating and sudden weight loss. She was subsequently admitted to the inpatient medical unit with very low heart rate and dehydration. A mental health assessment revealed that Sarah had dramatically reduced her dietary intake over the past 6 months in an effort to lose weight. She had also increased her exercise and was secretly weighing herself three times a day. She had not menstruated for 3 months, reported feeling dizzy upon standing and was unable to concentrate on her schoolwork. She was diagnosed with anorexia nervosa and, once medically stable, was discharged and referred for FBT and medical follow-up. Katie and her mother attended the hospital outpatient clinic for FBT. Katie's parents had divorced when she was 3 years old and she had no contact with her father. Her mother worked full time but arranged for time off to provide treatment for Katie.*

Treatment sessions were extremely difficult as they were typically disrupted by Katie's overwhelming distress. Upon coming into sessions with the therapist, Katie would start to sob uncontrollably. When her mother and the therapist tried to talk, she would pull violently at her hair, hit her arms and legs against the furniture or bang her head against the wall. She would lash out at anyone that came near her, and several times a medical team had to be called to sedate her. On one occasion Katie had to be restrained from running out of the clinic and onto the road. Once calm, Katie explained that she had no intention to kill herself, but that she could not stand to hear her mother and therapist talk about her need to eat and gain weight.

Staying on task with weight restoration became increasingly difficult for both the FBT therapist and for Katie's mother. Sessions were overtaken with managing Katie's distress, rather than focusing on recovering from her eating disorder. It very soon became clear that Katie would benefit from meeting with the team psychiatrist with a view towards pharmacotherapy in conjunction with learning more about relaxation and distress tolerance. The therapist also recommended that while the team member would assist Katie and her mother in learning these skills, FBT should continue but with the therapist meeting with Katie's mother alone in separate sessions. The goal of these meetings was not altered. That is, the therapist reviewed with Katie's mother how she was progressing with restoring Katie's weight and of course helped her manage Katie's self-injurious behaviours. FBT was able to progress more smoothly through these separated sessions, and in the meantime, Katie's wild mood swings became less frequent and severe through medication and skills training.

In this type of situation, meeting with parents separately from the adolescent can enable the therapist to review intersession progress without the adolescent's behaviour derailing the sessions. Patient in-session behaviour can be quite disruptive and make it difficult for the therapist to remain on task (e.g. continuously interrupting the therapist and/or parents). Consequently, the limited therapy hour is spent trying to focus on intersession parental strategies to help their offspring, but little time can practically be devoted to this endeavour given the adolescent's behaviours in-session. Therefore, meeting with the adolescent first, albeit briefly, to get an idea of how the week has been and make a brief assessment of their mental status, is followed by a separate session with only the parents present. This should allow the therapist to focus more exclusively on parental strategies for the upcoming week. Separated forms of FBT have been shown to be as effective in the treatment of AN as conjoint FBT (Eisler et al., 2000; Le Grange et al., 1992). Indeed, separated sessions may be preferable in situations like this where the adolescent's presence frequently derails sessions and also in situations where parents express high levels of criticism regarding their child (Eisler et al., 2000, 2007).

Conclusion and Future Directions

NSSI is common in eating disorders and may escalate during treatment, at least during the initial period when parents are focusing their efforts on weight restoration. Working with families, however, provides an opportunity for the therapist to help parents find healthy ways to address and contain these behaviours. The skills parents acquire, or that are reinforced by the therapist during FBT, should readily translate to supporting their child in the domain of NSSI behaviour as well. For example, setting firm boundaries around self-starvation enables parents to appreciate, anew, that following their parental instincts by taking care of their child is the "right thing to do". Similarly then, the parents' skills around refeeding generalise to other areas of problematic behaviour such as NSSI. Many parents' response to FBT is that they have been given "permission to be parents", and if they can rescue their child in one domain, then surely they can also do so in another.

Once the eating disorder has remitted, NSSI may also be better contained or even remitted as a function of improved physical health, mental status and the family's capacity to manage crisis behaviour. When NSSI remains an issue after remittance of the eating disorder, subsequent individual therapy may help to address this. Likewise, in many instances the NSSI is resolved, but the eating disorder symptoms remain in place or return once resolved. Standard FBT is currently not set up to contain typical "booster" sessions. Instead, the therapist will advise the family to remain focused on the eating disorder symptoms until such time as everyone concerned is convinced that the eating disorder has fully abated. This may very well mean that for some families, treatment is extended beyond the typical 20 sessions as per the treatment manual. In fact, what sets FBT apart from structural family therapy for anorexia nervosa (Minuchin et al., 1975), or behavioural family systems therapy (Robin & Le Grange, 2010), is that in FBT the therapist stays with the issue of self-starvation until it is resolved. In practice, this may mean that the treatment focus sits squarely in Phase I, and progress to the next phase is only embarked upon, once the eating disorder symptoms have abated.

While FBT first and foremost addresses the acute impact of self-starvation and binge eating and purging, most adolescents with an eating disorder present with comorbid psychiatric disorders and behaviours, e.g. NSSI. Managing these comorbidities alongside the eating disorder is also part of FBT, although this is typically done by another team member rather than the FBT therapist himself/herself. Augmenting FBT to incorporate other treatment modalities to address NSSI, such as DBT (Federici & Wisniewski, 2012), has been proposed. However, pursuing this avenue, as well as other adaptations of FBT to better accommodate serious coexisting psychiatric diagnoses, is in its infancy and should be a priority for more systematic treatment development efforts.

References

Ahren-Moonga, J., Holmgren, S., von Knorring, L., & Af Klinteberg, B. (2008). Personality traits and self-injurious behaviour in patients with eating disorders. *European Eating Disorders Review, 16*(4), 268–275.

American Psychiatric Association. (2000). *Diagnostic and statistical manual of mental disorders (4th ed., text revision)*. Washington, DC: American Psychiatric Press.

Botta, R. A., & Dumlao, R. (2002). How do conflict and communication patterns between fathers and daughters contribute to or offset eating disorders? *Health Communication, 14*(2), 199–219.

Burkhouse, K., Uhrlass, D., Stone, L., Knopik, V., & Gibb, B. (2012). Expressed emotion-criticism and risk of depression onset in children. *Journal of Clinical Child and Adolescent Psychology, 41*(6), 771–777.

Button, E. J., Chadalavada, B., & Palmer, R. L. (2010). Mortality and predictors of death in a cohort of patients presenting to an eating disorders service. *International Journal of Eating Disorders, 43*(5), 387–392.

Canavera, K. E., Ollendick, T. H., May, J. T., & Pincus, D. B. (2010). Clinical correlates of comorbid obsessive-compulsive disorder and depression in youth. *Child Psychiatry and Human Development, 41*(6), 583–594.

Claes, L., Soenens, B., Vansteenkiste, M., & Vandereycken, W. (2012). The scars of the inner critic: Perfectionism and nonsuicidal self-injury in eating disorders. *European Eating Disorders Review, 20*(3), 196–202.

Claes, L., & Vandereycken, W. (2007). Is there a link between traumatic experiences and self-injurious behaviors in eating-disordered patients? *Eating Disorders, 15*(4), 305–315. Brunner-Mazel eating disorders Monograph Series.

Claes, L., Vandereycken, W., & Vertommen, H. (2003). Eating-disordered patients with and without self-injurious behaviours: A comparison of psychopathological features. *European Eating Disorders Review, 11*(5), 379–396.

Claes, L., Vandereycken, W., & Vertommen, H. (2004). Family environment of eating disordered patients with and without self-injurious behaviors. *European Psychiatry: The Journal of the Association of European Psychiatrists, 19*(8), 494–498.

Eisler, I., Dare, C., Hodes, M., Russell, G. F. M., Dodge, E., & Le Grange, D. (2000). Family therapy for adolescent anorexia nervosa: The results of a controlled comparison of two family interventions. *Journal of Child Psychology and Psychiatry, and Allied Disciplines, 41*(6), 727–736.

Eisler, I., Simic, M., Russell, G. F., & Dare, C. (2007). A randomised controlled treatment trial of two forms of family therapy in adolescent anorexia nervosa: A five-year follow-up. *Journal of Child Psychology and Psychiatry, and Allied Disciplines, 48*(6), 552–560.

Federici, A., & Wisniewski, L. (2012). *Integrating dialectical behaviour therapy and family-based treatment for multidiagnostic adolescent patients. A collaborative approach to eating* (pp. 177–188). New York, NY: Routledge.

Frost, R. O., Marten, P., Lahart, C., & Rosenblate, R. (1990). The dimensions of perfectionism. *Cognitive Therapy and Research, 14*, 449–468.

Frye, A. A., & Garber, J. (2005). The relations among maternal depression, maternal criticism, and adolescents' externalizing and internalizing symptoms. *Journal of Abnormal Child Psychology, 33*(1), 1–11.

Fujimori, A., Wada, Y., Yamashita, T., Choi, H., Nishizawa, S., Yamamoto, H., et al. (2011). Parental bonding in patients with eating disorders and self-injurious behavior. *Psychiatry and Clinical Neurosciences, 65*(3), 272–279.

Gonzalez-Pinto, A., de Azua, S. R., Ibanez, B., Otero-Cuesta, S., Castro-Fornieles, J., Graell-Berna, M., et al. (2011). Can positive family factors be protective against the development of psychosis? *Psychiatry Research, 186*(1), 28–33.

Hay, C., & Meldrum, R. (2010). Bullying victimization and adolescent self-harm: Testing hypotheses from general strain theory. *Journal of Youth and Adolescence, 39*(5), 446–459.

Helgeland, M. I., & Torgersen, S. (1997). Maternal representations of patients with schizophrenia as measured by the Parental Bonding Instrument. *Scandinavian Journal of Psychology, 38*(1), 39–43.

Herzog, D. B., Greenwood, D. N., Dorer, D. J., Flores, A. T., Ekeblad, E. R., Richards, A., et al. (2000). Mortality in eating disorders: A descriptive study. *International Journal of Eating Disorders, 28*(1), 20–26.

Jacobi, C., Hayward, C., de Zwaan, M., Kraemer, H. C., & Agras, W. (2004). Coming to terms with risk factors for eating disorders: Application of risk terminology and suggestions for a general taxonomy. *Psychological Bulletin, 130*(1), 19–65.

Klonsky, E. D., & Moyer, A. (2008). Childhood sexual abuse and non-suicidal self-injury: Meta-analysis. *British Journal of Psychiatry, 192*(3), 166–170.

Konstantellou, A., Campbell, M., & Eisler, I. (2012). *The family context: Cause, effect or resource. A collaborative approach to eating disorders* (pp. 5–18). New York, NY: Routledge.

Krug, I., Treasure, J., Anderluh, M., Bellodi, L., Cellini, E., Collier, D., et al. (2009). Associations of individual and family eating patterns during childhood and early adolescence: A multicentre European study of associated eating disorder factors. *British Journal of Nutrition, 101*(6), 909–918.

Le Grange, D., Crosby, R. D., Rathouz, P. J., & Leventhal, B. L. (2007). A randomized controlled comparison of family-based treatment and supportive psychotherapy for adolescent bulimia nervosa. *Archives of General Psychiatry, 64*(9), 1049–1056.

Le Grange, D., Eisler, I., Dare, C., & Russell, G. F. (1992). Evaluation of family treatments in adolescent anorexia nervosa: A pilot study. *International Journal of Eating Disorders, 12*(4), 347–358.

Le Grange, D., & Lock, J. (2007). *Treating bulimia in adolescents: A family-based approach.* New York, NY: Guilford.

Le Grange, D., & Lock, J. (2010). Family-based treatment for adolescents with bulimia nervosa. In J. E. Mitchell (Ed.), *The treatment of eating disorders: A clinical handbook* (pp. 372–387). New York, NY: Guilford.

Lock, J., Agras, S., Bryson, S., & Kraemer, H. (2005). A comparison of short- and long-term family therapy for adolescent anorexia nervosa. *Journal of the American Academy of Child and Adolescent Psychiatry, 44*(7), 632–639.

Lock, J., & Le Grange, D. (2013). *Treatment manual for anorexia nervosa: A family-based approach* (2nd ed.). New York, NY: Guilford.

Lock, J., Le Grange, D., Agras, W. S., Moye, A., Bryson, S. W., & Jo, B. (2010). Randomized clinical trial comparing family-based treatment with adolescent-focused individual therapy for adolescents with anorexia nervosa. *Archives of General Psychiatry, 67*(10), 1025–1032.

Lopez, S. R., Nelson Hipke, K., Polo, A. J., Jenkins, J. H., Karno, M., Vaughn, C., et al. (2004). Ethnicity, expressed emotion, attributions, and course of schizophrenia: Family warmth matters. *Journal of Abnormal Psychology, 113*(3), 428–439.

Mehler, P. S. (2011). Medical complications of bulimia nervosa and their treatments. *International Journal of Eating Disorders, 44*(2), 95–104.

Mehler, P. S., Crews, C., & Weiner, K. (2004). Bulimia: Medical complications. *Journal of Women's Health, 13*(6), 668–675.

Meites, T. M., Ingram, R. E., & Siegle, G. J. (2012). Unique and shared aspects of affective symptomatology: The role of parental bonding in depression and anxiety symptom profiles. *Cognitive Therapy and Research, 36*(3), 173–181.

Minuchin, S., Baker, L., Rosman, B. L., Liebman, R., Milman, L., & Todd, T. C. (1975). A conceptual model of psychosomatic illness in children. *Archives of General Psychiatry, 32*, 1031–1038.

Moos, R. H., & Moos, B. S. (1986). *The family environment scale*. Palo Alto, CA: Consulting Psychologists.

Muehlenkamp, J. J., Claes, L., Smits, D., Peat, C. M., & Vandereycken, W. (2011). Non-suicidal self-injury in eating disordered patients: A test of a conceptual model. *Psychiatry Research, 188*(1), 102–108.

Murray, C. D., Macdonald, S., & Fox, J. (2008). Body satisfaction, eating disorders and suicide ideation in an Internet sample of self-harmers reporting and not reporting childhood sexual abuse. *Psychology, Health and Medicine, 13*(1), 29–42.

Parker, G., Tupling, M., & Brown, C. (1979). A parental bonding instrument. *British Journal of Medical Psychology, 52*, 1–10.

Paul, T., Schroeter, K., Dahme, B., & Nutzinger, D. O. (2002). Self-injurious behavior in women with eating disorders. *The American Journal of Psychiatry, 159*(3), 408–411.

Peebles, R., Wilson, J. L., & Lock, J. D. (2011). Self-injury in adolescents with eating disorders: Correlates and provider bias. *Journal of Adolescent Health, 48*(3), 310–313.

Robin, A. L., & Le Grange, D. (2010). Treating adolescents with anorexia nervosa using behavioral family systems therapy. In J. R. Weisz & A. E. Kazdin (Eds.), *Evidence-based psychotherapies for children and adolescents* (2nd ed., pp. 345–358). New York, NY: Guilford.

Robin, A. L., Siegel, P. T., Koepke, T., Moye, A. W., & Tice, S. (1994). Family therapy versus individual therapy for adolescent females with anorexia nervosa. *Journal of Developmental and Behavioral Pediatrics, 15*(2), 111–116.

Robinson, P., & Serfaty, M. (2008). Getting better byte by byte: A pilot randomised controlled trial of email therapy for bulimia nervosa and binge eating disorder. *European Eating Disorders Review, 16*(2), 84–93.

Ross, S., Heath, N. L., & Toste, J. R. (2009). Non-suicidal self-injury and eating pathology in high school students. *American Journal of Orthopsychiatry, 79*(1), 83–92.

Russell, G. F., Szmukler, G. I., Dare, C., & Eisler, I. (1987). An evaluation of family therapy in anorexia nervosa and bulimia nervosa. *Archives of General Psychiatry, 44*(12), 1047–1056.

Stein, D., Lilenfeld, L. R. R., Wildman, P. C., & Marcus, M. D. (2004). Attempted suicide and self-injury in patients diagnosed with eating disorders. *Comprehensive Psychiatry, 45*(6), 447–451.

Svirko, E., & Hawton, K. (2007). Self-injurious behavior and eating disorders: The extent and nature of the association. *Suicide and Life Threatening Behavior, 37*(4), 409–421.

Treasure, J., Claudino, A. M., & Zucker, N. (2010). Eating disorders. *Lancet, 375*(9714), 583–593.

Viner, R. M., Coffey, C., Mathers, C., Bloem, P., Costello, A., Santelli, J., et al. (2011). 50-year mortality trends in children and young people: A study of 50 low-income, middle-income, and high-income countries. *The Lancet, 377*(9772), 1162–1174.

Wildman, P., Lilenfeld, L. R. R., & Marcus, M. D. (2004). Axis I comorbidity onset and parasuicide in women with eating disorders. *International Journal of Eating Disorders, 35* (2), 190–197.

Wright, F., Bewick, B. M., Barkham, M., House, A. O., & Hill, A. J. (2009). Co-occurrence of self-reported disordered eating and self-harm in UK university students. *British Journal of Clinical Psychology, 48*(4), 397–410.

10 Mentalisation-Based Therapy of Non-suicidal Self-Injury and Eating Disorders: MBT-ED

Paul H. Robinson

Abstract

Mentalisation-based therapy (MBT) has been suggested as a rational approach to patients with eating disorders, and its success in reducing non-suicidal self-injury (NSSI) in patients with borderline personality disorder (BPD) suggests its use in those with eating disorders and NSSI. In fact, patients with eating disorders, and some with NSSI, often have problems with mentalising, and many have attachment issues which are addressed in MBT. MBT-ED (MBT for eating disorders) was developed and tested during a randomised controlled trial. Experiences during the study using a combination of weekly group and individual therapy suggested that the approaches used during MBT in BPD could be adapted to address eating disorder symptoms. Breaks in mentalisation due to increasingly unbearable emotional states can often be linked to the onset, worsening or recrudescence of eating disorder symptoms, while in BPD treatment, such breaks in mentalisation have long been familiar antecedents to NSSI. It was also found that symptoms could often be traced back to problems in relationships, and tracing these sequences, if present, was found to be helpful by patients. Because of its intuitively relevant theoretical basis, the straightforward training and the increasing evidence base, MBT may well prove a useful approach in the treatment of eating disorders and NSSI.

P.H. Robinson (✉)
Mental Health Sciences Unit, University College London, London, UK

Research Department, Barnet, Enfield & Haringey Mental Health Trust, St Ann's Hospital, London, UK
e-mail: p.robinson@ucl.ac.uk

L. Claes and J.J. Muehlenkamp (eds.), *Non-Suicidal Self-Injury in Eating Disorders*, DOI 10.1007/978-3-642-40107-7_10, © Springer-Verlag Berlin Heidelberg 2014

10.1 Introduction

Mentalisation-based therapy (MBT) is a model of therapy which has its roots in psychoanalytic thinking, especially object relations and attachment theories. It has been found to be helpful in patients with borderline personality disorder (BPD) and has been suggested as possibly appropriate for use with eating disorders, especially if BPD features or NSSI are present. Its defining feature is the concentration on enhancing mentalising, which is the capacity to explore and become aware of one's own mental processes (thoughts and feelings) and those of other people.

In the present chapter, MBT, and a description of a form of MBT specifically tailored for the patient with eating disorders and NSSI developed during the NOURISHED study[1] between 2010 and 2014, will be introduced. It is the first randomised controlled trial to test MBT in patients with both eating disorders and BPD/NSSI symptoms. Because all the participants have eating disorders, MBT was adapted so that ED symptoms were addressed, and the adapted therapy has been termed MBT-ED. Later in this chapter an outline of MBT-ED is presented reflecting how it has been used during the NOURISHED study in patients with ED and NSSI.

10.2 Why Use MBT in Eating Disorders?

MBT has been found to reduce NSSI and other symptoms in patients with BPD (Bateman & Fonagy, 2009). This suggests that in patients with eating disorders who also have NSSI (23–25 % of ED patients; Sansone & Levitt, 2002), MBT might be a useful treatment. Patients who have eating disorders combined with NSSI could be offered MBT on the basis that the approach does reduce the rate of NSSI amongst patients with BPD. Thus, in the NOURISHED study referred to above, it would not be surprising to find that MBT reduced the rate of NSSI. As described below, patients with eating disorders have difficulties in both attachment and mentalisation, and MBT aims to provide an experience of attachment within which the patient learns to identify and describe correctly, as far as possible, the thoughts and feelings they and others experience, giving at least some rationale for its use in eating disorders. It is also likely that the defining symptoms of eating disorders, body image disturbance, restriction, weight loss and bulimic symptoms have deeper roots in emotional difficulties, and it is a reasonable postulate that those roots may be usefully addressed by a therapy that targets problems in attachment and mentalisation.

[1] Nice OUtcomes for Referrals with Impulsivity, Self Harm and Eating Disorders: a Randomised Controlled Trial of MBT-ED versus Specialist Supportive Clinical Management. http://www.controlled-trials.com/ISRCTN51304415. Supported by RfPB grant PB PG 0408 15183 from the National Institute for Health Research.

MBT has in fact been used extensively in patients with eating disorders in Norway and other parts of Scandinavia (Skårderud, 2007a, 2007b, 2007c), and the latter author has shown that eating disorders can usefully be viewed through the mentalising prism. Extensive clinical experience and training has had positive results in those countries, although no randomised trial has yet been published.

10.2.1 Cognitive Changes in ED Indicating Compromised Mentalisation

Many symptoms observed in eating disorders can have a major impact on mentalising. Patients often say that their starving, bingeing and vomiting have the desirable effect of blocking out unpleasant thoughts and feelings that they would otherwise endure. This may constitute a level of motivation which comes after the symptoms have become established. The primary motivation for, say, restriction may be simply to lose weight. Once it is in place, the patient finds that in the restricted state, the mind becomes full of thoughts of food and weight, and this effectively blocks out thoughts about difficulties occurring, for example, in family relationships. In addition, some of the changes found in patients with eating disorders, especially anorexia nervosa, might also be expected to influence mentalising capacity. Poor set shifting (Tchanturia et al., 2004) reduces the ability to move between different viewpoints and may encourage the patient to stick with the idea that he or she is too fat rather than explore other possibilities. Similarly, enhanced detail focus (Oldershaw, Hambrook, Tchanturia, Treasure, & Schmidt, 2010) may fix the patient even more firmly on one small aspect of his or her world (often that covering body size), and poor central coherence (Oldershaw et al., 2010) means that viewing alternatives, the bigger picture, becomes increasingly difficult. These cognitive changes occur partly as a result of malnutrition but also occur in eating disorders irrespective of current weight. Patients with anorexia nervosa also have difficulty in judging people's emotional state, represented by the appearance of their eyes in photographs (Harrison, Sullivan, Tchanturia, & Treasure, 2009) or of their recorded voices (Oldershaw et al., 2010). Moreover, there is evidence that amongst patients with bulimia nervosa, there is a group who scores poorly on the Reflective Function Questionnaire, rating themselves as below average in their capacity to judge their own and others' mental states (Pedersen, Lunn, Katznelson, & Poulsen, 2012).

10.2.2 Attachment Styles in ED

Patients with NSSI have raised attachment anxiety (Stepp et al., 2008), while those with BPD have been found to have an attachment pattern that suggests that they are insecure, fearful and preoccupied (Barone, 2003). Moreover, adolescent patients with NSSI were found to have raised attachment avoidance which improved with MBT, along with a reduction in NSSI (Rossouw & Fonagy, 2012). Patients with eating disorders are also found to have insecure attachment (Ward, Ramsay, & Treasure, 2000), and those with bulimia nervosa are, in addition, more dependent (Pollack & Keaschuk, 2008). In describing their own primary attachments, patients with a variety of eating disorders were found to perceive their parents and being more overprotecting but to show less care than controls. Troisi, Massaroni, and Cuzzolaro (2005) found that body dissatisfaction was predicted by early separation anxiety and high levels of anxiety about rejection and abandonment. Attachment is therefore found to be disturbed in NSSI, BPD and in eating disorders, and this supports the testing of MBT in patients with eating disorders, especially if they also have NSSI.

10.3 An Outline of the Use of MBT in Patients with ED and NSSI

10.3.1 Key Aspects of MBT

The essential elements of MBT can be summarised as follows:

- Therapy occurs within a relatively intensive clinical context.
- MBT provides both individual and group treatment.
- Therapy begins with a didactic presentation of the principles of MBT.
- As MBT proceeds the therapist provides a safe context which facilitates the patient's exploration of his own mind, that of the therapist and those of other individuals, especially in the group.
- The intention is to provide an attachment experience within which the patient learns to mentalise.
- Behaviours and thinking styles which militate against mentalising are identified and, as far as possible, brought under control, in order to optimise mentalising.
- Transference is utilised in the approach, particularly as it applies to the therapist's emotional responses to the patient within therapy.
- The therapist's mental life, as it relates directly to the relationship with the patient, may be shared with the patient, and this can form an important part of therapy.

10.3.2 Structure of Treatment

MBT may be provided in a number of ways. In the NOURISHED study five introductory group sessions (introductory MBT or iMBT) were followed by 1 year of one group session and one individual session weekly. The approach was based in a team including the individual and group therapists and a responsible senior clinician, generally a psychiatrist, and other involved professionals. A risk strategy was developed with each patient, a formulation of the relevant issues that had emerged in the first few sessions was written and a copy given to the patient and the treatment was reviewed midway through therapy by the patient together with the team. All treatment notes were recorded on a computerised medical records system available to all involved professionals. In the following discussion, the different elements of treatment are reviewed and discussed.

10.3.3 Introductory MBT Group Therapy

In MBT-ED in the NOURISHED study, the initial iMBT phase was five sessions of 1½ h. iMBT is didactic and when a patient raises emotionally difficult issues, the approach is supportive, but not exploratory, in order to keep the session more like a class than a therapy group. The sessions were structured as follows:

- *Session 1: What is mentalising and a mentalising stance?*
  These terms are defined and the group invited to consider scenarios in which mentalising could be successful or might fail. They are asked to consider their own experience of mentalising and, in the gap before the next group, to pay attention to how they and other people appear to be mentalising or not. The explicit aims of MBT are described. The group members are given relevant information sheets.
- *Session 2: What does it mean to have problems with mentalising?*
  What did they notice about their own and others' mentalising since the last group? The group is provided with more scenarios in which mentalising may be challenged and asked to discuss them. Ideas such as different levels of mentalising, poor mentalising, good mentalising and misunderstandings and the consequences of each are discussed. The negative impact of arousal (e.g. anxiety) on mentalising is described and the group asked to comment from their own experience.
- *Session 3: Attachment*
  Secure and insecure attachments are described. The group is asked to consider a scenario involving someone neglecting a partner. They are then asked to think about important relationships in their lives and what sort of attachment pattern they have. The idea of a mentalising culture in a family is described and group members asked to describe their own family culture.
- *Session 4: Why is mentalising important in relationships with other people?*
  Group members are asked to describe what they would like help with, to discuss times they had difficulty mentalising, the benefits and other consequences of mentalising including the difficulties of facing reality. Links are made with both eating and self-injury. The group discusses their experiences of how failure of mentalising led to eating disorder symptoms such as restriction or NSSI symptoms such as an episode of cutting.
- *Session 5: Overview*
  The group is asked to view photographs of people expressing a variety of emotions, and each group member is asked to comment on the emotional state of a person in one of the photographs. Other members and the facilitators give their own views. A photograph illustrating an ambiguous scenario is handed around. Participants are asked to create a brief story describing the situation and what might be going on in the minds of the individuals. Group members are

asked to discuss times that they had mentalised effectively, and times when it failed, and to make the link if possible with symptoms.

10.3.4 MBT-ED: Qualities of Effective Interventions

10.3.4.1 The Therapist's General Approach or Stance

Bateman and Fonagy (2012) define a mentalising stance as follows (this author's notes in italics):

- Maintaining humility from a sense of not knowing
  The "not-knowing stance" is a critical element of MBT. It is also a very hard one to adopt, especially from the professions of medicine and psychoanalysis which have tended to a stance of omniscience, although, at least in medicine, well informed patients as well as publicised failings of doctors have led to this stance being tempered with some welcome humility. In MBT, we do not tell the patient how they are feeling or the interpretation of a particular behaviour or dream. We adopt the approach of "not knowing" or "curiosity", faced with a mind that we describe in the psycho-education (iMBT) phase as "opaque" and we ask questions until we have a better idea of what the patient is describing. The concept is also in use in family therapy, in which the Milan group (Cecchin, 1987*) also employ the term "curiosity". The not-knowing stance is a partial defence against "Teleological Mode".*[2] *This describes a patient-therapist relationship in which what the therapist does is what is important: giving out blood forms and letters to take to college, rescheduling sessions, providing extra sessions. All this may be perfectly reasonable, but the therapist needs to watch out that the practical activities that he or she engages in do not overshadow the changes in mentalizing that the patient needs to achieve. Eating disorder symptoms themselves are very much in Teleological Mode, "I'm only OK if I've managed to lose weight." NSSI has similar characteristics: "I can only calm myself by cutting and seeing blood flow."*
- Taking time to identify differences in perspective when possible
  This can be very helpful in group therapy, taking into account the possibly differing views of other group members and the therapist(s), while in individual therapy the therapist's views, and the patents reports of other people can introduce interesting and liberating differences of opinion. Underweight patients may be forced to agree that amongst everyone they have met, including people with eating disorders, nobody except the patient him or herself thinks weight loss is a good idea. While this may not change the patient's views, becoming aware of the thoughts of other people (i.e., mentalizing) may well introduce something new.

[2] Teleological Mode: Causality in which the effect is explained by an end (Gr: *telos*) to be realised.

- Legitimising and accepting different perspectives
  It is true that an individual has the right to live at a low BMI or manage tension using NSSI, in either case as long as the behaviour does not directly threaten life. The therapist adopts a pragmatic attitude which contains an assumption that as the patient is in therapy, some aspects of this lifestyle are not completely satisfactory, but nevertheless leaves it to the patient to decide whether or not to opt for change.
- Actively questioning the patient about his or her experience, asking for detailed descriptions ("what" questions) rather than explanations ("why" questions)
  This follows naturally from the not-knowing stance. As noted above in relation to Milan Family therapy, the therapist displays curiosity about the mind of the patient.
- Eschewing the need to understand what makes no sense (i.e. saying explicitly that something is unclear)
  While the therapist may have an idea on why the patient is pursuing a low body weight, or engaging in self-harm to manage emotions, it is often honest to express confusion about the behaviour: "You told me that you want to be really thin, but also you said that this pursuit is destroying your life, and thirdly, that you will definitely choose thinness. How does that work?"

The principle themes in the approach have been outlined by Bateman and Fonagy (2012):

- Constantly attempt to establish an attachment relationship with the patient.
- Aim to use this to create an interpersonal context in which understanding of mental states becomes a focus.
- Attempt (mostly implicitly) to recreate a situation in which understanding of the patient's self as intentional and real is a priority and ensure that this endeavour and aim is clearly perceived by the patient.

In addition, there are certain interventions which should be avoided, because they may militate against the above principle themes. Examples are telling the patient what he or she is thinking and encouraging detailed description of historical material without attention to the here and now mental state and the contemporary relational and affective concomitants of those events.

10.3.4.2 Approach to Symptoms Using MBT

Bateman and Fonagy (2012) helpfully define an intervention in therapy that is "on model":

- The therapist identifies a break in mentalising.
- Patient and therapist rewind to the moment before the break in subjective mentalisation.
- The current emotional context for the break in the session is explored by identifying and by exploring the momentary affective state between patient and therapist.
- The therapist explicitly identifies and owns up to his or her own contribution to the break in mentalisation.
- The therapist seeks to help the patient understand the mental states implicit in the current state of the patient-therapist relationship (mentalising the transference).

Mentalising itself is a term that causes concern in professionals and patients. In brief it is the capacity to explore and become aware of one's own mental processes (thoughts and feelings) and those of other people. It is normally done constantly and unconsciously. As noted in the next section, it is highly sensitive to arousal. Imagine you are in a room at a party and a new person comes in. You may well be aware of interest, attraction, dislike and other mental processes in yourself, while you may also register that the new person is a bit lost, puzzled, looking for someone, shy, etc. You would be, largely unconsciously, mentalising. However, if instead of a person, a hungry lion escaped from a zoo were to pad into the room in search of a canapé, which might be you, your anxiety level could well shoot off the scale and your fight or, more likely, flight mode would kick in as would your autonomic system which would limit your attention to matters of survival. It is very unlikely that you would stop to wonder how the lion was feeling. So level of arousal is one determinant of mentalising.

10.3.4.3 Application of MBT Principles to ED Symptoms and NSSI

Breaks in mentalisation happen frequently in ED patients. Simply asking to weigh a patient as part of risk management can cause the patient to have a flood of thoughts about weight, shape, greed and unworthiness, and the patient may find it very difficult to concentrate on anything else. Following the above sequence, the therapist might:

- Point out that the conversation appears to have changed abruptly when the issue of weight was raised.
- The therapist might say, "let's stop and think about this for a while".
- The therapist rewinds to what was being discussed before the mention of weight.
- Examine what feelings have developed in the room since the break. The patient might describe anxiety and self-loathing, and the therapist may describe puzzlement as to what happened.
- The therapist says that asking the patient to be weighed did seem to have a marked effect.
- The mental state of the patient is explored as well as that of the therapist (concern about the patient's health, concern about how powerful mention of weighing was), and the question of how to move forward in a safe way is discussed.
- The break in mentalising is explored. Rising anxiety or arousal (due to the mention of weight) can cause mentalising to fail (Fig. 10.1). This break should be identified and explored. It is also possible to suppress mentalisation through too little concern, also depicted in Fig. 10.1.

Using a similar approach in the case of NSSI, a patient comes to a session and describes an episode of self-cutting the day before:

- The therapist checks that the medical aspects of the injury have been dealt with and assesses the current risk of self-injury.
- The therapist asks the patient to rewind back to before thoughts of self-harming occurred: what were the feelings? What was going on? Who was around? What was the patient thinking or worrying about?

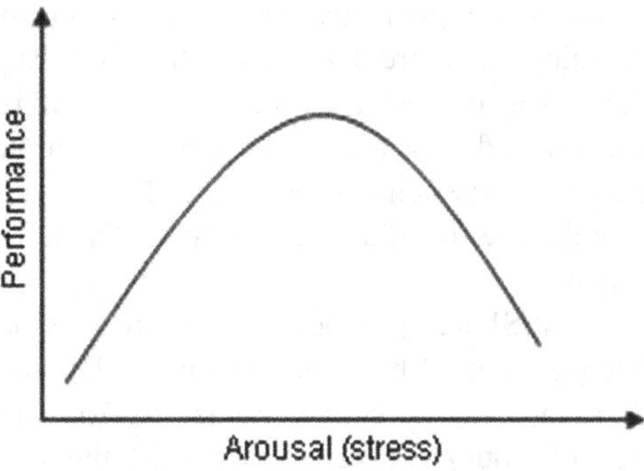

Fig. 10.1 Arousal *curve* showing the theoretical changes in performance (in this case mentalisation) with decreasing arousal (e.g. depersonalisation or denial) and increasing arousal (e.g. anxiety)

- The aim is to make some sense of the NSSI (to have a theory of why it happened) and to identify when mentalising failed (at what point did anxiety or stress get so high that mentalising became more difficult).
- The episode of NSSI might be linked to the failure of mentalising. For example, a rise in tension could be traced to a phone call with a parent. Unbearable feelings of anxiety, guilt and anger might have risen to a point at which mentalising failed and NSSI ensued. The aim of the therapist is to identify, clarify and name this process so that the sequence becomes familiar to the patient and potentially liable to interruption at a stage before mentalising fails.

10.4 Treatment of Specific Symptoms in Patients with ED and NSSI Using MBT

In general, symptoms are of two types: those that occur episodically (such as NSSI or bingeing) and those that are more or less continuous such as body image disturbance or restriction. As will be seen, the former type of symptom is approached in MBT by asking the patient to hold it just there ("stop and stand") to examine what occurred, to identify the break in mentalising, to "rewind" to before the break and to slowly track thoughts and especially feelings forward through the break in mentalising, reaching the onset of the symptom. The patient learns that it is usually possible to make sense of an apparently senseless behaviour and to associate the behaviour with a break in mentalising. For the more continuous symptoms, it is still possible sometimes to identify points at which they changed (such as increasing the dose of laxatives or resuming a severely restrictive diet after attempts to relax restriction) and hence to subject that change to the same inquiry.

10.4.1 NSSI

Research using MBT in patients with BPD suggests that the approach to NSSI used in MBT has a beneficial effect (Bateman & Fonagy, 2009). NSSI in eating disorders can be managed in the same way as that in other contexts, with a prior risk management plan, dealing with current risk, making appropriate referrals and deciding on current urgency. In MBT-ED, NSSI is managed in varied ways, depending on recent events. If the NSSI is historical, it should be discussed in therapy and appear in the formulation, along with an idea of how it fits into the patient's experiences and needs. If it is very rare, it may not have much or any prominence. If it has occurred recently, it is managed as described in the previous section.

If NSSI has just occurred, or if it is actively threatened, then the approach becomes one of harm minimisation. The therapist should establish what has been done and decide whether another opinion, say medical, is urgently required, or if the patient should be asked to wait while the therapist calls an ambulance. If the patient is describing plans to commit suicide, the therapist needs to assess the risk, and it may well be appropriate to call for help in assessing the risk and in judging whether the patient is safe to leave the clinic. A plan of what to do in such an emergency should be formulated well before it occurs, complete with relevant and current phone numbers.

10.4.2 Dietary Restriction

Food restriction amongst patients with AN is conceptualised by some as a type of indirect NSSI that if taken to extremes can lead to death. It is also an effective way to block mentalising. Starvation fills the mind with thoughts of food, and the accompanying fear of weight gain generates preoccupying anxieties that occupy any remaining space. In MBT a powerful approach is to track back from an incident (i.e. an act of NSSI or intentional restriction) to establish the antecedent thought processes and assess the role of mentalising in that series of events. This is sometimes referred to as "stop, stand and rewind". This may not be possible in the case of starvation which is often a more or less continuous process if not always successful. However, sometimes the approach can be used: a woman with a history of anorexia nervosa continues to restrict at times. On the latest occasion her husband told her that he was to work late on an urgent project for 2 weeks. The next day she started restricting and lost 2 kg over the following 2 weeks. In therapy the connection between her restriction and the anticipated absence of her husband was reasonably established, although she remained rather sceptical. It was also reported that she had been severely abused and neglected as a child, and it was noted that in therapy she alternated between not turning up and at times being extremely dependent. The therapist commented that working with her was sometimes confusing, and this linked in her mind with her ambivalence in all relationships, including that with her husband.

In other cases, attempts to restrict are fairly constant and form an essential part of the patient's capacity to cope with feelings. Another patient, underweight and anorexic, only felt, as she put it, "clean" when she was severely restricting, and when she ate anything calorific, she felt "disgusting, fat and dirty", and she said that it was obvious that other people could see that she was "enormous". It was apparent to the therapist that there were a number of cognitive distortions that might be addressed by attempting to enhance mentalising. She continually drew attention to the perceptual inaccuracies, assumptions and distortions, adding that she herself felt confused by the extreme statements that did not seem to fit the reality that she, the therapist, was able to observe. In addition, she was challenged by group members, who shared some distorted body perceptions but who nevertheless were shocked at the extreme nature of her statements. The continued challenges did have some impact. Towards the end of therapy, she said "This process has been so damaging. I had my way of dealing with things and now I'm not sure, they seem crazy to me. With the end of therapy coming up, I just need to put it all back in place so I can be a bit more in control". In fact she was not able to "put it all back in place' and at follow-up remained distressed, but more optimistic about being able to make changes.

10.4.3 Weight Loss

Loss of weight in someone of low or low normal weight may be a communication that signals distress. In order to be aware of this, however, we have to be weighing the patient. Hence, it is usually advisable in MBT-ED to make sure that you know the patient's weight each week. This may not be essential if the patient is in the upper part of the normal weight range or overweight, but it may be if BMI is below 20. This may not fit comfortably with every therapist's view of what their role is, but in an eating disorder, weight loss may be what will eventually kill the patient, and clearly it can only be addressed in therapy if it is known before it becomes so obvious that emergency measures become necessary. Agreement for you to weigh the patient needs to be accompanied by the means to do so, generally available in an eating disorders clinic, often not in other contexts. The solution is to obtain a set of digital scales and bring them to the session.

A patient with anorexia or bulimia nervosa who is losing weight may be in "pretend mode". The patient has a script and is not really in contact with his or her feelings or those of people around. "I'm losing weight so everything's fine and anyone who interferes with me is jealous". This arises because of the immensely powerfully ego-syntonic (meaning "this is really me!") nature of weight loss for patients with eating disorders.

The therapist needs to bear in mind the BMI ranges associated with different risks of collapse (>15 low risk, <15 moderate risk, <13 high risk) and to be aware that rapid weight loss (over 1 kg per week) at any weight can be dangerous.

Weight change can otherwise be regarded as a communication. The therapist investigates how the weight loss occurred: did something trigger a reduction in diet, or an increase in exercise, vomiting or laxative abuse? The feelings associated with the shift are explored, and the therapist tries to help the patient get in touch with ambivalence: yes, you enjoy the feeling weight loss gives you, but do you remember what happened last year, when you ended up in A and E? Is weight loss totally positive?

MBT-ED recommends an affect focus, so the feeling states that preceded and followed the change in diet or behaviour are explored. It may be possible to introduce a transference tracer "I must say I'm feeling really concerned about this change, and how it could affect your health and your capacity to mentalize. I wonder what it will do to our ability to work together?" Unfortunately, weight loss can cause food and weight preoccupations, detail focus and loss of central coherence, all potent anti-mentalising cognitive changes. Hence, it is important to start to address it as early as possible, before those changes have set in, a good reason to weigh the patient regularly.

If weight is being lost rapidly, or if you suspect the patient may be falsifying weight by using concealed weights or drinking water, then an urgent medical consultation, possibly with the therapist present, is arranged, and necessary tests, observations and treatment are instituted. Patients may lose most of their mentalising capacity during this process, and their mental states may become extremely opaque to the therapist and to themselves.

10.4.4 Body Image Distortion

The conviction that one is fat even though no one else shares that view is a powerful example of "psychic equivalence" in eating disorders, the process in which the patient believes that if he or she thinks something, then that becomes reality. "I feel fat; therefore, I am fat". The belief is held so strongly that it has been compared to psychotic delusions, and medication, known to loosen delusions in psychosis, has been used to try and shake the beliefs. Sadly, the medications used for schizophrenia have little effect on beliefs in anorexia nervosa (McKnight & Park, 2010). Consider this: an inpatient with anorexia nervosa asserts that she is the biggest person in the ward. The psychiatrists asked her to measure her waist with a tape measure and then measure the waist of the (informed and consenting) nurse in the room. The patient discovered that her waist is 15 cm less than that of the nurse. "OK", she says, "I'm thinner than her now, but as soon as I have a mouthful of that disgusting meal you're planning for me, I'll be bigger than her. I'll be enormous". This shows us that the belief in her own fatness is quite unlike the delusion of a psychotic patient, which would not shift in the face of evidence. This type of thought is termed, by psychiatric phenomenologists, an "overvalued idea". In MBT it is termed psychic equivalence.

Addressing psychic equivalence in MBT is an important and difficult task. The therapist needs to discuss the experience that the patient has, expressing interest in the belief that entertaining a thought is equivalent to carrying out the action, but maintaining respect and asking the patient to explain what is going on in her mind as best he or she can. In MBT the matter is discussed in detail, as would occur in CBT, to pay attention to the emotions which accompany the discussion and in a group, to invite other members (who may well have similar beliefs) to comment. The aim is to help the patient transform psychic equivalence into symbolic representation. The experience is not diminished by this, but it becomes confined to the intrapsychic realm. In psychic equivalence, inner reality and the external world (including the body) are fused. Skårderud (2007a, 2007b, 2007c) and Bateman and Fonagy (2012) have helpfully introduced the idea of "embodied mentalisation":

> Mentalizing the body means stimulating the patient to investigate her or his concrete experience with body and food and to connect them with emotional, cognitive and relational experiences in order to translate them into a language that reflects them both as physical reality and as metaphor for mind (Bateman & Fonagy, 2012, p. 371).

Changing a deeply held belief system such as that underlying body image distortion is, to say the least, challenging. However, we may be able to influence two important characteristics: salience and attribution. By challenging the beliefs, it may be possible to encourage the patient to consider alternative thinking. In this way, the belief in her fatness becomes less salient, simply because the patient allows in another, alternative, belief. A patient after a course of MBT-ED, describing how she had dealt with the feeling of fatness said: "I still have these thoughts and feelings, but now, I just say to myself 'Ignore that, it's just wrong". She has changed the attribution of the thought from "That's my firmly held and correct belief" to "That's a belief that I hold, but others profoundly disagree". This result could have emerged from CBT and is a good example of the way similar techniques can be used helpfully within different therapy models.

10.4.5 Binge Eating

Bingeing is a highly complex behaviour that can have many determinants, some of which will be summarised here. In treating the patient with bulimic symptoms, it is important that the therapist understands what underlies the binges, and, given that the mind is opaque, the only way to find out is to ask. Only by establishing what is going on can the therapist attempt to place the symptom in context. Bingeing can sometimes be viewed as a behaviour which follows an interpersonal event. Generally the intervening behaviour is restriction. The patient is in the clinic because he or she wishes to reduce bingeing, so the restriction comes at a cost he or she would prefer not to pay. The discussion then becomes about the bad feelings that his or her symptoms are causing and how to deal with them in a different way. Note how, in MBT-ED, the key is to locate a behavioural problem in its affective context. The affect (feeling) focus is an extremely important principle to be aware of in therapy sessions. If the affect is not there, the patient, and sometimes the therapist, might be in pretend mode.

Yet another way in which bingeing can be understood is in its capacity to block both mentalising and social interaction. A patient who, perhaps as a result of previous traumas, is subject to distressing thoughts and images may need to have a way of suppressing them for a while. Overeating is quite an effective way to block out thoughts perhaps due to its release of endorphins (Mercer & Holder, 1997). The task of the therapist is to help the patient address the feelings that are being blocked, i.e. that are leading to behaviour which is causing a break in mentalising. Secondly, patients may find meeting people very difficult, in part because of their feelings of disgust at their own bodies and general appearance. They may, therefore, have an evening of bingeing which effectively precludes any social engagement. The therapist should in this case identify the feelings that meeting other people elicits and focus on those while helping the patient enhance mentalising about these issues. Lastly, it should not be forgotten that bingeing is a normal response to undernutrition and is experienced, for example, by people fasting for religious reasons (Albawaba, 2013).

10.4.6 Compensatory Behaviours

Like bingeing, compensatory behaviours also have diverse antecedents. They often occur as a planned sequel to bingeing, in order to limit the weight-gaining effects of the latter. However, they can also be habitual weight-maintenance behaviours in the absence of overeating, especially in someone who has lost weight and wishes to maintain the new low weight, while the set-point mechanisms in the brain are pushing weight up to its prior level. Moreover, vomiting, or another compensatory behaviour, can follow a socially determined episode of eating (such as a meal out or a celebration dinner) that the patient finds it hard to refuse and subsequently compensates for secretly.

The principles in MBT-ED are to identify a discontinuity in the behaviour if it is there and to help the patient become aware of the emotional factors that may have led to that discontinuity. Thus, a patient who has successfully reduced laxatives from say ten tablets per day to four is shocked when a work colleague comments how well she is looking. This could well be related to the fact that she is less dehydrated and so looking healthier. However, the patient's immediate assumption is that it means she is looking fat and the laxatives go up to their previous level again. In MBT-ED the therapist "stops and stands" and "rewinds" to before the increase in the laxatives. The patient is encouraged to relate the story, the therapist maintaining an affect focus by asking about how she was feeling at each stage, and mentalisation is optimised so that, for example, the assumption about the work colleague's thoughts is challenged and may be modified in the patient's mind. This may be an opportunity to introduce questions relating to how the therapist thinks about the patient's appearance.

Compensatory behaviours are not always episodic and may be constant for an extended period, although the patient coming off laxatives had been taking them for years, so that the therapy had induced a change which proved helpful to investigate. It may be possible, however, to challenge some of the ideas about vomiting or laxatives that the patient may have. One patient said, about laxatives: "They are harmless, why are you bothered?" Almost always, the patient has information which refutes this statement, so it is not usually needed to cite examples of low potassium, cardiac arrest, dehydration, kidney failure and colon paralysis that can occur with laxative abuse, but a therapist should be able to fill in knowledge gaps and it may be useful to access a hand-out which gives the information. Once the facts are established, the questions change. Why is the patient taking such risks? What bad feelings might come if she changed her behaviour? In MBT-ED, rather than an expert position (although that might need to be taken to inform the patient of the risks), the therapist's stance is quizzical: "I'm not sure I follow why you would take laxatives when they put you at such risk, and don't work anyway. Could you explain?"

The patient might actually be in a vicious cycle. If she does stop laxatives or vomiting (known collectively as purging), her dehydration would reverse, and she may gain weight due to water and salt retention, which makes her resume the behaviour in a panic about continued weight gain. The information the therapist might wish to impart (or provide in a hand-out) is that such changes in the water content of the body frequently occur when purging stops and may take some time to reach a balance. Issues to address in therapy are then the emotional effects of weight gain, which may be very substantial, but which the patient may be willing to bear (just as an addict may be willing to bear the effects of drug or alcohol withdrawal) in order to improve their state of health.

Management of risk is essential in relation to compensatory behaviours, especially vomiting and laxative abuse which can lead to dehydration and low potassium levels, amongst other problems. Unlike weight loss, there is little evidence that changing electrolytes affects mentalising capacity. However, patients often deny the severity of the problem, and if potassium level comes back as abnormal (under 3.5 mmol/l), a medical consultation should be arranged and a decision made on the need for an electrocardiogram (ECG), the frequency of monitoring and the need for oral potassium supplements. Moving between the not-knowing stance recommended in MBT and the expert position in which misunderstandings about physical aspects of eating disorders are explained and risk management performed can demand a fair amount of agility on the part of the therapist.

Conclusions

In MBT-ED the focus is on emotions which arise in the patient, usually in relation to interpersonal contacts. These feelings become unbearable and result in eating disorder symptoms and NSSI which may be by cutting, burning, starving, bingeing, vomiting or any of the other self-damaging behaviours to which patients are subject.

We know that in one form of NSSI, that which occurs in association with BPD, mentalisation-based therapy is helpful and can significantly reduce the episodes of NSSI to which patients with BPD are subject.

Patients with eating disorders engage in different forms of harmful behaviour, including direct acts of self-injury (e.g. cutting, burning) and nutritional harm, and the fact that they have been shown to have difficulties in mentalisation suggests that therapy in which the improvement of mentalising is the primary focus could well have a role in treatment. While we naturally await the controlled studies that evaluate different therapies in different groups of patients, we can assert that mentalisation-based therapy has characteristics that make it particularly suitable for treatment of patients with either eating disorders, NSSI or both:

1. Theoretical considerations
    - MBT has a firm basis in object relations and attachment theory, in both of which areas the patients have been shown to have difficulties.
    - It has a proven record of effectiveness in treatment of BPD patients, many of whom have ED and the majority NSSI.
    - Using MBT we can hope to test hypotheses linking changes in attachment patterns, mentalisation and emotional theory of mind with clinical changes during therapy.
2. Practical considerations
    - MBT can be undertaken by any suitably talented mental health professional.
    - Training is much less onerous that for other treatments for these conditions. A suitable professional without former therapy training can be MBT trained within 6 months (4-day workshops followed by a probationary 6-month supervised therapy.) Hence, MBT can be "rolled out" in a service within a fairly short time.
    - Perhaps because MBT therapists are encouraged to disclose, appropriately, their own emotions arising during treatment, power relationships can be more equal than they often are in therapy, which is welcomed by therapists and patients.

Mentalisation-based therapy is a fairly recently conceived therapy which has its origins in Freudian psychoanalysis, object relations and, more recently, attachment theory. This genealogy is an attractive one to mental health workers who look to developmental processes to yield aetiological clues in the immensely damaging mental disorders suffered by patients and ideas for interventions that might change their course. With its combination of an intuitively relevant theory, straightforward training and improving evidence base, MBT may well be a significant option in the therapeutic choices available to clinicians in the future.

References

Albawaba. (2013). *Don't overeat in Ramadan, warn doctors*. Retrieved from http://www.albawaba.com/dont-overeat-ramadan-warn-doctors-386723

Barone, L. (2003). Developmental protective and risk factors in BPD: A study using the Adult Attachment Interview. *Attachment and Human Development, 5*(1), 64–77.

Bateman, A. W., & Fonagy, P. (2009). Randomized controlled trial of outpatient mentalization-based treatment versus structured clinical management for borderline personality disorder. *American Journal of Psychiatry, 166*(12), 1355–1364.

Bateman, A. W., & Fonagy, P. (2012). *Handbook of mentalizing in mental health practice*. Arlington, VA: American Psychiatric Association.

Cecchin, G. (1987). Hypothesizing, circularity, and neutrality revisited: An invitation to curiosity. *Family Process, 26*(4), 405–413.

Harrison, A., Sullivan, S., Tchanturia, K., & Treasure, J. (2009). Emotion recognition and regulation in anorexia nervosa. *Clinical Psychology and Psychotherapy, 16*(4), 348–356.

McKnight, R. F., & Park, R. J. (2010). Atypical antipsychotics and anorexia nervosa: A review. *European Eating Disorders Review, 18*, 10–21.

Mercer, M. E., & Holder, M. D. (1997). Food cravings, endogenous opioid peptides, and food intake: A review. *Appetite, 29*(3), 325–352.

Oldershaw, A., Hambrook, D., Tchanturia, K., Treasure, J., & Schmidt, U. (2010). Emotional theory of mind and emotional awareness in recovered anorexia nervosa patients. *Psychosomatic Medicine, 72*(1), 73–79.

Pedersen, S. H., Lunn, S., Katznelson, H., & Poulsen, S. (2012). Reflective functioning in 70 patients suffering from bulimia nervosa. *European Eating Disorders Review, 20*(4), 303–310.

Pollack, D. L., & Keaschuk, R. A. (2008). The object relations of bulimic women in context: An integration of two studies. *Eating Disorders, 16*(1), 14–29.

Rossouw, T. I., & Fonagy, P. (2012). Mentalization-based treatment for self-harm in adolescents: A randomized controlled trial. *Journal of the American Academy of Child and Adolescent Psychiatry, 51*(12), 1304–1313.

Sansone, R. A., & Levitt, J. L. (2002). Self-harm behaviors among those with eating disorders: An overview. *Eating Disorders, 10*(3), 205–213.

Skårderud, F. (2007a). Eating one's words, part I: 'Concretised metaphors' and reflective function in anorexia nervosa—An interview study. *European Eating Disorders Review, 15*(3), 163–174.

Skårderud, F. (2007b). Eating one's words, part II: The embodied mind and reflective function in anorexia nervosa—Theory. *European Eating Disorders Review, 15*(4), 243–252.

Skårderud, F. (2007c). Eating one's words: Part III. Mentalisation-based psychotherapy for anorexia nervosa: An outline for a treatment and training manual. *European Eating Disorders Review, 15*(5), 323–339.

Stepp, S. D., Morse, J. Q., Yaggi, K. E., Reynolds, S. K., Reed, L. I., & Pilkonis, P. A. (2008). The role of attachment styles and interpersonal problems in suicide-related behaviors. *Suicide and Life-Threatening Behaviors, 38*(5), 592–607.

Tchanturia, K., Morris, R. G., Anderluh, M. B., Collier, D. A., Nikolaou, V., & Treasure, J. (2004). Set shifting in anorexia nervosa: An examination before and after weight gain, in full recovery and relationship to childhood and adult OCPD traits. *Journal of Psychiatry Research, 38*(5), 545–552.

Troisi, A., Massaroni, P., & Cuzzolaro, M. (2005). Early separation anxiety and adult attachment style in women with eating disorders. *The British Journal of Clinical Psychology, 44*, 89–97.

Ward, A., Ramsay, R., & Treasure, J. (2000). Attachment research in eating disorders. *British Journal of Medical Psychology, 73*(1), 35–51.

The Use of Interpersonal Psychotherapy for Non-suicidal Self-Injury and Eating Disorders

11

Jon Arcelus, Walter Pierre Bouman, and Jonathan Baggott

Abstract

Interpersonal psychotherapy (IPT) is an effective treatment for depressive disorder. Over the last two decades, IPT has been modified to treat different mental health problems, including eating disorders. When working with patients presenting with eating disorder psychopathology, the eating disorder behaviour is used as a marker of "abnormality" that is linked to the person's interpersonal difficulty. Non-suicidal self-injury behaviour (NSSI) within the eating disorder individual can be treated in the same way as the eating disorder behaviour. Within IPT, the therapist firstly aims to identify the interpersonal focus associated with the unhealthy behaviour, in order to work through this focus to reduce the behaviour. This chapter describes the modified version of IPT for eating disorders. It also makes suggestions how IPT may be used in a population of patients with eating disorders and NSSI, by including NSSI in addition to eating disorder behaviour as a marker of distress.

11.1 Interpersonal Problems and Mental Health

The term "interpersonal" describes the pattern of interaction between the individual and others. These interactions are internalised and form part of the self-image (Sullivan, 1953). A positive interpersonal functioning is an extremely reliable indicator of happiness and well-being. Being involved in secure and fulfilling relationships is perceived by most individuals as critical to well-being and happiness (Berscheid & Peplau, 1983). Humans appear to be happiest when they have (1)

J. Arcelus (✉) • J. Baggott
Leicester Eating Disorders Service, Bennion Centre, Leicester Glenfield Hospital, Leicester LE3 9DZ, UK
e-mail: j.arcelus@lboro.ac.uk

W.P. Bouman
Nottingham Gender Clinic, Mandala Centre, Gregory Boulevard, Nottingham NG7 6LB, UK

L. Claes and J.J. Muehlenkamp (eds.), *Non-Suicidal Self-Injury in Eating Disorders*, DOI 10.1007/978-3-642-40107-7_11,

pleasure in life such as good food; (2) when they are involved in an enjoyable, yet challenging activity; (3) when they have a sense of accomplishment; and, finally, (4) when they have strong relationships and a sense of belonging to something bigger (Seligman, 2002).

Maladaptive interpersonal functioning is therefore central to unhealthy mental health and has been found to be co-morbid to several psychiatric disorders, including depression (e.g. Petty, Sachs-Ericsson, & Joiner, 2004), anxiety (e.g. Montgomery, Haemmerlie, & Edwards, 1991), schizophrenia (e.g. Sullivan & Allen, 1999) and eating disorders (e.g. Arcelus, Haslam, Farrow, & Meyer, 2013). For some psychiatric disorders, interpersonal difficulties may not only cause vulnerability to developing mental health problems, but they may also play a role in maintaining these. This is clearly highlighted in disorders, such as the eating disorders and non-suicidal self-injury behaviour (NSSI), where the unhealthy behaviour (bingeing, purging, self-harming) can become entangled with interpersonal communication difficulties.

Theories of the function of NSSI have emphasised the role of intrapersonal and interpersonal problems. Klonsky (2007) reviews the function of NSSI and identified seven functions: affect regulations, anti-dissociations, antisuicide, interpersonal boundaries, interpersonal influence, self-punishment and sensation seeking. Two of these functions are connected to the person's interpersonal world. The Interpersonal Influence Model (Bearden, Netemeyer, & Teel, 1989) stipulates that the self-injury behaviour is used to influence or communicate with people, as a cry for help, a means of avoiding abandonment and a means to influence other people's behaviour (Nock, 2009). This function is clearly demonstrated by the reduction of NSSI behaviour when it is followed by increased support and attention, which may alleviate loneliness and fear of abandonment. The interpersonal boundary function described by Klonsky (2007) describes the role of self-injury as a way to define the boundary between self and others. Suyemoto's review reaches a similar conclusion (Suyemoto, 1998). This claim is underpinned by research that has been able to identify a lack of normal sense of self due to insecure maternal attachment in people who engage in self-injury behaviour (Adrian, Zeman, Erdley, Lisa, & Sim, 2011; Di Pierro, Sarno, Perego, Galluci, & Madeddu, 2012; Friedman, Glasser, Laufer, Laufer, & Wohl, 1972). Social isolation including loneliness, social withdrawal and lack of satisfaction with social support have been found to be reliable predictors of NSSI as well as of suicide attempts (Dervic, Brent, & Oquedo, 2008; Joiner & Van Orden, 2008; Wichstrom, 2009). All of the aforementioned literature indicates that interventions aiming at improving interpersonal functioning may be effective for some people with NSSI. There is a strong relationship between eating disorders and NSSI (as described in this book). Moreover, interpersonal psychotherapy (IPT) has proven its efficacy in the treatment of people with eating disorders (Arcelus et al., 2009; Fairburn, 1997). Hence, we propose the use of IPT in the treatment of people with eating disorders and NSSI in this chapter.

11.2 The Development of Interpersonal Psychotherapy for Depression

IPT was developed in the 1970s by Gerald Klerman, Myrna Weissman and Eugene Paykel (Klerman, DiMascio, Weissman, Prusoff, & Paykel, 1974). Initially IPT was designed to reflect clinical practice as closely as possible in order to be used in a research study for the treatment of depression. The psychotherapy developed at that time was modelled after what was considered high-quality supportive psychotherapy. IPT was defined as "high contact" to describe the fact that it took place weekly. Whilst studying the efficacy of antidepressants, alone or paired with this psychotherapy, IPT was surprisingly found to be effective, leading to the further development of this therapy (Klerman, Weissman, Rounsaville, & Chevron, 1984).

The development of IPT has been influenced by the medical model of disability (WHO, 1980), the attachment theory (Bowlby, 1969), the communication theory (Craig, 1988) and the interpersonal theory (Sullivan, 1953). The IPT developed in 1984 has now been updated (Weissman, Markowitz, & Klerman, 2000, 2007), and several modifications have been developed for use in different populations and for the treatment of a variety of mental health problems. This includes IPT for depressed adolescents (Mufson, Dorta, Moreau, & Weissman, 2004), older adults (Hinrichsen & Clougherty, 2006), perinatal women (Weissman et al., 2000), bipolar disorder (Frank, 2005), social phobia (Hoffart et al., 2007), dysthymic disorder (Markowitz, 1998), bulimia nervosa (Fairburn, 1993) and bulimic disorders (Whight et al., 2011).

11.3 The Use of Interpersonal Psychotherapy for the Treatment of People with Eating Disorders

Research studies have clearly identified that people with eating disorders (ED) present with interpersonal problems (Ambwani & Hopwood, 2009; Arcelus et al., 2013; Hopwood, Clarke, & Perez, 2007) independent of whether they suffer from anorexia nervosa (O'Mahony & Hollwey, 1995) or bulimic-like disorders (Hopwood et al., 2007). One could hypothesise that this association may be explained by the high frequency of affective disorder, particularly major depression, found among patients with bulimia nervosa (BN) (Walsh, Roose, Glassman, Gladise, & Sadik, 1985). There is good evidence that after controlling for depressive disorders, this association is still maintained (Geller, Cockell, & Hewitt, 2000). Consequently, there is a clear rationale to modify IPT for use to treat patients with eating disorders.

IPT was firstly modified to be used in patients with BN by Fairburn (1993). He developed IPT-BN by adapting the IPT for depression in a clinical research study investigating the effectiveness of a cognitive-behavioural treatment (Fairburn et al., 1991). For this first adaptation and in order to measure the effectiveness of the cognitive-behavioural approach in the treatment of bulimia nervosa, the author removed non-specific factors associated with IPT, such as role play and problem solving.

IPT was not adapted specifically for the treatment of BN in this particular treatment trial, and beyond limited initial psycho-education, eating problems were not addressed during the treatment. The study found that whilst CBT was considered most effective, IPT also resulted in the improvement of eating disorder symptoms. This discovery led to the further development of IPT-BN as a viable treatment option, and it was subsequently manualised in 1993 (Fairburn, 1993). Since its conception, IPT-BN has been compared to CBT for BN with equally positive results in both individual (Agras, Walsh, Fairburn, Wilson, & Kraemer, 2000; Fairburn, 1997; Fairburn, Wilson, & Kraemer, 2000) and group settings (Roth & Ross, 1988; Wilfley et al., 1993; Wilfley, Stein, & Welch, 2003). For example, Agras et al. (2000) found that whilst CBT was superior to IPT at the end of treatment, there was no significant difference between the two treatments at 1-year follow-up. IPT was modified further by Whight et al. (2011) (IPT BNm) and evaluated through a case series study (Arcelus et al., 2009). Whight et al. (2011) brought back the original components of IPT (psycho-education, directive techniques, problem solving, modelling, role play and symptom review), which appear to produce early change in eating disorder psychopathology (Arcelus et al., 2009). These findings have also suggested that there may be a scope to develop a shorter form of therapy for mild eating disorders (Arcelus, Whight, Brewin, & McGrain, 2012). At present, there is no modification of IPT for treatment of patients with anorexia nervosa.

11.4 Description of IPT to Treat Patients with Bulimia-Like Disorders

IPT uses a time frame of 12–20 weekly sessions, although the usual number of sessions tends to be 16. IPT is generally divided into three parts: assessment sessions (first four sessions), middle sessions (following ten sessions) and termination sessions (last two sessions).

11.4.1 The Assessment Sessions: Sessions 0–4

The initial assessment sessions for IPT for bulimia nervosa are described in the original IPT manual for depression (Klerman et al., 1984) and are specifically adapted to collect information regarding the individual's eating disorder. In addition, there is a psycho-educational element specifically related to eating disorders throughout the sessions. The therapist aims, using food diaries, to stop the complex vicious circle of bingeing and restricting behaviour in order to help regulating the diet. During the second and third session, the therapist aims to get a clear picture of the current problems along with a history of previous difficulties and interpersonal events. This enables the therapist and patient to identify areas of current difficulty.

The areas for assessment include mood, interpersonal network, timeline of interpersonal events (for instance, new relationships, separations, deaths, changes in life events.) and eating disorder symptomatology. At the end of session 4, the therapist and the patient agree the treatment goals of therapy and select a focus for the remaining ten sessions of therapy. The main task of the first sessions is to help the patient gain some understanding of the relationship between their presenting eating disorders difficulties and their interpersonal world, which may explain the maintaining factors of their symptoms. At the end of the assessment sessions, the therapist will have a good understanding of the capacity of the patient to work with this model. The patient is informed that the style of the therapy will change after the assessment sessions from an inquisitive one, where the therapist takes the responsibility for the content of the therapy and actively asks questions to the patient, to a more passive style, where the patient is expected to take charge for their change as well as for identifying solutions to their problems.

As in the original manual of IPT for depression (Klerman et al., 1984), there are four clear focus areas in IPT for bulimia-like disorders:

- *Interpersonal role disputes*: The hypothesis of this focal area is that eating disorder symptoms occur when the patient has nonreciprocal expectations from a significant other.
- *Interpersonal role transitions*: Difficulties occur when the patient has difficulty adjusting or adapting to changes in their life.
- *Interpersonal deficits*: Difficulties occur when there are problems making or sustaining relationships with people.
- *Complicated Bereavement*: Difficulties can occur when a patient is not able to resolve the death of a significant figure.

The therapist uses the collected information to formulate the individuals' problems within the interpersonal framework. The task of the therapist is to find the most appropriate focus together with the patient. IPT does not seek to understand the dynamics underlying the eating disorder/depression but rather aims to reduce the interpersonal maintaining factors in order to allow the patient to make changes to their life. The formulation for IPT is therefore simple, pragmatic and collaborative (Arcelus, Whight, & Haslam, 2011).

11.4.2 The Middle Sessions: Sessions 5–14

During these sessions, the therapist helps the patient to link the symptomatology to the focal area. The patient is asked to bring in their own material from the week to work within therapy. The therapist helps the patient to link the changes in symptoms to the focus area and then works with patient at active problem solving, contingency planning and/or practising new skills. Each week the therapist reviews the eating disorder symptoms in order to maintain the focus. The therapist identifies changes and encourages and supports the patient. Halfway through IPT (session 8) therapy is reviewed. This review is planned from the beginning. It highlights a time to see how things have progressed thus far, ensuring that the right focal area is being targeted and worked on and allowing room for change if needed by the patient or the therapist.

11.4.3 Termination Sessions: 15–16

The end of therapy should not come as a surprise to the patient; the therapist will have been counting down sessions and will have planned the dates of the final session with the patient. Nevertheless, it can still come as a shock to some patients. The last two sessions are explicitly about ending therapy, about recognising and maintaining changes made, acknowledging that which has not changed and exploring feelings about ending. This can feel very positive for a patient who has recovered or more anxiety provoking for one who has not. One of the most powerful motivators for change can be the duration of treatment and working to a defined timescale. It is expected that patients will continue to use the skills learnt in therapy, with the support and help, where necessary, of their interpersonal network. This is the time when patients need to take responsibility for looking after themselves, physically and emotionally. If felt to be appropriate, the number of sessions can be increased, but this should never come as a surprise to the patient. It should be discussed and planned beforehand, preferably at the beginning or at the review (session 8) of therapy. To extend, sessions may be an avoidance of ending, either by the patient or by the therapist (Arcelus et al., 2011).

11.5 Interpersonal Difficulties in Patients with NSSI

There is good evidence to suggest that, as some eating disorder behaviours (bingeing or purging), NSSI also has an emotion-regulation function. For example, Nock and Prinstein (2005) found that many adolescents reported engaging in NSSI for automatic positive (to feel something) and negative (to stop bad feelings) reinforcement. Studies investigating the interpersonal function of NSSI have also identified the role of NSSI in improving interpersonal relationships; for example, following an act of NSSI, some people may increase their support network, reducing the fear of abandonment and isolation, which generally tends to maintain NSSI behaviour. This suggests that, as with eating disorder behaviour, interventions aiming at improving interpersonal relationships could potentially reduce NSSI.

However, IPT may not be successful for every individual with NSSI with or without eating disorder. Research examining the function of NSSI found that depressive symptoms, borderline personality features, suicidal ideation and engaging in NSSI when alone are more strongly associated with intrapersonal rather than interpersonal functions (Klonsky & Glenn, 2009). Interpersonal problems in NSSI, on the other hand, have been associated with several social concerns, including loneliness, socially prescribed perfectionism and peer victimisation (Hilt, Cha, & Nolen-Hoeksema, 2008). Turner, Chapman, and Layden (2012) explore the interpersonal role of NSSI further by examining 162 females with a history of this self-harm behaviour. The authors found that some specific affective traits, emotion-regulation deficits and interpersonal styles render a person more likely to engage in NSSI in order to achieve specific goals. They also identify the important role that NSSI has in communicating with others. These findings suggest that for these patients, increasing effective emotional expression and enhancing effective communication skills could potentially help to reduce NSSI.

NSSI and eating disorder behaviours such as bingeing and purging appear to have similar functions. Rieger et al. (2010) have suggested that eating disorders are triggered by negative feedback regarding an individual's social worth due to its negative effect on self-esteem and associated mood. Eating disorder behaviours often begin as a result of this negative social evaluation, and over time, such behaviours may become a more reliable source of self-esteem and mood regulation than social interactions. As NSSI in many patients has a similar role, it is therefore not surprising to find high levels of NSSI in patients with eating disorders.

Despite the clear association between NSSI and interpersonal difficulties and the frequent co-morbidity found between NSSI and eating disorders, there is a lack of research in the field of IPT and NSSI. Few studies have described the use of a very brief (four sessions) IPT intervention for people following a deliberate self-harm episode and showed that such an intervention can be a valuable treatment for this population (Guthrie et al., 2001). Another study using 16 weeks of IPT also showed a similar effect, although the group of patients studied presented with severe depression and the intervention was aimed at targeting the depression rather than being specifically focused on NSSI (Rucci et al., 2011).

The following section describes how IPT could be used in patients with NSSI with co-morbid eating disorders. It is important to bear in mind that this is not a description of a new modification of IPT but a suggestion regarding the modifications that the current IPT for eating disorders will require in order to be used in this population.

11.6 IPT for NSSI and Eating Disorders: Some Suggestions

The overall aim of IPT is to help the patient to develop positive, healthy relationships which replace the eating disorder and the NSSI behaviour in the attainment of positive esteem and affect. Patients' psychopathology is used as a marker of distress to track the interpersonal difficulties and the identification of the focus of therapy.

11.6.1 Pretreatment

Two main issues need to be considered before therapy commences. Firstly, the therapist' attitude towards the patient and their NSSI behaviours needs to be considered. The patient is presenting with problems of which NSSI is one component. Although the reasons for NSSI are often more complex than they appear at first and are often complicatedly rewarded, overall NSSI represents a problem to the patient. Therefore, the therapist needs to take a non-judgmental attitude towards the patient. Low self-esteem is not an unusual component of most patients presenting with ED and NSSI, and a positive and non-judgmental attitude towards the patient improves engagement and allows and facilitates a collaborative working relationship with the patient. First impressions are essential: it is not unusual to lose this type of patients before therapy even begins.

Secondly, the therapist needs to take into consideration the risk that the patient may present with. This risk will need to be assessed during each session. Patients with NSSI are at a significantly increased risk of serious self-injury and suicide. The therapist has to feel comfortable and competent working with people who self-harm; it follows that the therapist has to be confident and competent in risk assessment and management. Therapists who do not feel competent in this risk management should not work with this particular patient group. Lack of confidence leads to inappropriate worry (and often inappropriate action), whilst over confidence may lead to unnecessary and inappropriate risk-taking behaviour.

11.6.2 The Assessment Sessions

The bulk of the initial sessions remain as described in Sect. 11.4 above. NSSI is incorporated into the *psycho-education* component, and this should be considered as a two-way process, i.e. the patient educates the therapist as to their self-harm and then the therapist teaches the patient about NSSI. So when being educated, the therapist allows the patient to "tell it how it is"—When do they do it? Why do they do it? How does it affect them? What do they get out of it? Is this really being in control? How does it affect the people around them? This information should be obtained in as much detail as possible. Commonly, the patient will start off with a lot of information but quickly reveal huge gaps. This then allows the therapist to reflect on these and tell the patient what they know about NSSI, its feedback loops, what may reinforce NSSI and hence why it is so difficult to stop. Doing it this way tends to foster and develop a collaborative and engaging approach. The therapist does not judge the patient; equally, the therapist does not tell the patient what they should do. Usually a person has a pattern to their NSSI, although this is not usually recognised by the patient in the early stages of treatment, and identifying this pattern becomes one of the aims of the therapy.

In the early sessions, risk should also be discussed with the patient in a collaborative way. The therapist needs to advise the patient as to what their limits are regarding the severity of NSSI; there is the expectation that the patient takes responsibility for the consequences of their NSSI. In other words, the patient ensures that any serious self-inflicted injuries receive medical attention. In addition, there is the expectation that if the therapist is working with the patient to reduce the NSSI as a problem area, then the patient must do so too. Trying is expected, success is not.

The timeline of the NSSI is collected as well as the eating disorders symptomatology and depressive symptoms. This demonstrates to the patient the link between interpersonal events and the onset of problems, highlighting the use of IPT to treat NSSI behaviour. Interpersonal events include separation from love ones, development of new relationships, deaths, divorces, break-up of friendships and relationships, changes in life routine affecting interpersonal relationships such as new jobs, retirement, starting college or university studies and moving to a new area. A weekly diary is introduced to collect information about the eating disorders abnormal behaviour as well as the NSSI and mood symptomatology. It is essential that at a very early stage of the therapy, the therapists and the patient agree on the main aim and goals of the therapy, whether this concerns the reduction of the eating disorders behaviour, the NSSI behaviour or both. The aim for therapy should be as objectively measurable and realistically achievable as possible. Having a clear aim for therapy does not exclude the monitoring of some unhealthy behaviours, such as laxative abuse or over-exercising, of which both are also known to have a mood regulatory role. It is not unusual to see an increase of these types of unhealthy behaviours whilst actively working towards reducing other unwanted behaviour. Therefore, the weekly diary should allow a realistic monitoring of:

- Unhealthy eating behaviour—bingeing, restricting, vomiting, compulsively exercising, purgative use, etc.
- NSSI behaviour—intentional cutting, burning, hitting, scratching, ingestion of harmful substance, etc.
- Depressive symptoms—low mood, poor sleep and poor concentration

11.6.3 The Identification of the Focus Area

The main aim of the final part of the assessment sessions is the identification of the focal area. Whether a patient presents with an eating disorders with or without NSSI the same four focus areas will be used. Adding additional focal areas to IPT in order to treat NSSI in patients with an eating disorder is unnecessary as the standard four focal areas encompass all that needs to be covered. It is not uncommon that some patients with NSSI and ED have a diagnosis of personality disorder. There are contrasting views regarding the need to add an additional focus area for patients with these co-morbid diagnoses. Some experts have advocated for the introduction of a fifth focal area that aims to tackle the self-image of the patient (Angus & Gillies, 1994), whilst others have suggested the use of “regulation of the self through self-image” (Bateman, 2012). Most views encompass the idea that the majority of patients with personality disorders have issues with role transitions and disputes and that these specific focal areas should be pursued rather than creating a fifth focal area (Markowitz, Skodol, & Bleiberg, 2006; Markowitz, 2012). Our view is to use the same focal areas as per standard IPT and IPT for eating disorders:

- *Interpersonal role disputes*: This could be an overt or covert dispute, and often there is a pattern of difficult relationships associated with the patient. It is important to focus on one key relationship that is current and of which the patient feels that change is possible. The literature in this area suggests that there is an intricate and complex relationship between NSSI and fear of abandonment, isolation and poor interpersonal *communication*, and as such, these themes should be explored.

- *Interpersonal role transitions*: As described above, this focus is selected when the patient has not adapted well to a change in a new situation; examples include a change at work, in living situation, in a relationship, in financial status or any other area.
- *Interpersonal deficits*: This focal area is selected when there are often repeated patterns of broken or failed relationships, and the patient has become socially isolated. The patient may be highly sensitive to their difficulties so it can be very helpful to use role play in the session to help practise new skills. In some patients, the relationship between the therapist and the patient can be used to understand the interpersonal deficits and to address the maintaining factors.
- *Complicated bereavement*: This area is selected when there is evidence of an abnormal grief reaction. The nature of the attachment with the deceased is an important consideration when working with grief as a focus area. Grief has already been found to be a predictor of NSSI and suicide behaviour.

11.6.4 The Middle Sessions

It is important that the therapist maintains the focus of the sessions when working with this patient group. Due to the existence of several symptoms that the patient displays (eating disorders, NSSI and mood), it is important to track each of these. It is relatively easy for the therapy to get pushed off track. The symptoms are tracked using the diary as described above, and these are linked with the specific interpersonal focus by linking the interpersonal events to the symptom. In practice, if the focal area is correct, this flows well.

The following example is a common occurrence: the patient cuts herself following a binge, which has been followed by feeling low, which in turn was directly linked to an interpersonal event (i.e. a phone call during which the patient felt criticised by her mother). Once the interpersonal event has been identified, the therapist works with the patient on the focal area (i.e. dispute with mother). This continual linking of the target events to the interpersonal is the essence of IPT.

11.6.5 Termination

The final two sessions are explicitly about ending therapy. Ending should not come as a surprise. Each session will have been counted down towards the final session. IPT is a focused and time-limited therapy, and this is essential to its potency. In patients that have difficulties with attachment, planning the ending is crucial. The sessions are used to recognise the changes that the patient has made whilst acknowledging those which have not changed, as well as to explore feelings about ending therapy. Future problems are anticipated, and much use is made of the interpersonal network and how it can be used to maintain progress and deal with future problems.

A note of caution—not ending because of an episode of self-harm or problematic ED behaviour would reinforce this behaviour. Consequently, it is paramount that ending is planned and adhered to.

Clinical Sample

Holly is a 19-year-old university student referred by her primary care doctor with a 1-year history of repeated episodes of bingeing and vomiting behaviour and a 6-month history of NSSI. Holly has moved from the south of the UK to live in a city in the English midlands in order to study psychology at university. She describes a past psychiatric history of depression, bingeing behaviour and NSSI when she was living at home with her family. Influenced by the *medical model*, the therapist assesses the current psychopathology and gives the disorder a "name": bulimia nervosa. He offers her psycho-education regarding bulimia and NSSI and introduces the concept of regular eating in order to reduce the physiological maintaining factor of her eating disorder. The therapist discusses with the patient the use of diaries, asking the patient to record her daily binges and self-induced vomiting as well as all her episodes of NSSI. The *sick role* is also introduced and tentatively conferred on her. She receives this with some surprise at first as she had thought her problems were all her fault. Her *timeline* indicates that previous episodes of bingeing behaviour and NSSI were associated with episodes of low mood and events connected to changes, such as moving schools, moving to a different city due to father's job and starting university. The *timeline* together with the *interpersonal inventory* indicates difficulties related to attachment. Influenced by the *attachment theory*, the therapist understands Holly's difficulties in developing relationships to be associated to an anxious attachment with its origins seemingly linked to a period of maternal postnatal depression. The *interpersonal inventory* is also used to understand and highlight the lack of a supportive social network in the new city. An agreement is made to use the *focus of "interpersonal transition"* to work throughout the middle sessions. During the *middle sessions*, the patient works on developing a healthy social network. By employing *communication analysis, the therapist works with Holly to* try to understand the difficulties that she has in developing a social support network, and this highlights poor communication skills as a barrier to developing this network. The patient acknowledges the lack of adaptive coping skills when feeling anxious and the use of NSSI behaviour as well as bingeing behaviour to deal with the stress and anxiety related to social situations. Holly and her therapist work together in identifying the positive parts of the new role as a university student and the

(continued)

(continued)

possibilities of the new city. Themes used during the therapy are the use of Holly's independence and the need to accept the responsibilities associated with being an independent adult, the use of her old social network such as her sister or her best friend living in the south of the UK and the use of adaptive behaviour techniques in order to break the vicious cycle of bingeing and NSSI related to social stress. The role of bingeing and NSSI is understood as a way of coping with difficult emotions, associated to feelings of judgement, rejection and loneliness. Some cognitive challenge techniques are also used to help with her anxiety when meeting people. Holly is helped to analyse her behaviour around eating and NSSI by looking at the physiological and psychological factors affecting their development. Links are made between how her interpersonal world influences her feelings and behaviour. To begin with much guidance is required by her therapist, but as sessions progress, she makes these links herself. Using this, Holly is able to generate solutions and test them out by putting them into practice and evaluating the impact. Holly and her therapist are aware of the risk of deterioration when finishing therapy due to past attachment difficulties. It is a further transition that is predictable. An agreement is made to end after 16 sessions but to have the last three sessions every 2–3 weeks. Over the course of the therapy, Holly is able to join the university badminton club and yoga club; she meets other students and begins to develop friendships. This progresses to being able to consider attending parties. Her social network is expanding, and the difficulties related to eating disorders and NSSI are improving. A relapse prevention plan is introduced which includes the use of her social network and other adaptive coping skills such as distraction techniques and using her increasing interest in mindful meditation and yoga. Therapy ends at session 16 as planned. There have been no significant eating disorders symptoms or NSSI behaviour for more than 2 months. A follow-up appointment at 3 months reveals further improvement and the beginning of a new romantic relationship.

Conclusions

NSSI behaviour has been identified as co-morbid to eating disorders, which is not surprising in view of the similar function that both behaviours have. Clinically it is not uncommon to observe an increase of NSSI behaviour when treating eating disorder symptoms, as one type of behaviour may replace another. It does make sense, therefore, that both behaviours are targeted together during therapy. IPT has been found to be successful in targeting eating disorders behaviour by improving interpersonal problems which maintain the eating disorder behaviour. In that respect, IPT can be used to treat patients with NSSI and eating disorders, although some small changes in the way this therapy is conducted may be necessary. Future studies should aim to demonstrate the validity of this modified intervention in patients with co-morbid NSSI and eating disorders.

References

Adrian, M., Zeman, J., Erdley, C., Lisa, L., & Sim, L. (2011). Emotional dysregulation and interpersonal difficulties as risk factors for nonsuicidal self-injury in adolescent girls. *Journal of Abnormal Child Psychology, 39*, 389–400.

Agras, W. S., Walsh, T., Fairburn, C. G., Wilson, G. T., & Kraemer, H. C. (2000). A multicenter comparison of cognitive-behavioral therapy and interpersonal psychotherapy for bulimia nervosa. *Archives of General Psychiatry, 57*, 459–466.

Ambwani, S., & Hopwood, C. (2009). The utility of considering interpersonal problems in the assessment of bulimic features. *Eating Behaviours, 10*, 247–253.

Angus, L., & Gillies, L. A. (1994). Counseling the borderline patient: An interpersonal approach. *Canadian Journal of Counseling, 28*, 69–82.

Arcelus, J., Haslam, M., Farrow, C., & Meyer, C. (2013). The role of interpersonal functioning in the maintenance of eating psychopathology: A systematic review and testable model. *Clinical Psychology Review, 33*, 156–167.

Arcelus, J., Whight, D., Brewin, N., & McGrain, L. (2012). Brief interpersonal psychotherapy for the treatment of Bulimic Disorders: A pilot study. *European Eating Disorders Review, 20*, 326–330.

Arcelus, J., Whight, D., & Haslam, M. (2011). Interpersonal problems in people with Bulimia Nervosa and the role of interpersonal psychotherapy. In H. Hay (Ed.), *New insights into the prevention and treatment of Bulimia Nervosa* (pp. 3–12). Rijeka, Croatia: InTech.

Arcelus, J., Whight, D., Langham, C., Baggott, J., McGrain, L., Meadows, L., et al. (2009). A case series evaluation of a modified version of Interpersonal psychotherapy (IPT) for the treatment of bulimic eating disorders: A pilot study. *European Eating Disorders Review, 17*, 260–268.

Bateman, A. W. (2012). Interpersonal psychotherapy for borderline personality disorder. *Clinical Psychology and Psychotherapy, 19*, 124–133.

Bearden, W. O., Netemeyer, R. G., & Teel, J. A. (1989). Measurement of consumer susceptibility to interpersonal influence. *Journal of Consumer Research, 15*, 472–480.

Berscheid, E., & Peplau, L. A. (1983). The emerging science of relationships. In H. H. Kelley, E. Berscheid, A. Christensen, J. H. Harvey, T. L. Huston, G. Levinger, E. McClintock, L. A. Peplau, & D. R. Peterson (Eds.), *Close relationships* (pp. 1–19). New York: W.H. Freeman & Co Ltd.

Bowlby, J. (1969). *Attachment and loss, Vol. 1: Attachment*. New York: Basic Books.

Craig, R. T. (1988). The handbook of communication science: A review. *Quarterly Journal of Speech, 74*, 487–497.

Dervic, K., Brent, D. A., & Oquedo, M. A. (2008). Completed suicide in childhood. *Psychiatric Clinics of North America, 31*, 271–291.

Di Pierro, R., Sarno, I., Perego, S., Galluci, M., & Madeddu, F. (2012). Adolescent nonsuicidal self-injury: The effects of personality traits, family relationships and maltreatment on the presence and severity of behaviours. *European Child and Adolescent Psychiatry, 21*, 511–520.

Fairburn, C. G. (1993). Interpersonal psychotherapy for bulimia nervosa. In G. L. Klerman & M. M. Weissman (Eds.), *New applications of interpersonal therapy* (pp. 353–378). Washington, DC: American Psychiatric Press.

Fairburn, C. G. (1997). Interpersonal psychotherapy for bulimia nervosa. In D. M. Garner & P. E. Garfinkel (Eds.), *Handbook of treatment for eating disorders* (2nd ed., pp. 278–294). New York: Guilford.

Fairburn, C. G., Jones, R., Peveler, R. C., Carr, S. J., Solomon, R. A., O'Connor, M. E., et al. (1991). Three psychological treatments for bulimia nervosa: A comparative trial. *Archives of General Psychiatry, 48*, 463–469.

Fairburn, C. G., Wilson, G. T., & Kraemer, H. C. (2000). A multi-center comparison of cognitive-behavioural therapy and interpersonal psychotherapy for bulimia nervosa. *Archives of General Psychiatry, 5*, 459–466.

Frank, E. (2005). *Treating bipolar disorder: A clinician's guide to interpersonal and social rhythm therapy*. New York: Guilford.

Friedman, M., Glasser, M., Laufer, E., Laufer, M., & Wohl, M. (1972). Attempted suicide and self-mutilation in adolescence: Some observations from a psychoanalytic research project. *International Journal of Psychoanalysis, 53*, 179–183.

Geller, J., Cockell, S., & Hewitt, P. L. (2000). Inhibited expression of negative emotions interpersonal orientation in anorexia nervosa. *International Journal of Eating Disorders, 28*, 8–19.

Guthrie, E., Kapur, N., Mackway-Jones, K. M., Chew-Granham, C. C., Moorey, J., Mendel, E., et al. (2001). Randomised controlled trial of brief psychological intervention after deliberate self-poisoning. *British Medical Journal, 323*, 135–138.

Hilt, L. M., Cha, C. B., & Nolen-Hoeksema, S. (2008). Non suicidal self-injury in young adolescent girls: Moderators of the distress-function relationship. *Journal of Consulting and Clinical Psychology, 76*, 63–71.

Hinrichsen, G. A., & Clougherty, K. F. (2006). *Interpersonal psychotherapy for depressed older adults*. Washington, DC: American Psychological Association.

Hoffart, A., Abrahamsen, G., Bonsaksen, T., Borge, F. M., Ramstad, R., Lipsitz, J., et al. (2007). *A residential interpersonal treatment for social phobia*. New York: Nova Science Publishers Inc.

Hopwood, C., Clarke, A., & Perez, M. (2007). Pathoplasticity of bulimic features and interpersonal problems. *International Journal of Eating Disorders, 40*, 652–658.

Joiner, T. E., & Van Orden, K. A. (2008). The interpersonal psychological theories of suicidal behaviour indicates specific and crucial psychotherapeutic targets. *International Journal of Cognitive Therapy, 1*, 80–89.

Klerman, G. L., DiMascio, A., Weissman, M. M., Prusoff, B. A., & Paykel, E. S. (1974). Treatment of depression by drugs and psychotherapy. *American Journal of Psychiatry, 131*, 186–191.

Klerman, G. L., Weissman, M. M., Rounsaville, B. J., & Chevron, E. S. (1984). *Interpersonal psychotherapy of depression*. New York: Basic Books.

Klonsky, E. D. (2007). The function of deliberate self-injury: A review of the evidence. *Clinical Psychology Review, 27*, 226–239.

Klonsky, E. D., & Glenn, C. R. (2009). Assessing the function of non-suicidal self- injury: Psychometric properties of the Inventory of Statement about Self-Injury (ISAS). *Journal of Psychopathology and Behavioural Assessment, 31*, 215–219.

Markowitz, J. C. (1998). *Interpersonal psychotherapy for dysthymic disorder*. Washington, DC: American Psychiatric Press.

Markowitz, J. C. (2012). Interpersonal psychotherapy for personality disorders. In T. A. Widiger (Ed.), *The Oxford handbook of personality disorders* (pp. 751–762). Oxford: Oxford University Press.

Markowitz, J. C., Skodol, A. E., & Bleiberg, K. (2006). Interpersonal psychotherapy for borderline personality disorder: Possible mechanisms of change. *Journal of Clinical Psychology, 62*, 431–444.

Montgomery, R. L., Haemmerlie, F. M., & Edwards, M. (1991). Social, personal, and interpersonal deficits in socially anxious people. *Journal of Social Behavior and Personality, 6*, 859–872.

Mufson, L., Dorta, K. P., Moreau, D., & Weissman, M. M. (2004). *Interpersonal psychotherapy for depressed adolescents*. New York: Guildford.

Nock, M. K. (2009). Why do people hurt themselves? New insights into the nature and functions of self-injury. *Current Directions in Psychological Science, 18*, 78–83.

Nock, M. K., & Prinstein, M. J. (2005). Contextual features and behavioral functions of self-mutilation among adolescents. *Journal of Abnormal Psychology, 114*, 140–146.

O'Mahony, J. F., & Hollwey, S. (1995). Eating problems and interpersonal functioning among several groups of women. *Journal of Clinical Psychology, 51*, 345–351.

Petty, S. C., Sachs-Ericsson, N., & Joiner, T. E. (2004). Interpersonal functioning deficits: Temporary or stable characteristics of depressed individuals? *Journal of Affective Disorders, 81*, 115–122.

Rieger, E., Van Buren, D. J., Bishop, M., Tanofsky-Kraff, M., Welch, R., & Wilfley, D. E. (2010). An eating disorder-specific model of interpersonal psychotherapy (IPT-ED): Causal pathways and treatment implications. *Clinical Psychology Review, 30*, 400–410.

Roth, D. M., & Ross, D. R. (1988). Long-term cognitive-interpersonal group therapy for eating disorders. *International Journal of Group Psychotherapy, 38*, 491–510.

Rucci, P., Frank, E., Scocco, P., Calugi, S., Miniati, M., Fagiolini, A., et al. (2011). Treatment emergent suicidal ideation during 4 months of acute management of unipolar major depression with SSRI pharmacotherapy or interpersonal psychotherapy in a randomised clinical trial. *Depression and Anxiety, 28*, 303–309.

Seligman, M. E. P. (2002). *Authentic happiness: Using the new positive psychology to realize your potential for lasting fulfillment*. New York: Free Press.

Sullivan, H. S. (1953). *The interpersonal theory of psychiatry*. New York: Norton.

Sullivan, R. J., & Allen, J. S. (1999). Social deficits associated with schizophrenia defined in terms of interpersonal Machiavellianism. *Acta Psychiatrica Scandinavica, 99*, 148–154.

Suyemoto, K. L. (1998). The functions of self-mutilation. *Clinical Psychology Review, 18*, 531–554.

Turner, B. J., Chapman, A. L., & Layden, B. K. (2012). Intrapersonal and interpersonal functions of non-suicidal self-injury: Association with emotional and social functioning. *Suicide and Life-Threatening Behaviour, 42*, 36–55.

Walsh, T., Roose, S. P., Glassman, A. H., Gladise, M., & Sadik, C. (1985). Bulimia and depression. *Psychosomatic Medicine, 47*, 123–131.

Weissman, M. M., Markowitz, J. C., & Klerman, G. L. (2000). *Comprehensive guide to interpersonal psychotherapy*. New York: Basic Books.

Weissman, M. M., Markowitz, J. C., & Klerman, G. L. (2007). *Clinicians quick guide to interpersonal psychotherapy*. New York: Oxford University Press.

Whight, D., McGrain, L., Baggott, J., Meadows, L., Langham, C., & Arcelus, J. (2011). *Interpersonal psychotherapy for bulimia nervosa (IPT BNm)*. London: Troubador Ltd.

Wichstrom, L. (2009). Predictors of non-suicidal self-injury versus attempted suicide: Similar or different? *Archives of Suicidal Research, 13*, 105–122.

Wilfley, D. E., Agras, W. S., Telch, C. F., Rossiter, E. M., Schneider, J. A., Cole, A. G., et al. (1993). Group cognitive-behavioral therapy and group interpersonal psychotherapy for the non-purging bulimic individual: A controlled comparison. *Journal of Consulting and Clinical Psychology, 61*, 296–305.

Wilfley, D., Stein, R., & Welch, R. (2003). Interpersonal psychotherapy. In J. Treasure, U. Smith, & E. van Furth (Eds.), *Handbook of eating disorders*. London: Wiley.

World Health Organisation (WHO). (1980). *International classification of impairments, disabilities and handicaps*. Geneva: WHO.

Pharmacological Treatment of Non-suicidal Self-injury and Eating Disorders 12

Paul L. Plener and Ulrike M. Schulze

Abstract

There is very little evidence for the psychopharmacological treatment of NSSI and eating disorders and no evidence for the treatment of a combination of both. However, often patients with NSSI and eating disorders present with comparable problems with regard to emotional dysregulation, the need to control urges (e.g., to cut or to binge or purge), and the need to treat comorbid mental disorders or psychiatric symptoms such as depression or anxiety. Based on the recent literature, this chapter aims to summarize the available literature and give recommendations for the psychopharmacological treatment of these conditions. Due to the limited evidence that is available for this kind of treatment, we strongly recommend to use psychopharmacological treatment only in addition to psychotherapeutic interventions.

Abbreviations

AA	Atypical antipsychotics
BPD	Borderline personality disorder
CBT	Cognitive behavioral therapy
DBT	Dialectical behavioral therapy
NDD	Neurodevelopmental disorders
NSSI	Non-suicidal self-injury

P.L. Plener (✉) • U.M. Schulze
Department of Child and Adolescent Psychiatry and Psychotherapy, University of Ulm, Ulm, Germany
e-mail: paul.plener@uniklinik-ulm.de

L. Claes and J.J. Muehlenkamp (eds.), *Non-Suicidal Self-Injury in Eating Disorders*, DOI 10.1007/978-3-642-40107-7_12, © Springer-Verlag Berlin Heidelberg 2014

OCD Obsessive-compulsive disorder
PDD Pervasive developmental disorder
PRN "Pro re nata" medication
RCT Randomized controlled trial
SSRI Selective serotonin reuptake inhibitor
TCA Tricyclic antidepressant

12.1 Introduction

Both non-suicidal self-injury (NSSI) and eating disorders are debilitating and often long-lasting conditions posing a challenge to patients, their relatives, and clinicians. Both conditions bear the potential for lasting bodily harm, which alerts clinicians as well as caretakers. It has been demonstrated that psychotherapeutic approaches can help overcome NSSI and eating disorder symptoms; however, in some cases, it might be justified to add a further treatment component: psychotropic drugs. This chapter intends to act as a road map in dealing with the psychopharmacological treatment of NSSI and eating disorders both separately and in combination. It might help the reader to develop an understanding about when psychopharmacological interventions might be warranted and also when they are not. Starting with the presentation of a rationale for psychopharmacological treatment based on a neurobiological understanding of NSSI and eating disorders, we will highlight the obstacles and future directions of research in this field. Following this, we discuss psychopharmacological treatment for NSSI and eating disorders separately and then describe a treatment approach for comorbid NSSI/eating disorders.

Psychopharmacological treatment approaches try to influence the neurobiology and chemistry of the neurotransmitter system in the brain. The rationale behind using a psychopharmacological approach is that several influences, such as negative life events (e.g., sexual or physical abuse, death of a loved one), environmental stressors (e.g., attachment problems, invalidating environment), genetic vulnerability, and the interaction of such factors, have an effect on the brain's neurobiology and its development and maturation. The interplay of these influences can increase or decrease the possibility of developing a mental health disorder or maladaptive behaviors, such as NSSI or eating disorders. Furthermore, they can increase or decrease one's ability to cope and adapt new strategies, which often are crucial in psychotherapeutic treatment. Trying to reestablish a more stable mental state on a neurobiological level can thus open the opportunity for new learning experiences (Libal & Plener, 2008). Although medication does not have the ability to stop NSSI or eating disorders by itself, it can help to influence underlying conditions or emotions, which may then enable the individual to get rid of these behaviors or states. Therefore it should be clear that we understand psychopharmacological interventions to be considered only in addition to psychotherapeutic interventions. Psychopharmacology, in this case, can be described best as a crutch that enables the individual to walk in times of injury but remains an additional agent, and not the one and only solution, within the healing process. Such an aid can be necessary when psychosocial treatment approaches have failed to diminish eating disorder symptoms or NSSI sufficiently or the individual presents as severely impaired and unable to master developmental goals within his/her life (e.g., school, work, relationships). Just as a crutch can be abandoned as soon as the leg is mended, so too can psychopharmacological interventions. It should be considered that the "leg" may need some time to regain its full function, and it is wise to plan a stabilization phase after symptoms have ceased before abandoning psychopharmacological treatment altogether. The duration of treatment should be "as short as possible but as long as necessary." In summing up this approach, clinicians are advised to follow "three golden rules":

1. Never use psychotropic medication as a single treatment approach to NSSI or eating disorders.
2. Always be aware of the "off-label" nature of a psychopharmacological approach to NSSI and (in most cases) to eating disorders and inform your patient accordingly.
3. Use medication for as short of a time as possible but as long as necessary to regain a stable level of functioning.

So far, there is no drug available for specifically treating NSSI or anorexia nervosa (AN). Both clinicians and patients (as well as their caregivers in case of young patients) should be well aware of the fact that every psychotropic intervention to specifically target NSSI or AN is prescribed "off-label" [i.e., no drug has been approved for this condition by the drug regulation agencies such as the Federal Drug Administration FDA or the European Medicines Agency (EMEA)]. Patients need not only to know this for legal reasons but also to be able to discuss the pros and cons of medication openly in order to foster treatment adherence. As medication is used off-label, it is advisable that medication trials should be made by medical professionals with an expertise in psychopharmacological treatment (e.g., child and adolescent psychiatrists). Every psychopharmacological treatment approach should be based on the "knowledge of the literature" and a "focused assessment of the individual client" (Harper, 2012, p. 203).

Furthermore, when discussing the use of psychopharmacological approaches as an adjunct to other treatment options for NSSI or eating disorders, we face an ethical dilemma. On the one hand, we use drugs with only limited knowledge about a beneficial outcome and some of these drugs can cause severe (even lasting) side effects in certain patients. On the other hand, individuals with NSSI or eating disorders often present with severe, often bodily, impairment being unable to meet their lives' goals. Applying the principle of "primum non nocere" ("first: do no harm") when dealing with this dilemma may lead to a reluctant attitude towards drug use. However, we as clinicians come to see that either way we decide—for or against a psychopharmacological treatment approach—there is the potential to harm the individual patient. Therefore, we think that it is our obligation to individualize the knowledge acquired from numerous studies in this field and use our best clinical judgement in applying the results of these studies to the treatment of our individual patients. As no practice guidelines are available for psychopharmacological treatments of NSSI to date and there is only limited evidence for the psychopharmacological treatment of eating disorders, the individual clinician has to develop a best practice model based on the evidence that does exist, for each individual patient by himself or herself.

12.2 NSSI

12.2.1 Searching for Evidence

In comparing studies to find evidence for a psychopharmacological treatment, one has to deal with the fact that NSSI has so far been considered only as a symptom or a condition, and therefore, it can hardly be found as an outcome measure of psychopharmacological treatment studies. However, there is literature available dealing with the psychopharmacological treatment of self-injuring individuals with pervasive developmental disorders (PDD), autism spectrum disorders, mental retardation, or genetically inherited syndromes (e.g., Lesch–Nyhan syndrome, Cornelia de Lange syndrome). There also is literature about the psychopharmacological treatment of self-injuring individuals with borderline personality disorder (BPD), whereas pharmacological treatments for NSSI in populations other than the ones mentioned above rarely have been carried out. This creates a situation such that the neurobiological understanding and our knowledge about treating NSSI are mainly based on two clinically separate subtypes of self-injurers: individuals with and without neurodevelopmental disorders (NDD) (Sandman, 2009). Given both the differences in the clinical picture and the knowledge about a genetic background in some NDDs, it seems far from obvious to try to provide a general conjunct model for the psychopharmacological treatment of NSSI in both developmentally "normal" people and those suffering from NDDs. In reviewing the literature (Plener, Libal, Fegert, & Kölch, 2013), it is interesting to see that some psychopharmacological interventions seem to be effective in NDD populations but fail to show the same results in a BPD population. The most prominent examples are the opioid antagonists naloxone and naltrexone hydrochloride, with several studies and reviews of treatment reporting an improvement in treating self-injuring individuals with NDD (Sandman, 1990/1991; Sandman et al., 1993; Symons, Thompson, & Rodriguez, 2004; Thompson, Hackenberg, Cerutti, Baker, & Axtell, 1994), whereas no such clear-cut results exist from studies in BPD populations. Given the extent of excellent reviews that have been published concerning the psychopharmacological treatment of NSSI in PDD or NDD populations, or in individuals with a genetic disorder (e.g., Parikh, Kolevzon, & Hollander, 2008; Sandman, 2009; Scahill & Koenig, 1999), our chapter tries to focus on research that has been done in "normally" developing individuals, especially since the focus of this chapter is both on NSSI and eating disorders.

12.2.2 Specific Psychopharmacological Interventions

It is only recently that attempts have been made to review the empirical literature with regard to psychopharmacological treatments of NSSI (Bloom & Holly, 2011; Plener et al., 2013; Plener, Libal, & Nixon, 2009; Sandman, 2009). Based on these reviews, and by drawing upon recently available studies, this part of the chapter aims to (1) focus on the studies offering the best available evidence for a certain treatment, (2) present the available knowledge for psychopharmacological interventions based on a neurobiological understanding for NSSI, and (3) draw conclusions and recommendations for clinical practice.

12.2.2.1 Antidepressants

There is some evidence for a dysfunction within the serotonergic system in NSSI (Groschwitz & Plener, 2012). Antidepressants try to influence the serotonergic system by inhibiting the reuptake of serotonin from the synaptic cleft back to the presynaptic terminal after its release of serotonin, which leads to an improved signal transmission. Newer SSRIs are more selective (as described by their name) for this mechanism, whereas older tri- and tetracyclic antidepressants influence multiple neurotransmitter systems. SSRIs have been recommended for the treatment of NSSI (Pies & Popli, 1995; Roberts, 2003). Studies from adult samples with suicidal attempts or BPD point out the efficacy of SSRIs in this context. Verkes et al. (1998) described a reduction of suicide attempts in a double-blind placebo-controlled study of paroxetine ($N = 91$). Further examining newer SSRIs, Simpson et al. (2004) performed a placebo-controlled trial of fluoxetine in a sample of 20 patients with BPD. Fluoxetine was used as an "add-on" to dialectical behavior therapy (DBT); no differences between the fluoxetine and placebo groups were reported, but NSSI was not addressed specifically. Additionally, Markovitz, Calabrese, Schulz, and Meltzer (1991) presented data from a 12-week open-label trial of 22 adult patients with BPD or schizotypal personality disorder with fluoxetine and showed a reduction of NSSI in 10 out of 12 self-injuring patients. However, Hawton et al. (2009) stated in their Cochrane review that the pooled odds ratios for studies of antidepressants versus placebo did not show sufficient evidence for the reduction of deliberate self-harm (including NSSI) under antidepressant treatment.

Another point that needs to be addressed, especially with regard to the treatment of adolescents and young adults with SSRIs, is the risk of suicidality as an adverse event, which led to FDA warnings in 2004 (Brent, 2004; Isacsson, Holmgren, & Ahlner, 2005; Whittington et al., 2004). Concerns about increasing NSSI when administering SSRIs in adolescents arose early in its use (Teicher, Glod, & Cole, 1993). Donovan et al. (2000) presented a prospective study of 2,776 deliberate self-harm (DSH) cases and found significantly more DSH events following SSRI prescriptions than tricyclic antidepressant (TCA) prescriptions. As DSH does include both self-injuries with and without suicidal intent, it remains unclear if there is a specific impact of SSRIs on NSSI. In the Adolescent Depression Antidepressant and Psychotherapy Trial (ADAPT) of 208 adolescents with moderate to major depression, the patients received an SSRI (mostly fluoxetine) in combination with either routine care or cognitive behavioral therapy (CBT). Following 28 weeks of treatment, rates of NSSI decreased in both treatment groups regardless of the accompanying psychosocial intervention (Goodyer et al., 2007). In the SSRI and routine care group, the number was reduced from 23 self-injuring patients, at the beginning, to 9 after the 28 weeks, and, in the SSRI + CBT group, the number was reduced from 30 to 12. Recently the Treatment of SSRI-Resistant Depression in Adolescents (TORDIA) study assessed the effects of switching treatment-resistant depressed adolescents ($N = 334$) from an SSRI treatment to either another SSRI or to venlafaxine (Brent et al., 2008, 2009). The group reported 50 events of NSSI in 31 participants. Interestingly, the authors described higher rates of NSSI in patients who also received benzodiazepines, a relationship that remained stable after controlling for a prior history of NSSI (Brent et al., 2009). However, due to the small numbers (four out of ten), this result should be interpreted with caution. It has been reported from a recent analysis of longitudinal, randomized controlled trials with fluoxetine and venlafaxine that rates of suicidal ideation and suicide attempts declined in adults with depression, whereas there was no such decline in adolescents and young adults (Gibbons, Brown, Hur, Davis, & Mann, 2012).

In summary, it can be concluded that despite the fact that SSRIs have been recommended as first-line treatment for NSSI, there is a need to be cautious especially in prescribing SSRIs to self-injuring adolescents. Although concerns have been raised about SSRI treatment in depressed youth, there is often a necessity of effective treatment for depression. The lower mortality of SSRI overdose rate compared to other antidepressant groups (e.g., TCAs) needs to be underscored. In conclusion, we recommend treating depressed adults and adolescents according to national guidelines, but the clinician needs to stay alert for possible suicidal and non-suicidal self-injury-related side effects.

12.2.2.2 Antipsychotics

The term “antipsychotics” describes a rather mixed class of psychotropic agents that were originally used to treat schizophrenia. All antipsychotic drugs work by blocking dopamine receptors at the neuron’s postsynaptic terminal. However, most of the components also act on other neurotransmitter systems (e.g., by blocking serotonin receptors or histaminergic receptors). The class of antipsychotics consists of the “older” conventional antipsychotics (e.g., haloperidol, flupenthixol) and the “newer” atypical antipsychotics (AA) (e.g., olanzapine, clozapine, risperidone, quetiapine, ziprasidone [and even newer developments such as], aripiprazole). Within the last few years, more and more AAs also have been used in the treatment of bipolar disorders and BPD. As it was pointed out in a review of AA treatment of BPD patients, a subgroup of BPD patients with “psychotic, impulsive, and suicidal complaints” seem to profit from an AA treatment (Grootens & Verkes, 2005). In a review of the psychopharmacological treatment of BPD, including 28 double-blind randomized controlled trials, Abraham and Calabrese (2008) pointed out that the AA olanzapine showed positive results in five trials including 100 patients. However, it has to be noted again that only very few studies with antipsychotics addressed NSSI as an outcome measure. A double-blind placebo-controlled trial, which compared

155 BPD patients treated with olanzapine to 159 BPD patients treated with placebo, showed a decrease of BPD symptomatology in both groups without significant group differences. Decreases on the suicidal/self-injury item of the Zanarini rating scale for BPD were greater in the placebo group, and one report of self-injury was stated as an adverse effect in the olanzapine group, but not in the placebo group (Schulz et al., 2008). Linehan, McDavid, Brown, Sayrs, and Gallop (2008) reported data from a double-blind placebo-controlled trial of 24 females with BPD, who received DBT in combination with either placebo or olanzapine. It was shown that in both groups NSSI decreased significantly over the 6-month course of the study, again with larger decreases in the placebo group (Linehan et al., 2008). For the majority of AAs, only case studies are available so far. Chengappa, Ebeling, Kang, Levine, and Parepally (1999) reported a reduction of NSSI from a case study of seven patients with BPD under clozapine treatment, and Hilger, Barnas, and Kasper (2003) reported reduction of NSSI in two BPD patients after administering quetiapine. Nickel et al. (2006) and Nickel, Loew, and Pedrosa (2007) presented one of the most thorough psychopharmacological studies so far with respect to NSSI outcome data. They reported data from a double-blind placebo-controlled trial of 52 patients with BPD and followed them up for 18 months. Before starting the intervention, 7 out of 26 people from the aripiprazole group and 5 out of 26 patients from the placebo group injured themselves. After 8 weeks of treatment, this rate was decreased to two persons in the aripiprazole group injuring themselves, compared to seven patients in the placebo group (Nickel et al., 2006). After 18 months the results remained stable with 4 out of 26 patients in the aripiprazole group engaging in self-injury but 11 of 26 patients in the placebo group still showing NSSI (Nickel et al., 2007). The positive findings for aripiprazole were further supported by a meta-analysis of randomized controlled trials for the psychopharmacological treatment of personality disorders, reporting a positive effect on aripiprazole on impulse and behavioral control (Ingenhoven et al., 2010), which indirectly implies that NSSI may be reduced as well.

In studies with adolescents, reduction of NSSI was reported after administration of quetiapine in two cases (Good, 2006) and from a retrospective chart review of ziprasidone therapy in eight cases (Libal et al., 2005). It has to be noted that AAs seem to have a decreased risk for producing extrapyramidal motoric symptoms (e.g., tremor, rigor, dyskinesias), but they share the risk for weight gain and developing glucose tolerance, even leading to diabetes (Correll, 2007; Kumra et al., 2008). This limits the recommendation of a treatment trial with antipsychotics to severe cases of NSSI.

12.2.2.3 Anticonvulsants/Mood Stabilizers

This class of drugs is comprised of many mood-stabilizing agents, most of which originated from the treatment of epileptic disorders. Examples include valproate, carbamazepine, and lithium. One of the first studies assessing a mood-stabilizing agent in BPD was done by Cowdry and Gardner (1988), who reported a reduction of behavioral dyscontrol in a 6-week double-blind study with 16 BPD patients using carbamazepine. These results were contradicted by a double-blind placebo-controlled study of 20 BPD patients, which did not yield significant results (De la Fuente &

Lotstra, 1994). In a case report of two bulimic females with NSSI, Cordàs et al. (2006) reported reduction of NSSI after treatment with oxcarbazepine. However, in an open-label trial of oxcarbazepine in 17 BPD patients, no changes in "parasuicidal behavior" could be observed (Bellino et al., 2005). Cassano et al. (2001) reported reduction of NSSI from a single case study of a BPD patient with topiramate; however, this result has not been further assessed in a larger study so far, as most of the studies on BPD patients treated with topiramate focused on reducing anger.

Lithium is a mood-stabilizing drug that is commonly used in the treatment of bipolar disorder (Burgess et al., 2001; Cipriani et al., 2005). Masters (2008) reported on the efficacy of this drug for decreasing suicidal ideation and NSSI in an adolescent residential treatment center. He reported a decrease of suicidal thinking beginning approximately 48 h after starting a lithium therapy and a decrease of cutting. In a separate study, Dickstein et al. (2009) performed a 6-week placebo-controlled double-blind trial of lithium in 25 adolescents (ages: 7–17) with "severe mood dysregulation," observing no differences in clinical outcomes between the two groups. It has to be noted that strict monitoring is necessary when using this drug. Due to a small therapeutic range, toxic doses can be reached rather easily, which underscores the need for cautious supervision, especially for patients with co-occurring suicidal ideation.

12.2.2.4 Antihypertensive Agents

The suggested use of antihypertensive agents (alpha-agonists) is based on the assumption that states of inner tension precede NSSI and that such states can be reduced by using an antihypertensive drug (Sandman, 2009). It has been shown in a pilot study of 14 women with BPD that urges to self-injure and inner tension were reduced by clonidine. This is an understudied area of pharmacological treatment of NSSI so use of such agents should be done cautiously.

12.2.2.5 Opiate Antagonists

The role of endogenous opiates for maintaining NSSI has been widely discussed (Osuch & Payne, 2009; Sandman, 2009; Sher & Stanley, 2009), and Nixon et al. (2002) have reported addictive properties of NSSI from their clinical sample of adolescent patients. Opiate antagonists are meant to work by blocking opiates, believed to be released after injuring oneself, from the receptor, thus diminishing the reinforcing effect of NSSI. Thorough reviews of the use of opiate antagonists (naloxone and naltrexone hydrochloride) have been undertaken in NDD populations and have shown good effects in reducing NSSI (Sandman, 1990/1991; Symons et al., 2004). Interestingly, in studies focusing on "normally" developed populations, the evidence for an effect of opiate antagonists for treating NSSI is much weaker. With regard to NSSI, Roth et al. (1996) reported a reduction of self-injury in an open-label trial of seven patients under naltrexone treatment, and Griengl et al. (2001) reported a reduction of NSSI in one BPD patient. Another case report of cessation of self-injury in a 28-year-old female BPD patient under naltrexone treatment was provided by McGee (1997). Sonne et al. (1996) reported decreased self-injurious thoughts and actions in four out of five BPD patients under naltrexone treatment. Therefore, it has to be assumed that although the evidence for opioid antagonist treatment in NDD population is rapidly increasing, evidence for the use in non-NDD populations with NSSI does not go beyond open-label trials. Though it may be warranted to start a therapeutic trial in an individual who shows strong "addictive" symptoms of NSSI, there is no support at the moment for opiate antagonists as the drug of choice in the treatment of NSSI in non-NDD patients.

12.2.2.6 Benzodiazepines

Benzodiazepines (e.g., diazepam, lorazepam, alprazolam) are used as anxiolytic agents. Studies have shown mixed results with regard to self-injury. An increase of NSSI under alprazolam was reported from a trial of alprazolam, carbamazepine, trifluoperazine, tranylcypromine, and placebo in patients with BPD (Cowdry & Gardner, 1988). Further, in a retrospective chart review of 323 psychiatric inpatients (Rothschild et al., 2000), no differences concerning acts of NSSI were reported for the benzodiazepines in the alprazolam group (1.9 %) and the clonazepam group (1.8 %), compared to the no-benzodiazepine group (2.9 %). Together with recently published reports of the TORDIA study (Brent et al., 2009), these data support recommendations that benzodiazepines should be used with caution in NSSI patients. Considering their addictive potentials, their use should be confined to short-term interventions, especially among adolescents (Libal & Plener, 2008).

12.2.2.7 Omega-3 Fatty Acids

The role of omega-3 fatty acids (eicosapentaenoic acid and docosahexaenoic acid) has been observed in different mental health disorders (e.g., Owen et al., 2008). Lower levels of omega-3 fatty acids in the blood have been reported from self-harming patients (Garland et al., 2007), and Zanarini and Frankenburg (2003) reported a reduction of aggression and depression from a trial of 30 BPD patients. In a RCT of 49 patients exhibiting NSSI and suicidal behaviors, scores of suicidality and depression were improved, but no differences in NSSI could be found between individuals receiving omega-3 fatty acids and placebo (seven in each group) (Hallahan et al., 2007). Therefore, the benefit of omega-3 fatty acids in reducing NSSI remains uncertain.

12.3 Eating Disorders

12.3.1 Specific Psychopharmacological Interventions

Pharmacotherapy in patients with eating disorders is a matter of high complexity. Patients are faced not only with weight loss or gain but also with symptoms like hunger, craving, loneliness, feelings of emptiness and helplessness, compulsion, anxiety, anger, depression and sadness, uncertainty, inner tension, panic, scruple, aggression, despair, and much more. Especially these perceptions may be adjunct to thought disorders related to somatic state, other psychiatric symptoms, and most notably to their disturbed emotion regulation.

As part of a multimodal treatment approach and following national guidelines, psychopharmacological treatment can be understood as an attempt to resolve various target symptoms. With a few exceptions, also depending on the eating disorder subtype, there is mostly no convincing evidence for a psychopharmacological treatment approach in this field. Therapists have to be aware that next to a sustainable therapeutic relationship, psychotherapy, and the patient's motivation to change, psychopharmacological treatment is only one component of a multimodal approach to help the patient to overcome the disorder. Usually, patients with an eating disorder are cautious against pharmacological treatment since they often have great ambitions to succeed on their own, without help from outside. Often these patients present with great ambivalence about whether they want to change their behavior (Herpertz et al., 2011) and it may take some time until the hope for symptom reduction outweighs the fear of side effects, allowing for a pharmacological treatment approach. Therefore, time to start medication should be convenient and patients have to be really convinced.

Considering pharmacological treatment, the clinician has to be aware of the "off-label" nature of most prescriptions (especially for children and adolescents) in the field of eating disorders and needs to inform the patient accordingly.

12.3.1.1 Antidepressants

Notwithstanding the fact that serotonin is involved in almost all of the behavioral changes observed in patients with anorexia nervosa (AN), supplementation or restoration of adequate levels of serotonin is a complex task. It has been shown that the use of SSRIs is unsuitable for attempts to gain weight and there is hardly any evidence for an antidepressant effect or an effect with regard to relapse prevention of SSRIs in children and adolescents (Flament et al., 2012; Haleem, 2012; Holtkamp et al., 2005). Nevertheless, the use of SSRIs could be considered in cases of treatment-resistant anorectic patients with comorbid depression or anxiety disorders as a closely monitored adjunctive treatment option. In adults, positive effects of fluoxetine and citalopram have been reported for relapse prevention and reduction of depressive and obsessive symptoms as well as impulsiveness (Fassino et al., 2002; Kaye et al., 2005). Claudino et al. (2009) reported no effect on weight gain when compared to placebo and no reduction of eating disorder psychopathology in comparison to placebo during the starvation state in their Cochrane review. Furthermore, there is no evidence for any specific antidepressant to be more effective in nourishing weight gain than any other antidepressant (Claudino et al., 2009). It has been discussed that in acute AN, there is a disturbance of serotonin function (Attia & Schroeder, 2005; Kaye et al., 2005), thus diminishing the effect of antidepressants before weight restoration is achieved (Kaye et al., 1998). However, antidepressants can be useful in treating comorbid depression after weight is restored (Claudino et al., 2009). Due to the low level of evidence, there is no general recommendation for the use of antidepressants in AN, especially since this patient group seems prone to develop adverse events (Greetfeld et al., 2012).

In patients with bulimia nervosa (BN), the administration of SSRIs has been recommended as adjunctive measure (Herpertz et al., 2011) to target depressive symptoms and binging as well as purging (Greetfeld et al., 2012). The use of an SSRI with a long half-life (such as fluoxetine with dosing up to 60 mg/day) has been recommended in order to provide rather constant plasma levels despite purging (Greetfeld et al., 2012), and a good risk-benefit ratio has been reported for fluoxetine (Aigner et al., 2011) as well as other SSRIs (Greetfeld et al., 2012). Although there is some evidence for the effectiveness of older tricyclic antidepressants, these should be avoided, especially in young patients (with AN), since there is a high lethality when overdosed and there is potential for fatal arrhythmia at low body weight (Flament et al., 2012).

12.3.1.2 Antipsychotics

Interpretation of trials of antipsychotics in eating disorders is often impaired due to inadequate sample sizes, high dropout rates, and short duration. A recent meta-analysis, involving eight controlled trials of the use of antipsychotics in AN, failed to report an effect on weight gain, depression, and anxiety (Kishi et al., 2012). There is stronger evidence for the use of olanzapine for gaining weight in AN than for other antipsychotics (Aigner et al., 2011); however, the outcomes in the literature with regard to weight gain are mixed, with some case reports and open-label studies reporting weight gain, while RCTs were often not able to provide evidence for such an effect (Greetfeld et al., 2012). However, there might be potential for the use of olanzapine in addressing compulsion, inner tension, anxiety, hyperactivity, delusion-like thinking, and adverse reactions on weight gain often encountered in the treatment of patients with AN. There is a need to closely monitor for adverse effects, especially for extrapyramidal motoric symptoms as well as changes of ECG. Besides olanzapine, there have been positive findings in studies on quetiapine and aripiprazole (Greetfeld et al., 2012). With regard to quetiapine, there have been both studies not describing any difference to placebo (Powers et al., 2012) and studies reporting effectiveness on psychopathology (Mehler-Wex et al., 2008). With regard to aripiprazole, there has been a case report describing a broad spectrum of positive effects (Trunko et al., 2011). Keeping in mind that the meta-analysis of controlled trials was not able to show an effect on core symptomatology and weight gain, the use of antipsychotics in AN needs to be restricted to closely monitored patients not responding adequately to other forms of therapy.

12.3.1.3 Other Agents

Despite the well-known adverse effect of weight gain, lithium is not recommendable for patients with eating disorders, due to sodium and fluid depletion in eating disorders which could result in intoxication (Flament et al., 2012). Particularly in case of comorbid depression, the application of omega-3 polyunsaturated essential fatty acids is also a matter of debate (Forbes & Pearsons, 2012; Swenne et al., 2011). With regard to bulimics, a small-scale RCT reported the effectiveness of the antiemetic drug ondansetron in BN (Faris et al., 2000) and two RCTs reported effectiveness of topiramate on binging and purging (Aigner et al., 2011;

Greetfeld et al., 2012), whereas one RCT revealed positive effects of baclofen on binge frequency and craving (Corwin et al., 2012). Results of trials with opiate antagonists in AN and BN are mixed, with effects reported on binging and purging in some studies, while others could not replicate these findings (Flament et al., 2012). Based on an eating disorder-related symptomatology in zinc deficiency, as well as on experiments with zinc-deficient rats, the idea of zinc supplementation was tested in three RCTs that showed mixed results (Aigner et al., 2011; Flament et al., 2012).

12.4 Recommendations for Combined Treatment of NSSI and Eating Disorders

Facing the fact that the literature about the pharmacological treatment of both NSSI and eating disorders is limited and mostly based on an individual off-label approach, it seems feasible to identify shared symptomatology. However, we agree with Nose et al. (2006) and Mercer et al. (2009) that in spite of low levels of evidence, psychopharmacological treatment can become necessary for severely impaired individuals and should be based on the best available evidence.

Despite the obvious bodily signs of both NSSI and eating disorders (such as scars, weight loss, purging, and binge eating), we often find these patients to report feelings of depression, emptiness, anxiety, anger, inner tension, despair, aggression, and much more. Both sets of behaviors encompass difficulties in regulating emotions. Due to the fact that evidence for treating NSSI directly is very limited [see Plener et al. (2009, 2013)], the approach proposed by Katz and Fotti (2005) for treating emotionally dysregulated behavior might seem more feasible, as regulation of negative affect is believed to be one of the main motivations behind engagement in NSSI (Kleindienst et al., 2008; Klonsky, 2007) and is also a crucial component in eating disorders. According to Katz and Fotti's (2005) model, in a first step, any possible underlying Axis I disorders should be treated according to national guidelines (such as national practice parameters or the UK National Institute for Health and Clinical Excellence [NICE] guidelines). Secondly, symptoms associated with NSSI (or in this case: also eating disorders) (e.g., tension, anxiety, anger, irritability, feelings of emptiness) should be targeted. The psychopharmacological agent is then chosen according to the presenting symptoms.

As far as psychopharmacological treatment choice, AAs can be recommended, if inner tension, impulse control deficits, affective lability, suicidal ideation, or anorectic symptomatology is within the focus of therapy. If obsessive-compulsive, bulimic, depressive symptoms, flashbacks, or anxiety is targeted, treatment with an SSRI as mono-strategy or as an augmentation strategy to the AA might be warranted. Chronic suicidality, aggression, affective lability, or impulse control deficits also can be targeted by using a mood-stabilizing agent (e.g., an anticonvulsant).

In addition to these treatment choices, it needs to be mentioned that situations exist wherein there is a strong urge to self-injure or a strong inner tension, or a strong urge to purge, and other behavioral treatments are not sufficient in reducing the situation. In these cases, it may prove necessary to administer a short-term medication ("pro re nata," PRN) in order to decrease tension. In this case, low-potency conventional antipsychotics as well as benzodiazepines can be used, but their use (especially of benzodiazepines—due to their addictive potential and the findings of the TORDIA study mentioned before) should be reduced to emergency situations.

12.5 Case Report

M., a 14-year-old female patient, was sent to inpatient psychiatric treatment by her general practitioner as her body mass index (BMI) was found to be below the second age-dependent BMI percentile. In addition to a restrictive anorexia nervosa, which has started at the age of 12, she presented with depressed mood, suicidal thoughts, and diminished social activity, all of which had been present for approximately 6 months before admission to inpatient care. She reported a history of NSSI, which had started at the age of 12 but had ceased after 6 months due to fears that her parents might notice the scars. M. was treated following a cognitive behavioral approach, with weight gain as the first treatment goal, supported by contingency management. Despite the severely depressed mood, which did not change for weeks after admission, and the wish of the parents for psychopharmacological support for their daughter, we abstained from the use of an SSRI, as long as M.'s BMI was below the tenth percentile. Since the depressive symptoms remained after an initial weight gain, it was decided together with M. and the caregivers to administer the SSRI fluoxetine. As suicidal thoughts were still present, the issue of a possible influence of SSRIs on suicidality was discussed with the patient and the parents. Twelve days after the first administration of fluoxetine, M. disclosed to her therapists that she was experiencing strong urges to self-injure, which she found hard to control. She reported feeling disappointed since she had thought that she had overcome NSSI in the past. Strategies for dealing with the upcoming urges were discussed and M. was told that she could ask for "pro re nata" medication (a low-potency conventional antipsychotic) if the urges to self-injure became unmanageable. She used this strategy only once in the following week and reported that the urges to self-injure decreased 3 weeks after the first administration of fluoxetine. This decrease was accompanied by an increase in social contacts towards other patients on the inpatient unit, as well as sufficiently elevated mood. Following this phase, M. seemed more open to the psychotherapy and was able to participate more actively. She was discharged from the inpatient service 2 months after admission, with a weight at the 15th BMI percentile.

12.6 Summary

The available literature on the psychopharmacological treatment of both NSSI and eating disorders can be summed up shortly: with the exception of SSRI use in bulimia, there is no clear-cut psychopharmacological solution to target both NSSI and/or anorexia nervosa. Despite several studies, which have focused on this issue, the evidence is still mixed, with a lot of studies showing contradictory results or having only very small sample sizes. Keeping in mind the low evidence on which treatment recommendations are built on, it seems best to first target comorbid mental disorders (such as depression), treating them according to national guidelines, when considering a psychopharmacological approach. A second step could be to address specific symptom clusters accompanying NSSI or eating disorders, such as symptoms of anxiety, affective dysregulation, or compulsion. As it has been stated before, both SSRIs as well as atypical antipsychotics and several other classes of drugs might play a role in this scheme. However, this can only be done as part of an individually tailored treatment scheme and clinicians are urged to consider the off-label nature of these approaches. Finally, the clinician has to keep in mind that psychopharmacological approaches can only be one element of a multimodal treatment scheme and should never be used without accompanying psychotherapy.

References

Abraham, P. F., & Calabrese, J. R. (2008). Evidence-based pharmacologic treatment of borderline personality disorder: A shift from SSRIs to anticonvulsants and atypical antipsychotics? *Journal of Affective Disorders, 111*, 21–30.

Aigner, M., Treasure, J., Kaye, W., Kasper, S., & WFSBP Task Force On Eating Disorders. (2011). World ion of Societies of Biological Psychiatry (WFSBP) guidelines for the pharmacological treatment of eating disorders. *World Journal of Biological Psychiatry, 12*, 400–443.

Attia, E., & Schroeder, L. (2005). Pharmacologic treatment of anorexia nervosa: Where do we go from here? *International Journal of Eating Disorders, 37*, S60–S63.

Bellino, S., Paradiso, E., & Bogetto, F. (2005). Oxcarbazepine in the treatment of borderline personality disorder: A pilot study. *Journal of Clinical Psychiatry, 66*, 1111–1115.

Bloom, C. M., & Holly, S. (2011). Toward new avenues in the treatment of nonsuicidal self-injury. *Journal Pharmacy Practice, 24*, 472–477.

Brent, D. A. (2004). Antidepressants and pediatric depression—The risk of doing nothing. *New England Journal of Medicine, 351*, 1598–1601.

Brent, D. A., Emslie, G. J., Clarke, G. N., Asarnow, J., Spirito, A., Ritz, L., et al. (2009). Predictors of spontaneous and systematically assessed suicidal adverse events in the treatment of SSRI-resistant depression in adolescents (TORDIA) study. *American Journal of Psychiatry, 166*, 418–426.

Brent, D. A., Emslie, G., Clarke, G., Wagner, K. D., Asarnow, J. R., Keller, M., et al. (2008). Switching to another SSRI or to venlafaxine with or without cognitive behavioural therapy for adolescents with SSRI-resistant depression: The TORDIA randomized controlled trial. *Journal of the American Medical Association, 299*, 901–913.

Burgess, S., Geddes, J., Hawton, K., Townsend, E., Jamison, K., & Goodwin, G. (2001). Lithium for maintenance treatment of mood disorders. *Cochrane Database of Systematic Reviews, 3*, CD003013.

Cassano, P., Lattanzi, L., Pini, S., Dell'Osso, L., Battistini, G., & Cassano, G. B. (2001). Topiramate for self-mutilation in a patient with borderline personality disorder. *Bipolar Disorders, 3*, 161.

Chengappa, K. N. R., Ebeling, T., Kang, J. S., Levine, J., & Parepally, H. (1999). Clozapine reduces severe self-mutilation and aggression in psychotic patients with borderline personality disorder. *Journal of Clinical Psychiatry, 60*, 477–484.

Cipriani, A., Pretty, H., Hawton, K., & Geddes, J. R. (2005). Lithium in the prevention of suicidal behaviour and all-cause mortality in patients with mood disorders: A systematic review of randomized trials. *American Journal of Psychiatry, 162*, 1805–1819.

Claudino, A. M., Slva de Lima, M., Hay, P. P. J., Bacaltchuk, J., Schmidt, U. U. S., & Treasure, J. (2009). Antidepressants for anorexia nervosa (review). *The Cochrane Library, 1*, 1–47.

Cordàs, T. A., Tavares, H., Calderoni, D. M., Stump, G. V., & Ribeiro, R. B. (2006). Oxcarbazepine for self-mutilating bulimic patients. *International Journal of Neuropsychopharmacology, 9*, 769–771.

Correll, C. U. (2007). Weight gain and metabolic effects of mood stabilizers and antipsychotics in pediatric bipolar disorder: A systematic review and pooled analysis of short term trials. *Journal of the American Academy of Child and Adolescent Psychiatry, 46*, 687–700.

Corwin, R. L., Boan, J., Peters, K. F., & Ulbrecht, J. S. (2012). Baclofen reduces binge eating in a double-blind, placebo-controlled, crossover study. *Behavioral Pharmacology, 23*, 616–625.

Cowdry, R. W., & Gardner, D. L. (1988). Pharmacotherapy for borderline personality disorder. *Archives of General Psychiatry, 45*, 111–119.

de la Fuente, J. M., & Lotstra, F. (1994). A trial of carbamazepine in borderline personality disorder. *European Neuropsychopharmacol, 4*, 479–486.

Dickstein, D. P., Towbin, K. E., Van Der Veen, J. W., Rich, B. A., Brotman, M. A., Knopf, L., et al. (2009). Randomized double-blind placebo-controlled trial of lithium in youths with severe mood dysregulation. *Journal of Child and Adolescent Psychopharmacology, 19*, 61–73.

Donovan, S., Clayton, A., Beeharry, M., Jones, S., Kirk, C., Waters, K., et al. (2000). Deliberate self-harm following antidepressant drugs. *British Journal of Psychiatry, 177*, 551–556.

Faris, P. L., Kim, S. W., Meller, W. H., Goodale, R. L., Oakman, S. A., Hofbauer, R. D., Marshall, A. M., Daughters, R. S., Banerjee-Stevens, D., Eckert, E. D., & Hartman, B. K. (2000). Effect of decreasing afferent vagal activity with Ondansetron on symptoms of bulimia nervosa: A randomised, double-blind trial. *Lancet, 355*, 792–797.

Fassino, S., Leombruni, P., Daga, G., Brustolin, A., Migliaretti, G., Cavallo, F., & Rovera, G. (2002). Efficacy of citalopram in anorexia nervosa: A pilot study. *European Neuropsychopharmacology, 12*, 453–459.

Flament, M. F., Bissada, H., & Spettigue, W. (2012). Evidence-based pharmacotherapy of eating disorders. *International Journal of Neuropsychopharmacology, 15*, 189–207.

Forbes, D., & Pearsons, H. (2012). Essential fatty acids: Food for mind and body. *Acta Paediatrica, 101*, 806–810.

Garland, M. R., Hallahan, B., McNamara, M., Carney, P. A., Grimes, H., Hibbeln, J. R., et al. (2007). Lipids and essential fatty acids in patients presenting with self-harm. *British Journal of Psychiatry, 190*, 112–117.

Gibbons, R. D., Brown, H., Hur, K., Davis, J. M., & Mann, J. J. (2012). Suicidal thoughts and behaviour with antidepressant treatment. *Archives of General Psychiatry, 69*, 580–587.

Good, C. R. (2006). Adjunctive Quetiapine targets self-harm behaviors in adolescent females with major depressive disorder. *Journal of Child and Adolescent Psychopharmacology, 16*, 235–236.

Goodyer, I., Dubicka, B., Wilkinson, P., Kelvin, R., Roberts, C., Byford, S., et al. (2007). Selective serotonin reuptake inhibitors (SSRIs) and routine specialist care with and without cognitive behaviour therapy in adolescents with major depression: Randomised controlled trial. *British Medical Journal, 335*, 142–150.

Greetfeld, M., Cuntz, U., & Vorderholzer, U. (2012). Pharmacotherapy for anorexia nervosa and bulimia nervosa. *Fortschritte Der Neurologie Psychiatrie, 80*, 9–16.

Griengl, H., Sendera, A., & Dantendorfer, K. (2001). Naltrexone as a treatment of self-injurious behavior: A case report. *Acta Psychiatrica Scandinavica, 103*, 234–236.

Grootens, K. P., & Verkes, R. J. (2005). Emerging evidence for the use of atypical antipsychotics in borderline personality disorder. *Pharmacopsychiatry, 38*, 20–23.

Groschwitz, R. C., & Plener, P. L. (2012). The neurobiology of non-suicidal self-injury (NSSI): A review. *Suicidology Online, 3*, 24–32.

Haleem, D. J. (2012). Serotonin neurotransmission in anorexia nervosa. *Behavioural Pharmacology, 23*, 478–495.

Hallahan, B., Hibbeln, J. R., Davis, J. M., & Garland, M. R. (2007). Omega-3 fatty acid supplementation in patients with recurrent self-harm. *British Journal of Psychiatry, 190*, 118–122.

Harper, G. (2012). Psychopharmacological treatment. In B. W. Walsh (Ed.), *Treating self-injury. A practical guide* (2nd ed., pp. 195–203). New York: The Guilford Press.

Hawton, K., Townsend, E., Arensmann, E., Gunnel, D., Hazell, P., House, A., & van Heeringen, K. (2009). Psychosocial and pharmacological treatments for deliberate self harm. *Cochrane Database of Systematic Reviews, 1999*(4). Art. No.: CD001764. doi:10.1002/14651858.CD001764.

Herpertz, S., Hagenah, U., Vocks, S., von Wietersheim, J., Cuntz, U., & Zeeck, A. (2011). Clinical practice guideline: The diagnosis and treatment of eating disorders. *Deutsches Ärzteblatt International, 108*, 678–685.

Hilger, E., Barnas, C., & Kasper, S. (2003). Quetiapine in the treatment of borderline personality disorder. *World Journal Biological Psychiatry, 4*, 42–44.

Holtkamp, K., Konrad, K., Kaiser, N., Ploenes, Y., Heussen, N., Grzella, I., & Herpertz-Dahlmann, B. (2005). A retrospective study of SSRI treatment in adolescent anorexia nervosa: Insufficient evidence for efficacy. *Journal of Psychiatric Research, 39*, 303–310.

Ingenhoven, T., Lafay, P., Rinne, T., Passchierj, J., & Duivenvoorden, H. (2010). Effectiveness of pharmacotherapy for severe personality disorders: Meta-analysis of randomized controlled trials. *Journal of Clinical Psychiatry, 71*, 14–25.

Isacsson, J., Holmgren, P., & Ahlner, J. (2005). Selective serotonin reuptake inhibitor antidepressants and the risk of suicide: A controlled forensic database study of 14 857 suicides. *Acta Psychiatrica Scandinavica, 111*, 286–290.

Katz, L. Y., & Fotti, S. (2005). The role of behavioral analysis in the pharmacotherapy of emotionally-dysregulated problem behaviors. *Child and Adolescent Psychopharmacology News, 10*, 1–5.

Kaye, W. H., Frank, G. K., Bailer, U. F., & Henry, S. E. (2005). Neurobiology of anorexia nervosa: Clinical implications of alterations of the function of serotonin and other neuronal systems. *International Journal of Eating Disorders, 37*, S15–S19.

Kaye, W. H., Gendall, K., & Strober, M. (1998). Serotonin neuronal function and selective serotonin reuptake inhibitor treatment in anorexia and bulimia nervosa. *Biological Psychiatry, 44*, 825–838.

Kishi, T., Kafantaris, V., Sunday, S., Sheridan, E. M., & Correll, C. U. (2012). Are antipsychotics effective for the treatment of anorexia nervosa? Results from a systematic review and meta-analysis. *Journal of Clinical Psychiatry, 73*, e757–e766.

Kleindienst, N., Bohus, M., Ludäscher, P., Limberger, M. F., Kuenkele, K., Ebner-Priemer, U. W., et al. (2008). Motives for non-suicidal self-injury among women with borderline personality disorder. *Journal of Nervous and Mental Disease, 196*, 230–236.

Klonsky, E. D. (2007). The functions of deliberate self-injury: A review of the evidence. *Clinical Psychology Review, 27*, 226–239.

Kumra, S., Oberstar, J. V., Sikich, L., Findling, R. L., McClellan, J. M., Vinogradov, S., et al. (2008). Efficacy and tolerability of second-generation antipsychotics in children and adolescents with schizophrenia. *Schizophrenia Bulletin, 34*, 60–71.

Libal, G., & Plener, P. L. (2008). Pharmakologische Therapie des selbstverletzenden Verhaltens im Jugendalter. In R. Brunner & F. Resch (Eds.), *Borderline-Störungen und selbstverletzendes Verhalten bei Jugendlichen* (pp. 165–195). Göttingen: Vandenhoeck & Ruprecht.

Libal, G., Plener, P. L., Ludolph, A. G., & Fegert, J. M. (2005). Ziprasidone as a weight-neutral treatment alternative in the treatment of self-injurious behavior in adolescent females. *Child and Adolescent Psychopharmacology News, 10*, 1–6.

Linehan, M. M., McDavid, J. D., Brown, M. Z., Sayrs, J. H., & Gallop, R. J. (2008). Olanzapine plus dialectical behaviour therapy for women with high irritability who meet criteria for borderline personality disorder: A double-blind, placebo-controlled pilot study. *Journal of Clinical Psychiatry, 69*, 999–1005.

Markovitz, P. J., Calabrese, J. R., Schulz, C., & Meltzer, H. Y. (1991). Fluoxetine in the treatment of borderline and schizotypal personality disorders. *American Journal of Psychiatry, 18*, 1064–1067.

Masters, K. J. (2008). Anti-suicidal and self-harm properties of lithium carbonate. *CNS Spectrums, 13*, 109–110.

McGee, M. D. (1997). Cessation of self-mutilation in a patient with borderline personality disorder treated with naltrexone. *Journal of Clinical Psychiatry, 58*, 32–33.

Mehler-Wex, C., Romanos, M., Kirchheiner, J., & Schulze, U. M. (2008). Atypical anti-psychotics in severe anorexia nervosa in children and adolescents—Review and case reports. *European Eating Disorders Review, 16*, 100–108.

Mercer, D., Douglass, A. B., & Links, P. S. (2009). Meta-analyses of mood stabilizers, antidepressants and antipsychotics in the treatment of borderline personality disorder: Effectiveness for depression and anger symptoms. *Journal of Personality Disorders, 23*, 156–174.

Nickel, M. K., Loew, T. H., & Pedrosa, G. F. (2007). Aripiprazole in treatment of borderline patients, part II: An 18-month follow-up. *Psychopharmacology, 191*, 1023–1026.

Nickel, M. K., Muehlbacher, M., Nickel, K., Kettler, C., Gil, F. P., Bachler, E., et al. (2006). Aripiprazole in the treatment of patients with borderline personality disorder: A double-blind, placebo-controlled study. *American Journal of Psychiatry, 163*, 833–838.

Nixon, M. K., Cloutier, P. F., & Aggarwal, S. (2002). Affect regulation and addictive aspects of repetitive self-injury in hospitalized adolescents. *Journal of the American Academy of Child and Adolescent Psychiatry, 41*, 1333–1341.

Nose, M., Cipriani, A., Biancosino, B., Grassi, L., & Barbui, C. (2006). Efficacy of pharmacotherapy against core traits of borderline personality disorder: Meta-analysis of randomized controlled trials. *International Clinical Psychopharmacology, 21*, 345–353.

Osuch, E. A., & Payne, G. W. (2009). Neurobiological perspectives on self-injury. In M. K. Nixon & N. L. Heath (Eds.), *Self-injury in youth* (pp. 79–111). New York: Routledge.

Owen, C., Rees, A. M., & Parker, G. (2008). The role of fatty acids in the development and treatment of mood disorders. *Current Opinion in Psychiatry, 21*, 19–24.

Parikh, M. S., Kolevzon, A., & Hollander, E. (2008). Psychopharmacology of aggression in children and adolescents with autism: A critical review of efficacy and tolerability. *Journal of Child and Adolescent Psychopharmacology, 18*, 157–178.

Pies, R. W., & Popli, A. P. (1995). Self-injurious behavior: Pathophysiology and implications for treatment. *Journal of Clinical Psychiatry, 56*, 580–588.

Plener, P. L., Libal, G., Fegert, J. M., & Kölch, M. G. (2013). Psychopharmacological treatment of non-suicidal self-injury. *Nervenheilkunde, 32*, 38–41.

Plener, P. L., Libal, G., & Nixon, M. K. (2009). Use of medication in the treatment of nonsuicidal self-injury in youth. In M. K. Nixon & N. L. Heath (Eds.), *Self-injury in youth* (pp. 275–309). New York: Routledge.

Powers, P. S., Klabunde, M., & Kaye, W. (2012). Double-blind placebo-controlled trial of quetiapine in anorexia nervosa. *European Eating Disorders Review, 20*, 331–334.

Roberts, N. (2003). Adolescent self-mutilatory behavior: Psychopharmacological treatment. *Child and Adolescent Psychopharmacology News, 8*, 10–12.

Roth, A. S., Ostroff, R. B., & Hoffman, E. R. (1996). Naltrexone as a treatment for repetitive self-injurious behaviour: An open-label trial. *Journal of Clinical Psychiatry, 57*, 233–237.

Rothschild, A. J., Shindul-Rothschild, J. A., Viguera, A., Murray, M., & Brewster, S. (2000). Comparison of the frequency of behavioural disinhibition on alprazolam, clonazepam, or no benzodiazepine in hospitalized psychiatric patients. *Journal of Clinical Psychopharmacology, 20*, 7–11.

Sandman, C. A. (1990/1991). The opiate hypothesis in autism and self-injury. *Journal of Child and Adolescent Psychopharmacology, 1*, 237–248.

Sandman, C. A. (2009). Psychopharmacologic treatment of nonsuicidal self-injury. In M. K. Nock (Ed.), *Understanding nonsuicidal self-injury. Origins, assessment, and treatment* (pp. 291–323). Washington, DC: American Psychological Association.

Sandman, C. A., Hetrick, W. P., Taylor, D. V., Barron, J. L., Touchette, P., Lott, I., et al. (1993). Naltrexone reduces self-injury and improves learning. *Experimental and Clinical Psychopharmacology, 1*, 242–258.

Scahill, L., & Koenig, K. (1999). Pharmacotherapy in children and adolescents with pervasive developmental disorders. *Journal of Child and Adolescent Psychiatric Nursing, 12*, 41–43.

Schulz, S. C., Zanarini, M. C., Bateman, A., Bohus, M., Detke, H. C., Trzaskoma, Q., et al. (2008). Olanzapine for the treatment of borderline personality disorder: Variable dose 12-week randomised double-blind placebo-controlled study. *British Journal of Psychiatry, 193*, 485–492.

Sher, L., & Stanley, B. (2009). Biological models of nonsuicidal self-injury. In M. K. Nock (Ed.), *Understanding nonsuicidal self-injury. Origins, assessment, and treatment* (pp. 99–117). Washington, DC: American Psychological Association.

Simpson, E. B., Yen, S., Costello, E., Rosen, K., Begin, A., Pistorello, J., et al. (2004). Combined dialectical behavior therapy and fluoxetine in the treatment of borderline personality disorder. *Journal of Clinical Psychiatry, 65*, 379–385.

Sonne, S., Rubey, R., Brady, K., Malcolm, R., & Morris, T. (1996). Naltrexone treatment of self-injurious thoughts and behaviours. *Journal of Nervous and Mental Disease, 184*, 192–195.

Swenne, I., Rosling, A., Tengblad, S., & Vessby, B. (2011). Omega-3 polyunsaturated essential fatty acids are associated with depression in adolescents with eating disorders and weight loss. *Acta Paediatrica, 100*, 1610–1615.

Symons, F. J., Thompson, A., & Rodriguez, M. C. (2004). Self-injurious behaviour and the efficacy of naltrexone treatment: A quantitative synthesis. *Mental Retardation and Developmental Disabilities Research Reviews, 10*, 193–200.

Teicher, M. H., Glod, C. A., & Cole, J. O. (1993). Antidepressant drugs and the emergence of suicidal tendencies. *Drug Safety, 8*, 186–212.

Thompson, T., Hackenberg, T., Cerutti, D., Baker, D., & Axtell, S. (1994). Opioid antagonist effects on self-injury in adults with mental retardation: Response from and location as determinants of medication effects. *American Journal of Mental Retardation, 99*, 85–102.

Trunko, M. E., Schwartz, T. A., Duvvuri, V., & Kaye, W. H. (2011). Aripiprazole in anorexia nervosa and low-weight bulimia nervosa: Case reports. *International Journal of Eating Disorders, 44*, 269–275.

Verkes, R. J., Van der Mast, R. C., Hengeveld, M. W., Tuyl, J. P., Zwinderman, A. H., & Van Kempen, G. M. (1998). Reduction by paroxetine of suicidal behavior in patients with repeated suicide attempts but not major depression. *American Journal of Psychiatry, 155*, 543–547.

Whittington, C. J., Kendall, T., Fonagy, P., Cottrell, D., Cotgrove, A., & Boddington, E. (2004). Selective serotonin reuptake inhibitors in childhood depression: Systematic review of published versus unpublished data. *The Lancet, 36*, 1341–1345.

Zanarini, M. C., & Frankenburg, F. R. (2003). Omega-3 fatty acid treatment of women with borderline personality disorder: A double-blind, placebo-controlled pilot study. *American Journal of Psychiatry, 160*, 167–169.

Part III

Specific Topics

Co-occurring Health-Risk Behaviors of Non-suicidal Self-injury and Eating Disorders

13

Jamie M. Duggan and Nancy L. Heath

Abstract

Health-risk behaviors represent a form of direct and indirect self-injury, and examples include behaviors such as suicide, non-suicidal self-injury (NSSI), alcohol misuse, nicotine use, illicit and licit drug use, disordered eating behaviors, unsafe sexual practices, and other forms of risky or reckless and thrill-seeking behaviors. NSSI and eating disorders (ED) frequently co-occur with other health-risk behaviors among youth and young adults. Studies examining the prevalence of various health-risk behaviors are reviewed from clinical and community NSSI, eating disorders (ED), and NSSI/ED populations of youth and young adults. Trends and patterns regarding the scope and nature of co-occurring health-risk behaviors and NSSI/ED are discussed. Concluding comments center on the implications for the researcher and practitioner with a focus on assessment of health-risk behaviors among at-risk populations.

13.1 Defining Health-Risk-Taking Behaviors

Scholars generally agree that self-destructive behaviors can be conceptualized as either direct (i.e., suicide and non-suicidal self-injury) or indirect (e.g., substance misuse, disordered eating behaviors, sexual-risk-taking behaviors) in form (Boudewyn & Liem, 1995; Hooley & St. Germain, 2009; Nock, 2010; St. Germain & Hooley, 2012). In general, both direct and indirect behaviors represent a risk to overall health; therefore, the term "health-risk behaviors" serves as an umbrella term. Within the literature, the nature of the act, including the immediacy, visibility, and directness of the bodily destruction assists in formally classifying behaviors as either direct or indirect (St. Germain & Hooley, 2012). For example, non-suicidal self-injury (NSSI) refers to

J.M. Duggan (✉) • N.L. Heath
Department of Educational and Counseling Psychology, McGill University, Montreal, QC, Canada
e-mail: jamie.duggan@mail.mcgill.ca

L. Claes and J.J. Muehlenkamp (eds.), *Non-Suicidal Self-Injury in Eating Disorders*, DOI 10.1007/978-3-642-40107-7_13,

highly overt, immediate, direct, and visible forms of tissue destruction, including cutting, picking, object insertion, and burning of the skin (Nock, 2010). Indirect self-injury refers to behaviors that result in the abuse or mistreatment of the body over an extended period of time, but the *nature of harm does not deliberately and directly result in the destruction of body tissue* (Boudewyn & Liem, 1995; Hooley & St. Germain, 2009). Examples of indirect self-injury include behaviors such as smoking tobacco, disordered eating behaviors, substance misuse (e.g., alcohol, nicotine, illicit and licit drugs), unsafe sexual practices, and other forms of risky or reckless and thrill-seeking behaviors (e.g., reckless or impaired driving; Nock, 2010).

Within the literature, indirect and direct self-injuries have been theorized to fall along a continuum, with suicidal behaviors marking an extremity and alternative forms of self-injury falling within the spectrum (e.g., Brausch & Gutierrez, 2010; Favaro, Ferrara, & Santonastaso, 2003; Favazza, DeRosear, & Conterio, 1989; Orbach, 1996; Silverman, Berman, Sanddal, Carroll, & Joiner, 2007). As summarized by Nock (2010) and Svirko and Hawton (2007), all self-destructive behaviors (both direct and indirect) commonly begin in adolescence, represent an individual's attempt to modify feelings and thoughts, result in a degree of bodily harm, and frequently co-occur, supporting the theoretical notion that both NSSI and disordered eating behaviors fall along the spectrum of self-injurious behaviors. One clear distinction concerns the degree of immediate damage done to the tissue, and individuals who engage in indirect health-risk behaviors may be unaware of, or neglect the potential long-term, harmful consequences of such actions (Boudewyn & Liem, 1995). Within the literature, it is argued that indirect behaviors can potentially serve as precursors to more severe, direct forms of self-injury (Nock, 2010). Given the indirect nature of certain health-risk behaviors, youth may be more prone to disclosing their engagement in risky, less overt self-injury (e.g., smoking cigarettes, alcohol misuse) compared to other harmful behaviors such as NSSI and disordered eating behaviors that can be easily concealed and often done in private. As such, knowledge regarding the scope and nature of an individual's engagement in health-risk behaviors can potentially serve as a possible behavioral marker for more severe forms of direct and indirect self-injury.

As the current chapter will illustrate, individuals who engage in NSSI, and/or disordered eating behaviors, also frequently engage in a multitude of other health-risk behaviors, suggesting that health-risk behaviors often co-occur. Although a substantial body of literature has documented this trend, the findings have been predominantly descriptive or correlational in nature. As such, the implications and consequences of these associations remain largely undetermined. For example, it remains unclear if less severe forms of self-injury (e.g., alcohol and drug misuse, sexual-risk-taking behaviors) serve as precursors or consequences of NSSI and/or disordered eating behaviors or arise from additional underlying causes that remain to be determined. The objective of the current review is to assist researchers and clinicians in understanding different behavioral profiles of youth and young adults who engage in both direct and indirect forms of self-injury. Identifying distinct and shared health-risk behavioral correlates represent an important step in further understanding the etiology underlying co-occurring NSSI and eating disorders.

13.2 NSSI and Co-occurring Health-Risk-Taking Behaviors

The available literature strongly suggests that individuals who engage in NSSI are also likely to engage in a wide range of additional health-risk behaviors. Among the spectrum of health-risk behaviors, substance use has received the majority of empirical attention, with studies reporting that almost 60 % of NSSI inpatient adolescents meet DSM-IV criteria for a substance-related disorder (Nock, Joiner, Gordon, Lloyd-Richardson, & Prinstein, 2006). This is substantially higher than prevalence rates (25 %) of substance-related disorders observed among non-NSSI adolescent inpatients (Wu, Gersing, Burchett, Woody, & Blazer, 2011). In addition to alcohol and substance misuse, self-asphyxiation, sexual-risk behaviors, cigarette smoking, and general reckless and risk-taking behaviors have been documented among youth and young adults with a history of NSSI at a higher rate than non-NSSI adolescents (e.g., Brausch, Decker, & Hadley, 2011; Brown, Houck, Grossman, Lescano, & Frenkel, 2008; Hilt, Nock, Lloyd-Richardson, & Prinstein, 2008; Laye-Gindhu & Schonert-Reichl, 2005; Lloyd-Richardson, Perrine, Dierker, & Kelley, 2007; Matsumoto & Imamura, 2008; Nock, Prinstein, & Sterba, 2009; Taliaferro, Muehlenkamp, Borowsky, McMorris, & Kugler, 2012). It is important to note that the association between NSSI and other health-risk behaviors remains a somewhat novel area of examination. As such, some behaviors have been studied substantially more than others. This makes it difficult to conclusively conclude if specific behaviors (i.e., self-asphyxiation, sexual risk taking) co-occur less frequently than others (i.e., substance use), or simply remain understudied. Thus, what follows is a review of the available literature among adolescents and young adults regarding the association between NSSI and other health-risk behaviors. Again, the review of the available literature does not necessarily reflect the strength of the relationship, but merely the state of the field of study.

13.2.1 NSSI and Health-Risk Behaviors in Adolescent Samples

Adolescence also represents a developmental period that confers particular risk for NSSI engagement. In addition to markedly elevated prevalence rates, the majority of youth who report engaging in NSSI describe the behavior as beginning between the ages of 12 and 15 years (Rodham & Hawton, 2009; Ross & Heath, 2002). Additionally, adolescence is a period where experimenting with certain health-risk behaviors (e.g., cigarette smoking, alcohol and substance use) represents a common developmental norm. Understanding the behavioral correlates of NSSI represents a step in identifying factors that can potentially contribute to the cause and maintenance of the behavior. Thus, a review of the relationship between NSSI and the engagement in other health-risk behaviors during adolescence offers a valuable opportunity to understand the temporal nature (i.e., emergence) and nature of the overlap between both indirect and direct self-injury.

A consistent pattern that emerges within the literature is that NSSI is associated with multiple health-risk behavioral correlates. For example, Laye-Gindhu and

Schonert-Reichl (2005) investigated the association between NSSI and other health-risk behaviors among a community sample of 425 adolescents aged 13–18. Adolescents who engaged in NSSI were more likely to report other health-compromising behaviors when compared to their non-NSSI peers, including suicidal ideation and behaviors, illicit drug use, and reckless and/or impaired driving. Only females who reported engaging in NSSI were more likely to report smoking. Additionally, adolescents who reported engaging in NSSI also endorsed higher levels of emotional distress (Laye-Gindhu & Schonert-Reichl, 2005). In a similar study, Hilt and colleagues examined health-risk behavioral correlates among a sample of over 500 high-school students from sixth to eighth grade. Their findings indicate that adolescents who reported engaging in NSSI were more likely than their non-NSSI peers to have engaged in hard drug use, nicotine use, sexual intercourse under the influence of a substance, and maladaptive eating behaviors, such as binging and fasting (Hilt et al., 2008). Taken together, both studies provide evidence that NSSI frequently co-occurs with additional health-risk behaviors, highlighting that NSSI youth are more at risk for a variety of health-risk behaviors during adolescence. More recently, Taliaferro et al. (2012) surveyed 61,330 youth in grades 9–12 in an attempt to understand health-risk behavior profiles of youth who reported engaging in NSSI. Results indicated that both male and female youth who reported engaging in NSSI were more likely to run away from home and engage in maladaptive dieting behaviors compared to their non-NSSI peers. Similar to the findings of Laye-Gindhu and Schonert-Reichl (2005), female NSSI youth were more likely to smoke cigarettes and engage in prescription drug misuse compared to NSSI males (Taliaferro et al., 2012). Such studies provide direct evidence regarding the variable nature of how "health-risk behaviors" are conceptualized and measured within the literature. For example, Laye-Gindhu and Schonert-Reichl (2005) used traditional behaviors (such as illicit drug use) and reckless and thrill-seeking behaviors (such as reckless or impaired driving) and included body modification (tattoos), whereas Taliaferro et al. (2012) included a wider range of behaviors, in addition to "skipping school" and "running away from home." Regardless, the three studies reported similar results regarding the co-occurring nature of both direct and indirect health-risk behaviors, highlighting the need to assess for a wide range of health-risk behaviors when examining behavioral correlates among NSSI youth. Future studies would benefit from taking a longitudinal approach in order to understand the temporal nature of this association (i.e., are certain health-risk behaviors precursors or consequences for other health-risk behaviors, or do they arise from additional underlying interpersonal causes not examined?).

Youth who engage in NSSI also report engaging in significantly more sexual-risk-taking behaviors. In one of the first studies to examine the association between NSSI and health and sexual-risk-taking behaviors, DiClemente, Ponton, and Hartley (1991) reported that 27 % of adolescent inpatients who reported engaging in NSSI also reported sharing cutting implements, an act that placed them directly at risk for human immunodeficiency virus (HIV; DiClemente et al., 1991). In a series of follow-up studies, Brown, Houck, Hadley, and Lescano (2005) and

Brown et al. (2008) reported that frequent NSSI was significantly associated with being sexually active and sharing cutting instruments among adolescent inpatient population with various psychiatric diagnoses. Interestingly, even though adolescents who engaged in NSSI were more knowledgeable about HIV than their non-NSSI peers, they were three and a half times more likely to use condoms inconsistently during intercourse. Additionally, risky sexual behaviors remained uniquely associated with NSSI after controlling for gender, sexual abuse history, and additional psychological variables, including impulsivity (Brown et al., 2005, 2008).

In one of the most recent studies examining NSSI and health-risk-related behaviors, Brausch et al. (2011) extended previous findings by included self-asphyxial risk-taking behavior (SAB) in their conceptualization of health-risk behaviors. SAB represents a form of indirect self-injury, and is commonly referred to as the "choking game," and results in a euphoric high through the act of self-asphyxiation (Brausch et al., 2011). Additional behaviors assessed included measures of direct self-injury (i.e., NSSI and suicidal behaviors) as well as indirect self-injury (i.e., alcohol/substance use and disordered eating behaviors). The sample included 4,693 adolescents in grades 9–12. Results indicated that 21 % of the students reported engaging in NSSI, 16.5 % reported engaging in SAB, and 6.5 % of youth reported engaging in both behaviors. Adolescents who endorsed both NSSI and SAB reported higher levels of additional health-risk behaviors, including substance use, suicidal ideation/attempts, and disordered eating behaviors, than adolescents who engaged in neither behavior, or only engaged in one of the behaviors. These findings add to current knowledge by identifying a new dangerous and potentially life-threatening health-risk behavior that appears to be quite prevalent among youth in general, as well as among those who engage in NSSI. It is possible that SAB represents a gateway behavior for additional health-risk behaviors that are more difficult to access at a young age (e.g., drugs and alcohol). It may also represent a clinically valuable marker that indicates that adolescents are more open and willing to partake in additional risk-taking behaviors, including alcohol and substance use and direct forms of self-injury, such as NSSI and suicidal behaviors and ideation (Brausch et al., 2011).

Beyond studies investigating prevalence rates and general behavioral correlates, preliminary evidence also supports an association between health-risk behaviors and the severity of NSSI behaviors. Lloyd-Richardson et al. (2007) examined the association between health-risk behaviors and NSSI characteristics (i.e., severity, methodology, and frequency) among a sample of 263 community adolescents. Participants who reported engaging in NSSI within the past year were grouped according to NSSI methodology. Minor NSSI included picking, hitting, pulling hair out, and inserting objects under nails and skin. Moderate/severe NSSI included cutting/carving skin, burning skin, self-tattooing, and scraping and erasing skin. Adolescents who engaged in moderate/severe NSSI were more likely to engage in NSSI under the influence of drugs and alcohol compared to those who engaged in minor NSSI. Additionally, those who reported moderate/severe NSSI reported using more types of self-injury and engaged in NSSI behaviors more often than the minor NSSI group. As suggested by the authors, it is likely that substance use prior to and during NSSI episodes reduces inhibition and impairs an adolescent's judgment, resulting in more severe tissue damage. Although preliminary, these findings indicate that the use of health-related risk behaviors during NSSI episodes appear to be indicative of a more severe NSSI profile and prognosis (Lloyd-Richardson et al., 2007).

To date, the bulk of the literature identifying an overlap between NSSI and other health-risk behaviors has used a similar methodology, relying mainly on retrospective, self-report data. Nock et al. (2009) took a novel approach by examining the overlap of self-injurious thoughts and behaviors (SITBI's) and health-risk behaviors using an ecological momentary assessment (EMA) measure. The EMA approach measures thoughts and behaviors as they in real time; participants were asked to complete event and signal-contingent assessments over a 14-day period on handheld computers (Nock et al., 2009). The community sample included 30 adolescents and young adults aged 12–19, with a recent history of NSSI. Results indicated that thoughts of alcohol and drug use and binging and purging co-occurred with thoughts of NSSI, 15–20 % of the time. However, the *use* of alcohol and drugs overlapped only 3–5 % with NSSI thoughts, suggesting that the majority of incidences occurred during sobriety, and none of the health-risk behaviors were significant predictors of actual NSSI behaviors. Although preliminary, such findings suggest that substance use may play a limited role in the transition between NSSI thoughts and behaviors, and other factors may be at play (Nock et al., 2009). Additionally, the methodology offers a unique and valuable approach for studying the overlap between health-risk behaviors and NSSI and warrants replication among community and clinical samples of youth and young adults.

In addition to examining health-risk behavioral correlates of NSSI, Matsumoto and Imamura (2008) tangentially investigated the degree of access to health-risk behaviors and social relationships among almost 3,000 Japanese high-school students. The investigators reported that NSSI was positively associated with the use of tobacco and alcohol, as well as illicit drug use, and that youth who reported engaging in NSSI were more likely to report having friends or acquaintances using illicit drugs. Participants also reported experiencing more temptations to engage in substance use than their non-NSSI peers. Building upon these findings, using an exploratory and qualitative approach, Deliberto and Nock (2008) examined family history of health-risk behaviors among a community sample of 64 adolescents with a history of NSSI. The authors reported that adolescents who reported engaging in NSSI were significantly more likely to have a family history of alcoholism and drug abuse compared to their non-NSSI peers. Taken together, such findings are of concern as they suggest that NSSI youth are more likely to be immersed in a social environment (i.e., home and school) in which high-risk health behaviors are easily accessible and available and can successfully access health risk-related behaviors more easily than non-NSSI youth (Deliberto & Nock, 2008; Matsumoto & Imamura, 2008).

In sum, the literature strongly supports an association between NSSI and the co-occurring engagement in numerous additional health-risk behaviors, including suicidal ideation and behaviors, alcohol and substance misuse, nicotine use, self-asphyxiation, sexual-risk-taking behaviors, and other reckless and thrill-seeking behaviors (e.g., running away from home). Further, the literature suggests a need to investigate the use of health-related risk behaviors, such as substance use, during NSSI incidences, due to the implications such health-risk behaviors can potentially have on NSSI episode outcomes. The use of health-related risk behaviors during NSSI episodes appears to be indicative of a more severe NSSI profile and prognosis among adolescents, although this area warrants further investigation. Additionally, although preliminary, a small body of literature suggests that the home and social environment may play a role in the association between NSSI and other co-occurring health-risk behaviors.

13.2.2 NSSI and Health-Risk Behaviors in Adult Samples

Despite reports that 80 % of adolescents typically stop engaging in NSSI within 5 years of the initial onset, the behavior can often persist into adulthood (Whitlock, Eckenrode, & Silverman, 2006). Moreover, the increased ease and relative access adults have to other health-risk behaviors compared to adolescents may play a role in the nature and types of health-risk behavior utilized. Thus, examining the association between NSSI and other health-risk behaviors in adulthood is important and may serve to provide information regarding the developmental trajectory of NSSI and other co-occurring health-risk behaviors. To date, a small but growing body of literature has documented that the association between health-risk behaviors and NSSI carries on into adulthood (e.g., Haw, Hawton, Casey, Bale, & Shepherd, 2005; Serras, Saules, Cranford, & Eisenberg, 2010; Williams & Hasking, 2010). In a wide-scale study, Serras et al. (2010) examined the extent to which NSSI was associated with different forms of health-risk behaviors among 5,689 undergraduate and graduate college students. The investigators reported that drug use and frequent binge drinking were associated with more frequent NSSI engagement. Although binge drinking was associated with an increased risk for NSSI, drug use (not limited to marijuana) was associated with nearly a threefold risk for NSSI engagement. College students who endorsed engaging in both NSSI and drug use also reported increased rates of depression, cigarette smoking, and binge eating. Furthermore, depression, cigarette use, and drug use were significant, independent predictors of past-year NSSI engagement, whereas binge drinking and binge eating were not (Serras et al., 2010). Extending upon these findings, Williams and Hasking (2010) examined the association between alcohol misuse, psychological distress, coping styles, and NSSI engagement among 289 young adults aged 18–30. Young adults who reported engaging in NSSI reported greater levels of psychological distress and were more likely to engage in frequent risky drinking. The authors suggest that the combination of increased psychological distress, poor coping skills, and risky drinking poses a risk for NSSI engagement. Both studies highlight the importance of taking into account the synergistic combination of health-risk behaviors and psychological distress when examining the relationship between health-risk behaviors and NSSI and are similar to previous findings among adolescent samples (Laye-Gindhu & Schonert-Reichl, 2005) suggesting that elevated levels of emotional distress and poor emotional coping are present in both youth and young adults who report simultaneous engagement in NSSI and other health-risk behaviors. Additionally, these findings lend validation to previous findings (Nock et al., 2009), which suggest that substance use may play a limited role in the transition between NSSI thoughts and behaviors and that other factors such as psychological distress and lack of appropriate coping strategies may play a role in explaining the frequent co-occurrence of NSSI and other health-risk behaviors (Nock et al., 2009).

Similarly, Haw et al. (2005) examined the trends of alcohol consumption before and during incidences of DSH among inpatients aged 15–24 between 1989 and 2002. It is important to note that DSH consists of a broad range of health risk-taking behaviors, both direct and indirect, such as hanging, self-poisoning, and deliberate substance abuse, and does not distinguish between behaviors with and without suicidal intent (Haw, Houston, Townsend, & Hawton, 2002). Results indicated that 8.6 % of DSH inpatients were diagnosed with alcohol dependence, and 23.4 % were diagnosed with excessive drinking. Additionally, more than one third of patients drank alcohol within 6 h of engaging in a DSH episode, and 18 % reported consuming alcohol while engaging in DSH. Rates of alcohol disorders and consumption were significantly higher in males who engaged in DSH but substantial increases were seen in females of all ages over time with respect to excessive drinking and alcohol consumption rates (Haw et al., 2005). These findings suggest that engaging in substance use is also related to self-destructive behaviors in adulthood and identifies potential gender differences with respect to the developmental trajectory of the association.

In sum, it appears that NSSI frequently co-occurs with a multitude of health-risk behaviors among both adolescents and young adults, highlighting the need to assess for a wide range of health-risk behaviors. Further, the literature suggests a need to investigate the use of health-related risk behaviors, specifically substance and alcohol use, during NSSI incidences and the implications such health-risk behaviors can potentially have on NSSI episode outcomes (e.g., exacerbating negative effect, reducing inhibition). In addition to identifying health-risk behavioral correlates, researchers have also documented the presence of elevated emotional distress and lack of appropriate coping skills among youth and young adults who engage in NSSI and other health-risk behaviors (Laye-Gindhu & Schonert-Reichl, 2005; Williams & Hasking, 2010). Given that NSSI is frequently cited as an emotion regulation strategy (Klonsky & Muehlenkamp, 2007), continuing to assess for levels of emotional distress and emotion dysregulation, as well as other factors such as impulsivity (Glenn & Klonsky, 2011; St. Germain & Hooley, 2012), represents an important avenue in elucidating as to why youth who engage in NSSI are at risk for engagement in a wide range of health-risk behaviors.

13.3 Eating Disorders and Co-occurring Health Risk-Taking Behaviors

A more extensive and comprehensive body of literature exists regarding the association between eating disorders (ED) and/or disordered eating behaviors and other health-risk behaviors. This is due to the heterogeneous nature of the ED population in general and the spectrum of subclinical eating behaviors that have been examined in the literature. In addition to the DSM-IV diagnosis of ED, subclinical diagnoses, including eating disorder not otherwise specified (EDNOS), and pathological eating behaviors (e.g., binge eating, purging behaviors, food restriction) have also been examined, as they serve as precursors to ED (Svirko & Hawton, 2007). As such, studies on the co-morbidity of eating disorders and substance use vary dramatically with respect to the conceptualization and definition of eating pathology. For example, some studies have used DSM-IV diagnostic criteria for eating disorders, whereas others use different scales of ED and disordered eating behavior symptom severity (Svirko & Hawton, 2007). Therefore, what follows is a brief and selective review of health-risk behaviors and a spectrum of pathological eating behaviors among adolescents and adults from clinical and community samples. For comprehensive reviews concerning the association between disordered eating behaviors and various health-risk behaviors, see Holderness, Brooks-Gunn, and Warren (1994) and Wolfe and Maisto (2000).

Similar to the NSSI/health-risk behavior literature, substance use disorders are the most extensively studied health-risk behavior in the ED literature. A large body of literature has successfully documented an association between ED and substance use among clinical samples of adolescents and young adults with a diagnosed ED. It is estimated that about 12–18 % of people with anorexia nervosa and 30–70 % of individuals with bulimia nervosa abuse alcohol, tobacco, or other substances [see Holderness et al. (1994)]. In general, individuals who binge eat or have bulimia nervosa (BN) tend to report a higher prevalence of alcohol problems than individuals with a diagnosis of restriction-type anorexia nervosa (Holderness et al., 1994). Studies in community-based samples of women indicate that the relationship between eating disorders and substance use extends beyond the limits of clinically diagnosed disorders to less severe levels and subclinical levels of disordered eating behaviors (e.g., Field et al., 2012; Krahn, Kurth, Gomberg, & Drewnowski, 2005).

13.3.1 ED and Health-Risk Behaviors in Adolescence Samples

Adolescence is the typical time of onset for the emergence of subclinical disordered eating behaviors, which serve as a developmental precursor to diagnosable eating disorders (Lock, Reisel, & Steiner, 2001). Factors that contribute to the transition of subclinical symptoms to a diagnosable eating disorder remain to be determined (Lock et al., 2001). As previously mentioned, engagement in other health risk-taking behaviors also emerge during this time, and it is possible that alternative forms of self-injury (e.g., substance use, sexual-risk-taking behaviors) contribute to this transition; thus, the association between disordered eating behaviors and health-risk behaviors warrants further investigation. A large body of literature has focused on patterns of covariation between a range of disordered eating behaviors and other health-risk behaviors and has successfully demonstrated that youth with disordered eating behaviors are at increased risk for engaging in an array of other health-risk behaviors (e.g., Fisher, Higgins-D'Alessandro, Rau, Kuther, & Belanger, 1996; Lock et al., 2001; Neumark-Sztainer, Story, Dixon, & Murray,

1998; Pisetsky, Chao, Dierker, May, & Striegel-Moore, 2008). In one of the first studies to examine the association between disordered eating behaviors and other health-risk behaviors, Fisher et al. (1996) reported that in a sample of 268 high-school students, students with abnormal eating attitudes and behaviors were more likely to smoke cigarettes, consume alcohol, use illicit substances, and engage in sexual activity with more partners, as well as report lower self-esteem and higher levels of emotional distress. Similarly, Neumark-Sztainer et al. (1998) examined the association between severity of disordered eating behaviors and engagement in alcohol use, marijuana use, and unprotected sexual activity, among 9th through 12th graders using a school-based survey. Results indicated that both male and female adolescents who reported engaging in extreme disordered eating behaviors (i.e., self-induced vomiting and diet pill use) were more likely to utilize all health risk-related behaviors when compared to their peers who engaged in less severe eating behaviors. Additionally, a strong association was documented between extreme weight control behaviors and suicidal thoughts and behaviors (Neumark-Sztainer et al., 1998). Both studies indicate that similar to the NSSI literature, health-risk behaviors tend to frequently co-occur, and an association exists between the severity/nature of disordered eating behaviors and health-risk behaviors, lending support to the notion that other health-risk behaviors can serve as a marker regarding severity of ED and disordered eating behaviors, which in turn may serve as an indicator of possible suicidal thoughts and behaviors (Fisher et al., 1996; Neumark-Sztainer et al., 1998).

Studies have also reported gender differences in relation to disordered eating behaviors and health-risk behaviors. For example, Lock et al. (2001) compared the health-risk behaviors of high-school adolescents with and without disordered eating behaviors. The investigators reported that regardless of gender, adolescents who reported engaging in disordered eating behaviors were more at risk for engaging in other health-risk behaviors when compared to their non-disordered eating peers. Co-occurring health-risk behaviors of boys and girls with disordered eating behaviors were mostly similar, but some gender differences did emerge. Boys with disordered eating behaviors were at equal risk to their non-disordered eating behavior peers for using drugs and drinking alcohol but were more at risk for smoking cigarettes. Females with disordered eating behaviors showed significant increased risk for engagement in all risk-taking behaviors compared to their female peers, including smoking cigarettes and marijuana, drinking alcohol, and sexually risk-taking behaviors. These findings suggest that females who engage in disordered eating behaviors engage in more externalizing health-risk behaviors (i.e., substance use and sexual-risk-taking behaviors) than their peers that do not display disordered eating behaviors and appear to be at greater risk for engaging in other health-risk behaviors than males with similar disordered eating behaviors. The authors suggest that adolescence may represent a salient period that leads to divergent developmental paths for males and females with disordered eating behaviors as females appear to be more at risk for engaging in more overall externalizing health-risk behaviors in addition to their disordered eating behaviors when compared to males with similar difficulties (Lock et al., 2001).

In a recent large study by Field et al. (2012), investigators examined the overlap between health risk-related behaviors (i.e., alcohol consumption and illicit drug use) among 8,594 female participants aged 9–15 over a 2-year period. Participants presented with eating disorder not otherwise specified (EDNOS), bulimia nervosa (BN), or non-disordered. Results indicated that females who presented with purging disorder (a subgroup of EDNOS) had significantly increased risk of binge drinking and using drugs. Such findings extend previous knowledge as they support an association between health-risk behaviors and less prevalent and studied forms of disordered eating that are classified as "subthreshold," specifically purging disorder.

One limitation within the ED/health-risk literature concerns how supplementary health-risk behaviors are often conceptually measured and defined. The majority of studies focus on alcohol and marijuana use and do not sufficiently examine various typologies of illicit substances. In one of the most large-scale studies to date examining disordered eating and health-risk behaviors among adolescents, Pisetsky et al. (2008) examined the association between gender, disordered eating (fasting, diet product use, or purging), and use of multiple substances (i.e., cigarette, alcohol, marijuana, cocaine, inhalants, heroin, methamphetamines, ecstasy, steroids, and hallucinogens) in a school-based study of over 13,000 students. Results indicated that disordered eating was significantly associated with the use of each substance. With regard to gender differences, for female students, associations between substance use and disordered eating were strongest for smoking, binge drinking, and inhalants. For male students, strong associations were found for marijuana, steroids, and inhalants. Such findings call attention to the necessity of also assessing multiple substances when examining health-risk behaviors among males and females who report disordered eating behaviors (Pisetsky et al., 2008) and again document gender differences with respect to substance used.

In sum, it appears that ED and disordered eating behaviors among youth are also associated with a multitude of other health-risk behaviors, including suicidal ideation and behaviors, illicit and licit substance use, alcohol consumption, nicotine use, and sexual risk-taking behaviors, highlighting the need to assess for a wide variety of health-risk behaviors when working with clinical and subclinical youth. Moreover, it appears that an association exists between the severity/nature of disordered eating behaviors and engagement in other health-risk behaviors, lending support to the notion that other health-risk behaviors can serve as a marker regarding severity of ED and disordered eating behavioral symptoms, which in turn may serve as an indicator of possible suicidal thoughts and behaviors.

13.3.2 ED and Health-Risk Behaviors in Adult Samples

It appears that substance use and disordered eating behaviors share a complex and intricate relationship that carries on into adulthood (e.g., Gadalla & Piran, 2007; Krahn et al., 2005; Piran & Robinson, 2006; Wiederman & Pryor, 1996). Piran and Robinson (2006) examined the association between disordered eating behaviors and substance use among a sample of over 500 female university students. Results indicated that 9 % of 15–24-year-old women at risk of eating disorders were identified as alcohol dependent, compared to 4.1 % of women who were not at risk of eating disorders. Additionally, results indicate that eating disordered behaviors are differentially related to the use of various substance classes. For example, purging behaviors were associated with stimulant use, whereas severe levels of alcohol consumption, tobacco use, and prescription medication usage were associated with binge eating. Furthermore, the investigators reported that as disordered eating behaviors increased in severity and frequency, the number of substance classes used increased. Extending these results to examine gender influences in a wide-scale Canadian study, Gadalla and Piran (2007) investigated disordered eating behaviors and health-risk behaviors among adolescents and young adults 15 years and older. Results indicated that alcohol use and amphetamine use were associated with disordered eating in both males and females. Among females, disordered eating was associated with illicit drug use and dependence, as well as with the number of substance classes used. Such findings highlight the intricate and complex nature of the relationship between particular types of eating disturbances and the use of numerous substances and highlight the need for further examination in order to understand the function of these co-occurring behaviors.

Broadening previous findings to include sexual risk-taking behaviors, Wiederman and Pryor (1996) examined health-risk behaviors among females aged 18–35 who met criteria for BN-purging type. The investigators categorized participants into two groups: BN who displayed impulsive behaviors and those who did not display impulsive behaviors. Results indicated that young females with BN/impulsivity reported an earlier age of BN onset, a greater number of overall sexual experiences, and a younger age of first sexual episode and had tried a greater number of illicit substances (Wiederman & Pryor, 1996). Such findings suggest that impulsivity may play a role in the decision to experiment with health-risk behaviors in addition to disordered eating behaviors. Extending these findings, Krahn et al. (2005) investigated negative consequences associated with alcohol use among 1,384 college women who reported engaging in dysfunctional eating behaviors and reported that severity of both dieting and binging behaviors were positively associated with the prevalence of negative consequences of alcohol use, including blacking out and unintended sexual activity and smoking cigarettes (Krahn et al., 2005). Moreover, dieting and binging severity was associated with binge drinking (e.g., heavy drinking, drinking to get drunk, prevalence of past-month alcohol use). Taken together, such findings suggest that particular eating disordered behaviors appear to be differentially related to the use of various substance classes and that the number of substance classes can potentially serve as a marker of the severity of disordered eating symptoms and sexual-risk behaviors (Krahn et al., 2005; Piran & Robinson, 2006; Wiederman & Pryor, 1996).

13.4 Overlap: Examining NSSI/ED and Additional Health-Risk Behaviors

Few studies have examined the existence of other health-related risk behaviors among individuals with co-occurring NSSI/ED despite arguments that risk-taking behaviors, NSSI, and ED are clinically, conceptually, and empirically linked (e.g., Glenn & Klonsky, 2011; Muehlenkamp, Peat, Claes, & Smits, 2012; Vrouva, Fonagy, Fearon, & Roussow, 2010). Such studies would assist in clarifying which health-risk behavioral correlates are specific and unique to NSSI/ED co-occurrence. To begin, examining the co-occurrence of NSSI, ED, and health-risk behaviors, Nagata, Oshima, Wada, Yamada, and Kiriike (2003) reported that repetitive self-injury was more prevalent among inpatients with co-occurring ED and drug abuse than in patients with drug abuse only. Similarly, Solano, Fernández Aranda, Aitken, López, and Vallejo (2005) reported that drug use was positively correlated with NSSI in a small sample of inpatients with ED (Solano et al., 2005). Moving beyond behavioral correlates, Claes, Vanderycken, and Vertommen (2003) examined the co-occurrence of health-risk behaviors among 70 ED female inpatients and reported that female ED inpatients who also reported engaging in NSSI reported higher levels of physical fighting and alcohol consumption compared to ED inpatients who did not report engaging NSSI. Moreover, results indicated that participants with both ED/NSSI reported higher levels of impulsivity and emotional distress (i.e., anxiety and depression) compared to participants who reported only engaging in ED. In a more recent study, Peebles, Wilson, and Lock (2011) retrospectively examined the prevalence of self-injurious behaviors in a large clinical sample of 1,432 adolescents with a diagnosed eating disorder. Results indicated that adolescents with both ED and NSSI were more likely to be older or female, have a longer ED diagnosis, and present with a history of substance misuse (e.g., alcohol, marijuana, prescription drugs). A recent study by Claes et al. (2012) investigated the presence of health-risk behaviors among an inpatient sample of 130 males with a diagnosed eating disorder. Results indicated that males with a history of NSSI reported more severe ED symptoms and similar to Claes et al. (2003), greater impulse-control problems and affective issues compared to males without an NSSI history. Specifically the NSSI/ED group reported greater suicidal ideation, aggression towards the self and others, and drug abuse. In sum, the literature suggests that a combination of NSSI/ED is associated with more severe ED symptomology and a greater likelihood of other health-risk behaviors. Future replication of these findings among clinical and community samples of males and females would contribute greatly to the current understanding of general and specific health-risk behaviors associated with co-occurring NSSI/ED.

13.5 Summary: Patterns and Trends of Health-Risk Behaviors in NSSI and ED

With regard to adolescent engagement in NSSI, the general consensus within the literature indicates that both clinical and community samples of youth who engage in NSSI are more likely to engage in a range of health-risk behaviors when compared to their non-NSSI peers. Such behaviors include alcohol misuse, cigarette smoking, maladaptive eating/dieting behaviors, illicit and licit substance use, sexual risk-taking behaviors, self-asphyxiation behaviors, and suicidal ideation and behaviors. Additionally, it appears that youth who engage in more severe forms of

NSSI are more likely to use drugs/alcohol during NSSI episodes. Furthermore, it appears that youth who engage in NSSI are more likely to have peers, acquaintances, and family members that engage in similar health-risk behaviors. A review of health-risk behaviors in adulthood suggests that similar trends carry on into adulthood, and adults who engage in NSSI are likely to engage in substance-related health-risk behaviors, including alcohol misuse, and licit and illicit substance misuse as well as cigarette smoking and risky sexual behaviors. Preliminary findings concerning gender differences also indicate that females may be at greater risk for engaging in NSSI and certain health-risk behaviors (i.e., cigarette smoking), although further investigation is warranted. The literature clearly suggests that NSSI engagement in adulthood is associated with increased substance use over time, alcohol dependence, and substance use disorder diagnoses. Among both adolescents and young adults, higher levels of both emotional distress and impulsivity were also documented among individuals who reported engaging in supplementary health-risk behaviors in addition to NSSI.

Similar to the NSSI literature, common health-risk behaviors that most often occur in youth and young adult clinical and community ED populations typically include cigarette smoking, alcohol and substance use, risky sexual behaviors, and suicidal ideation/behaviors. With regard to gender differences, it appears that females are more likely to smoke, binge drink, and use inhalants, whereas males are more likely to use marijuana, steroids, and inhalants in addition to their clinical and subclinical disordered eating behaviors. Moreover, different substance classes appear to be related to various levels of disordered eating behaviors, highlighting the need for assessing multiple substances as well as examining clinical and subclinical levels of disordered eating behaviors. Studies reporting on the co-occurrence of NSSI/ED suggest that similar additional health-risk behaviors are evident among this population, although it remains much less studied. Studies suggest that individuals who present with both NSSI and ED are more likely to report greater ED symptom severity, engage in alcohol and illicit substance use, and report higher levels of aggression towards the self and others than those who do not present with NSSI/ED. Individuals who present with co-occurring NSSI/ED and engage in supplementary health-risk behaviors tend to report higher levels of impulsivity and emotional distress (i.e., anxiety and depression) compared to individuals who present with either NSSI or ED. Such findings offer an important step in understanding the specific risk factors associated with the co-occurrence of NSSI/ED and highlight the need for assessing multiple health-risk behaviors as well as specific intrapersonal risk factors in order to further understand the complex association.

13.6 Clinical Implications: Assessment and Intervention

In light of the conclusions of the current literature, simply stated, all self-injurers (indirect and direct) should be screened for suicide risk and for the presence of other risky or health-compromising behaviors. Knowledge of the frequency and severity of the health-risk behaviors can provide valuable insight regarding NSSI and ED severity. Additionally, the co-occurrence of health-risk behaviors suggests that youth and young adults who engage in one health-risk behavior are more likely to experiment with additional behaviors. It is possible that certain behaviors serve as a catalyst for other, more severe, and potentially life-threatening behaviors. Assessment should include inquiring about frequency and timing of risk behaviors, given the behavioral influences of alcohol and certain illicit substances and the potential danger of using them while engaging in NSSI and ED behaviors (e.g., severe restricting, binging, and purging).

In order to effectively assist youth and young adults in developing adaptive coping strategies, it is necessary for clinicians to accurately understand the scope and nature of the health-risk behaviors in which the individual is engaging. Thus, it is suggested that a basic functional analysis be completed with the individual in order to understand health-risk thoughts and behaviors as they occur naturally. As described elsewhere [see Lewis, Heath, Michal, and Duggan (2012)], clinicians should ask youth and young adults to keep a weekly log to record health-risk behaviors and NSSI and ED episodes. Specifically, the individual should record health-risk behaviors and thoughts and feelings that precede, occur during, and follow NSSI and ED episodes. A detailed log will assist in documenting the nature, scope, and frequency of both the health-risk behavior(s) and NSSI/ED episodes. Additionally, such information will provide insight concerning the temporal nature and association between the behaviors, as well as which behavior takes precedence with regard to treatment and intervention efforts.

An additional topic that should be addressed when working with NSSI and ED populations concerns the social environment and access that the individual has to health-risk behaviors. As evidenced, NSSI youth can access health risk-related behaviors more easily than non-NSSI youth and are more likely to be immersed in a social environment in which high-risk health behaviors are easily accessible and available (Deliberto & Nock, 2008; Matsumoto & Imamura, 2008). Clinicians would benefit from inquiring about peer relationships and social networks to further understand the social environment that the individual may be exposed to and the influence such interactions have on the engagement in health-risk behaviors.

The reviewed literature suggests that adolescents and young adults who have difficulty regulating emotions and present as impulsive and distressed may be more likely to experiment with high risk-taking behaviors in an attempt to manage overwhelming affect. Interventions that focus on decreasing health-risk behaviors and impulsivity and promote the development of self-regulation, build adaptive coping strategies for managing overwhelming affect, and foster communication skills (i.e., dialectic behavioral therapy) represent valuable avenues (Miller, Muehlenkamp, & Jacobson, 2009).

13.7 Case Vignette

13.7.1 Presentation of Co-occurring Health-Risk Behaviors

Stephanie is a 14-year-old female who attends public high school. The principal has recently contacted her parents because Stephanie was caught drinking alcohol in the parking lot during school hours. A school meeting is held with the parents, school psychologist, and principal. Stephanie's father and mother express concern with Stephanie's change in overall affect and report that she seems unhappy and won't talk to them about anything, spending almost all of her time at home alone in her room. The parents report that they suspect that Stephanie is also engaging in binge eating at home, as they have found food wrappers in Stephanie's closet. According to her mother, Stephanie's eating has alternated between excessively healthy and restrictive eating with night binges that she tries to hide. All parent efforts to talk to Stephanie about her behavior have resulted in Stephanie refusing to speak and withdrawing to her room. Her parents turn to the school for assistance.

During the first meeting with the psychologist, Stephanie is withdrawn, but eventually discloses that she has been binge eating and purging for more than 6 months and feels it is out of control. When asked about the drinking during school hours, she admits that she has begun to drink to calm herself during the day, and on weekends with her peers she will often binge drink to "stop feeling everything for a while." The school psychologist responds by probing in the following manner: "Sometimes we use alcohol or food to dull or escape our feelings. I know that lots of times teenagers who do this also use other unhealthy coping behaviours … are there other ways you try to manage your feelings?" After some hesitation, Stephanie responds by disclosing that she also occasionally cuts herself. She reports that she often doesn't feel like getting out of bed and feels that although she has a group that she spends time with, she doesn't feel they really know her at all; she feels she is really alone. She feels that her binge eating and purging are out of control and is worried that more and more she needs to turn to alcohol and even cutting to cope.

13.7.2 Plans for Assessment and Intervention

Based on the Stephanie's presentation and initial assessment, the school psychologist plans on further inquiring about the frequency and timing of Stephanie's alcohol use, cutting and engagement in additional health-risk behaviors, illicit and licit drug use, and conduct a brief suicide-risk assessment. The psychologist also plans to inquire about the nature of Stephanie's peer relationships, to further understand the social climate that she is exposed to and the influence such interactions have on her access to and engagement in health-risk behaviors. The psychologist also plans developing a log with Stephanie, so she can record her thoughts, feeling, and frequency of engagement in health-risk behaviors. Following the initial assessment, the psychologist refers Stephanie to an outpatient adolescent dialectic behavioral therapy program at a local hospital, which focuses primarily on decreasing Stephanie's engagement in health-risk behaviors and promotes the development of her self-regulation, adaptive coping strategies, and communication skills.

13.8 Directions for Future Research

The relatively novel state of the literature results in limitations and need for future research. To begin, certain health-risk behaviors (i.e., substance use) have been examined substantially more than others (e.g., self-asphyxiation, reckless driving, sexual-risk behaviors); therefore, it is difficult to conclude whether certain health-risk behaviors occur more than others or have simply been studied more. Studies also typically assess health-risk behaviors retrospectively and rely heavily on self-report. Future research would benefit from conceptualizing health-risk behaviors from a broader lens to provide a more holistic and comprehensive picture of the spectrum of behaviors that youth and young adults who present with NSSI, ED, and NSSI/ED are utilizing. Additional studies are needed to examine the unique and shared correlates of risk, along with longitudinal research to determine the onset, course, and interrelationship between DE and NSSI.

The reviewed literature has identified many shared risk correlates related to the co-occurrence of NSSI/DE and engagement in other health-risk behaviors, including factors such as impulsivity, presence of emotional distress, and difficulty regulating emotions (Claes et al., 2003; Claes, Klonsky, Muehlenkamp, Kuppens, & Vandereycken, 2010; Glenn & Klonsky, 2011; Muehlenkamp et al., 2012). However, such correlates are not specific to the co-occurrence of NSSI/ED and are collectively and/or independently associated with other maladaptive behaviors (i.e., pathological gambling) that do not represent a health-risk (Hopley & Nicki, 2010). This suggests that other factors warrant investigation when attempting to identify specific risk factors associated with the frequent co-occurrence and overlap between direct and indirect forms of self-injury. One critical, defining feature that is shared across both indirect and direct forms of self-injury concerns the predominant body-oriented nature and focus of self-injury. As suggested by scholars, how an individual experiences the body may play a role in the decision to engage in both indirect and direct forms of self-injury (e.g., Duggan, Toste, & Heath, 2012; Muehlenkamp, Swanson, & Brausch, 2005; Muehlenkamp et al., 2012; Nelson & Muehlenkamp, 2012; Orbach, 1996; Ross et al., 2009), suggesting that inclusion of body image and related constructs represents a logical area of investigation in understanding specific risk factors related to NSSI/ED and engagement in other health-risk behaviors. Based on the available literature, it is likely that a combination of factors such as impulsivity, emotional distress, difficulty regulating emotions, and an overall lack of investment/care towards the body facilitate an individual's propensity to engage in maladaptive coping strategies that center on forms of direct and indirect self-injury (Duggan et al., 2012; Muehlenkamp et al., 2005, 2012; Nelson & Muehlenkamp, 2012).

In sum, the existing literature strongly supports an association between NSSI/ED, and the co-occurring engagement in numerous health-risk behaviors, including suicidal ideation and behaviors, alcohol and substance use (both illicit and licit), nicotine use, self-asphyxiation, sexual-risk-taking behaviors, and other reckless and thrill-seeking behaviors in both male and female adolescents and young adults from community and clinical samples. Such findings should encourage awareness regarding the spectrum of health-risk behaviors that co-occur with NSSI and ED, among mental health professionals, and assist assessment, prevention, and early intervention efforts. Future research is clearly needed in order to gain a more comprehensive understanding of the relationships between multiple risk factors that contribute to the overlap between indirect and direct forms of self-injury.

References

Boudewyn, A. C., & Liem, J. H. (1995). Psychological, interpersonal, and behavioral correlates of chronic self-destructiveness: An exploratory study. *Psychological Reports, 77*, 1283–1297.

Brausch, A. M., Decker, K. M., & Hadley, A. G. (2011). Risk of suicidal ideation in adolescents with both self-asphyxial risk-taking behavior and non-suicidal self-injury. *Suicide and Life-Threatening Behavior, 41*, 424–434.

Brausch, A. M., & Gutierrez, P. M. (2010). Differences in non-suicidal self-injury and suicide attempts in adolescents. *Journal of Youth and Adolescents, 39*, 233–242.

Brown, L. K., Houck, C. D., Grossman, C. I., Lescano, C. M., & Frenkel, J. L. (2008). Frequency of adolescent self-cutting as a predictor of HIV risk. *Journal of Developmental and Behavioral Pediatrics, 29*, 161–165.

Brown, L. K., Houck, C. D., Hadley, W. S., & Lescano, C. M. (2005). Self-cutting and sexual risk among adolescents in intensive psychiatric treatment. *Psychiatric Services, 56*, 216–218.

Claes, L., Jiménez-Murcia, S., Agüera, Z., Castro, R., Sánchez, I., Menchón, J. M., & Fernández-Aranda, F. (2012). Male eating disorder patients with and without non-suicidal self-injury: A comparison of psychopathological and personality features. *European Eating Disorders Review, 20*, 335–338.

Claes, L., Klonsky, E. D., Muehlenkamp, J., Kuppens, P., & Vandereycken, W. (2010). The affect-regulation function of non-suicidal self-injury in eating-disordered patients: Which affect states are regulated? *Comprehensive Psychiatry, 51*, 386–392.

Claes, L., Vanderycken, W., & Vertommen, H. (2003). Eating-disordered patients with and without self-injurious behaviours: A comparison of psychopathological features. *European Eating Disorders Review, 11*, 379–396.

Deliberto, T. L., & Nock, M. K. (2008). An exploratory study of correlates, onset, and offset of non-suicidal self-injury. *Archives of Suicide Research, 12*, 219–231.

DiClemente, R. J., Ponton, L. E., & Hartley, D. (1991). Prevalence and correlates of cutting behavior: Risk for HIV transmission. *Journal of the American Academy of Child and Adolescent Psychiatry, 30*, 733–739.

Duggan, J. M., Toste, J. R., & Heath, N. L. (2012). An examination of the relationship between body image factors and non-suicidal self-injury in young adults: The mediating influence of emotion dysregulation. *Psychiatry Research, 1996*, 1–9.

Favaro, A., Ferrara, S., & Santonastaso, P. (2003). The spectrum of eating disorders in young women: A prevalence study in a general population sample. *Psychosomatic Medicine, 65*, 701–708.

Favazza, A. R., DeRosear, L., & Conterio, K. (1989). Self-mutilation and eating disorders. *Suicide and Life-Threatening Behavior, 19*, 352–361.

Field, A. E., Sonneville, K. R., Micali, N., Crosby, R. D., Swanson, S. A., Laird, N. M., Treasure, J., et al. (2012). Prospective association of common eating disorders and adverse outcomes. *Pediatrics, 130*, 289–295.

Fisher, C. B., Higgins-D'Alessandro, A., Rau, J., Kuther, T., & Belanger, S. (1996). Referring and reporting research participants at risk: Views from urban adolescents. *Child Development, 67*, 2086–2100.

Gadalla, T., & Piran, N. (2007). Co-occurrence of eating disorders and alcohol use disorders in women: A meta analysis. *Archives of Women's Mental Health, 10*, 133–140.

Glenn, C. R., & Klonsky, E. D. (2011). Prospective prediction of non-suicidal self-injury: A 1-year longitudinal study in young adults. *Behavior Therapy, 42*, 751–762.

Haw, C., Hawton, K., Casey, D., Bale, E., & Shepherd, A. (2005). Alcohol dependence, excessive drinking and deliberate self-harm: Trends and patterns in Oxford, 1989–2002. *Social Psychiatry and Psychiatric Epidemiology, 40*, 964–971.

Haw, C., Houston, K., Townsend, E., & Hawton, K. (2002). Deliberate self-harm patients with depressive disorders: Treatment and outcome. *Journal of Affective Disorders, 70*, 57–65.

Hilt, L. M., Nock, M. K., Lloyd-Richardson, E. E., & Prinstein, M. J. (2008). Longitudinal study of non-suicidal self-injury among young adolescents: Rates, correlates, and preliminary test of an interpersonal model. *The Journal of Early Adolescence, 28*, 455–469.

Holderness, C. C., Brooks-Gunn, J., & Warren, M. P. (1994). Co-morbidity of eating disorders and substance abuse: Review of the literature. *International Journal of Eating Disorders, 16*, 1–34.

Hooley, J. M., & St. Germain, S. A. (2009). Expanding the conceptualization of self-injurious behavior. In M. K. Nock (Ed.), *Oxford handbook of suicide and self-injury*. New York: University Press.

Hopley, A. A. B., & Nicki, R. M. (2010). Predictive factors of excessive online poker playing. *Cyberpsychology, Behavior and Social Networking, 13*, 379–385.

Klonsky, E. D., & Muehlenkamp, J. J. (2007). Self-injury: A research review for the practitioner. *Journal of Clinical Psychology, 63*, 1045–1056.

Krahn, D. D., Kurth, C. L., Gomberg, E., & Drewnowski, A. (2005). Pathological dieting and alcohol use in college women-a continuum of behaviors. *Eating Behaviors, 6*, 43–52.

Laye-Gindhu, A., & Schonert-Reichl, K. A. (2005). Non-suicidal self-harm among community adolescents: Understanding the "whats" and "whys" of self-harm. *Journal of Youth and Adolescence, 34*, 447–457.

Lewis, S. P., Heath, N. L., Michal, N. J., & Duggan, J. M. (2012). Non-suicidal self-injury, youth, and the Internet: What mental health professionals need to know. *Child and Adolescent Psychiatry and Mental Health, 6*, 13.

Lloyd-Richardson, E. E., Perrine, N., Dierker, L., & Kelley, M. L. (2007). Characteristics and functions of non-suicidal self-injury in a community sample of adolescents. *Psychological Medicine, 37*, 1183–1192.

Lock, J., Reisel, B., & Steiner, H. (2001). Associated health risks of adolescents with disordered eating: How different are they from their peers? Results from a high school survey. *Child Psychiatry and Human Development, 31*, 249–265.

Matsumoto, T., & Imamura, F. (2008). Self-injury in Japanese junior and senior high-school students: Prevalence and association with substance use. *Psychiatry and Clinical Neurosciences, 62*, 123–125.

Miller, A. L., Muehlenkamp, J. J., & Jacobson, C. M. (2009). Special issues in treating adolescent non-suicidal self-injury. In M. K. Nock (Ed.), *Understanding non-suicidal self-injury: Origins, assessment, and treatment* (pp. 251–270). Washington, DC: APA.

Muehlenkamp, J. J., Peat, C. M., Claes, L., & Smits, D. (2012). Self-injury and disordered eating: Expressing emotion dysregulation through the body. *Suicide and Life-Threatening Behavior, 42*, 416–425.

Muehlenkamp, J. J., Swanson, J. D., & Brausch, A. M. (2005). Self-objectification, risk taking, and self-harm in college women. *Psychology of Women Quarterly, 29*, 24–32.

Nagata, T., Oshima, J., Wada, A., Yamada, H., & Kiriike, N. (2003). Repetitive self-mutilation among Japanese eating disorder patients with drug use disorder: Comparison with patients with methamphetamine use disorder. *The Journal of Nervous and Mental Disease, 191*, 319–323.

Nelson, A., & Muehlenkamp, J. J. (2012). Body attitudes and objectification in non-suicidal self-injury: Comparing males and females. *Archives of Suicide Research, 16*, 1–12.

Neumark-Sztainer, D., Story, M., Dixon, L. B., & Murray, D. M. (1998). Adolescents engaging in unhealthy weight control behaviors: Are they at risk for other health-compromising behaviors? *American Journal of Public Health, 88*, 952–955.

Nock, M. K. (2010). Self-injury. *Annual Review of Clinical Psychology, 6*, 339–363.

Nock, M. K., Joiner, T. E., Gordon, K. H., Lloyd-Richardson, E., & Prinstein, M. J. (2006). Non-suicidal self-injury among adolescents: Diagnostic correlates and relation to suicide attempts. *Psychiatry Research, 144*, 65–72.

Nock, M. K., Prinstein, M. J., & Sterba, S. K. (2009). Revealing the form and function of self-injurious thoughts and behaviors: A real-time ecological assessment study among adolescents and young adults. *Journal of Abnormal Psychology, 118*, 816–827.

Orbach, I. (1996). The role of body experience in self-destruction. *Clinical Child Psychology and Psychiatry, 1*, 607–619.

Peebles, R., Wilson, J. L., & Lock, J. D. (2011). Self-injury in adolescents with eating disorders: Correlates and provider bias. *The Journal of Adolescent Health, 48*, 310–313.

Piran, N., & Robinson, S. R. (2006). Associations between disordered eating behaviors and licit and illicit substance use and abuse in a university sample. *Addictive Behaviors, 31*, 1761–1775.

Pisetsky, E. M., Chao, Y. M., Dierker, L. C., May, A. M., & Striegel-Moore, R. H. (2008). Disordered eating and substance use in high-school students: Results from the Youth Risk Behavior Surveillance System. *The International Journal of Eating Disorders, 41*, 464–470.

Rodham, K., & Hawton, K. (2009). Epidemiology and phenomenology of non-suicidal self-injury. In M. Nock (Ed.), *Understanding non-suicidal self-injury: Origins, assessment, and treatment* (pp. 37–62). Washington, DC: APA Books.

Ross, S., & Heath, N. (2002). A study of the frequency of self-mutilation in a community sample of adolescents. *Journal of Youth and Adolescence, 31*, 67–77.

Ross, S., Heath, N. L., & Toste, J. R. (2009). Non-suicidal self-injury and eating pathology in high school students. *American Journal of Orthopsychiatry, 79*, 83–92.

Serras, A., Saules, K. K., Cranford, J. A., & Eisenberg, D. (2010). Self-injury, substance use, and associated risk factors in a multi-campus probability sample of college students. *Psychology of Addictive Behaviors: Journal of the Society of Psychologists in Addictive Behaviors, 24*, 119–128.

Silverman, M. M., Berman, A. L., Sanddal, N. D., Carroll, P. W. O., & Joiner, T. E. (2007). Rebuilding the tower of Babel: A revised nomenclature for the study of suicide and suicidal behaviors Part 2: Suicide-related ideations, communications, and behaviors. *Suicide and Life-Threatening Behaviors, 37*, 264–277.

Solano, R., Fernández Aranda, F., Aitken, A., López, C., & Vallejo, J. (2005). Self-injurious behaviour in people with eating disorders. *European Eating Disorders Review, 13*, 3–10.

St. Germain, S. A., & Hooley, J. M. (2012). Direct and indirect forms of non-suicidal self-injury: Evidence for a distinction. *Psychiatry Research, 197*, 78–84.

Svirko, E., & Hawton, K. (2007). Self-injurious behaviour and eating disorders: The extent and nature of the association. *Suicide and Life-Threatening Behavior, 37*, 409–421.

Taliaferro, L. A., Muehlenkamp, J. J., Borowsky, I. W., McMorris, B. J., & Kugler, K. C. (2012). Factors distinguishing youth who report self-injurious behavior: A population-based sample. *Academic Pediatrics, 12*, 205–213.

Vrouva, I., Fonagy, P., Fearon, P. R. M., & Roussow, T. (2010). The risk-taking and self-harm inventory for adolescents: Development and psychometric evaluation. *Psychological Assessment, 22*, 852–865.

Whitlock, J., Eckenrode, J., & Silverman, D. (2006). Self-injurious behaviours in a college population. *Pediatrics, 117*, 1939–1948.

Wiederman, M. W., & Pryor, T. (1996). Multi-impulsivity among women with bulimia nervosa. *International Journal of Eating Disorders, 20*, 359–365.

Williams, F., & Hasking, P. (2010). Emotion regulation, coping and alcohol use as moderators in the relationship between non-suicidal self-injury and psychological distress. *Prevention Science, 11*, 33–41.

Wolfe, W. L., & Maisto, S. A. (2000). The relationship between eating disorders and substance use: Moving beyond co-prevalence research. *Clinical Psychology Review, 20*, 617–631.

Wu, L. T., Gersing, K., Burchett, B., Woody, G. E., & Blazer, D. G. (2011). Substance use disorders and comorbid Axis I and II psychiatric disorders among young psychiatric patients: Findings from a large electronic health records database. *Journal of Psychiatric Research, 45*, 1453–1462.

14 Experience of the Body

Amy M. Brausch and Jennifer J. Muehlenkamp

Abstract

Both eating disorders and non-suicidal self-injury involve some type of harm, either indirectly or directly, inflicted on the body. Individuals who perceive and experience their body in a negative manner may be more able to cause harm to the body. Therefore, the body represents an important variable to consider when understanding both eating disorders and self-injury. This chapter explores how an individual's experience of his or her body may increase risk for engaging in self-injury and eating disorder behaviors. The concept of body regard is reviewed along with theoretical and empirical data describing how a negative relationship with the body can potentially facilitate engagement in NSSI and disordered eating. The importance of including body experiences in treatment is presented along with suggestions for how to integrate and address bodily experiences within standard treatments for NSSI and eating disorders.

14.1 Case Example

Lucy is an 18-year-old Caucasian female college student who recently visited the University Counseling Center for feelings of depression. She is a student-athlete and competes on the university volleyball team. Upon questioning, Lucy also notes that some of her friends are concerned that she is "obsessed" with volleyball and are worried about her exercise and eating habits. She admits to working out more than the team requires and sometimes skips meals or tries to restrict calories. She talks about the volleyball uniforms as being "horrible." She notes that she and other teammates worry about how they look in their uniforms. "We have to wear these small, Spandex bottoms that look like bikini bottoms and because they are Spandex they show everything. Sometimes when I'm out on the court I find myself thinking about how awful I must look." Lucy thinks she is depressed because she is

A.M. Brausch (✉) • J.J. Muehlenkamp
Department of Psychology, University of Wisconsin - Eau Claire, Eau Claire, WI, USA

Department of Psychology, Western Kentucky University, Bowling Green, KY, USA
e-mail: amy.brausch@wku.edu

L. Claes and J.J. Muehlenkamp (eds.), *Non-Suicidal Self-Injury in Eating Disorders*, DOI 10.1007/978-3-642-40107-7_14, © Springer-Verlag Berlin Heidelberg 2014

away from home and misses old friends. She is also very busy with school and volleyball practice, has little time to socialize, and finds herself feeling discouraged and crying frequently. She recalls being an "emotional" kid and noting that even minor events felt like "huge deals" and a small inconvenience could ruin her day. When asked about how she copes with her negative feelings, she responds that exercising and fasting take her mind off her feelings. She notes a feeling of pride for being able to tolerate strenuous exercise and extreme hunger pains. She reluctantly also admits that sometimes she cuts herself when negative feelings are especially strong. "It's weird that it doesn't really hurt that much, but I feel better after doing it, as least for a little while." When asked how she feels about herself, Lucy responds, "I'm a mess. I love volleyball, but I know I get obsessed with exercising and practicing. I want everything to be perfect – my game, my body, school – but it's not. I hate myself sometimes and think I deserve the grueling workouts. But I want to appear normal so I have to do something to release all of that bad stuff inside. At least with cutting I can get that stuff out when I'm alone and still seem normal on the outside."

Lucy represents a growing population of youth and young adults who present with both NSSI and eating disorder behaviors. As described in earlier chapters in this volume, eating disorders and NSSI co-occur rather frequently. This co-occurrence signals the importance of examining shared factors that appear to underlie and contribute to the onset and maintenance of both behaviors. While already established as a salient risk factor for eating disorders, body experiences (e.g., body image, body dissatisfaction, dissociation) also appear to be relevant to understanding risk for engaging in NSSI. Both behaviors involve treating the body as an object of mistreatment and/or self-inflicted pain, further underscoring the importance of the body to both of these behaviors. Additionally, an individual's experience of the body is intimately tied with one's self-concept and emotional functioning. Lucy provides a clear example of how concerns about her body are contributing to early eating disorder symptoms as well as exacerbating her depression, or emotional distress, which triggers acts of self-injury. The goal of this chapter is to highlight how an individual's experience of the body is relevant and essential to understanding risk for both eating disorders and NSSI, as well as to offer some treatment suggestions that incorporate elements of the body experience.

To best understand how the body becomes a salient risk factor for both eating disorders and NSSI, it is important to recognize the multidimensional nature of the concepts linked to the body. Numerous terms have been used to describe how an individual experiences his or her body, including body image, body satisfaction, and body esteem. A quick review of the literature reveals that the term "body image" is used frequently in the context of eating disorders. Body image has been defined in simplistic ways such as "a person's perceptions, thoughts, and feelings about his or her body" (Grogan, 1999, p. 1), while comprehensive definitions recognize that body image is a multidimensional construct (Cash, 2004). Body image disturbance is a term used to describe negative thoughts and feelings toward the body. According to Bergstrom and Neighbors (2006), body image disturbance can be further divided into two independent categories. The first category of disturbance is body-size distortion, which involves inaccurate perceptions of one's body size. Body-size distortion is included as a diagnostic criterion for anorexia nervosa and is commonly exhibited as individuals perceiving their overall body size or specific body parts as being larger than they are objectively. The second type of body disturbance is "body dissatisfaction" which can be exhibited through cognitive, affective, and/or attitudinal avenues. Whether one subscribes to the simple or comprehensive definition of body image, the construct is largely defined as an individual's perceptions of their body shape, size, and outward appearance.

The term "body regard" has been used in recent literature to broaden the conceptualization of body image so that it extends beyond physical appearance. Body regard is also a multifaceted construct to describe an individual's perception of the body and includes the relationship with, attitudes toward, and experience of the body (Muehlenkamp, 2012). Comprehensively defined, body regard includes aspects of body protection, body esteem, body competence, interoceptive awareness, and body integrity. Body protection includes protective attitudes, actions, and feelings toward the body, the extent to which an individual protects his or her body from harm. Body esteem includes feelings of perceived attractiveness and subjective satisfaction with the body, the extent to which an individual feels content with the body. Body competence includes perceived health, physical abilities, and level of physical coordination, the extent to which an individual feels their body is healthy and capable of participating and excelling in sports, exercise, and general physical work. Interoceptive awareness is an individual's awareness of their own physiological functioning, the extent to which an individual is aware of their body's sensations and cues. Lastly, body integrity refers to an individual's sense of ownership and understanding of the body, the extent to which an individual feels connected to his or her body. While body regard has recently emerged in the literature as being salient to NSSI, it is not a term widely used when discussing disordered eating.

Within the literature on disordered eating behaviors and clinically significant eating disorders, the terms of body image and body dissatisfaction are more likely to be used. This trend is understandable considering the diagnostic importance of bodily distortion and intense dislike for the body shape, size, and weight found in eating disorders. For both anorexia nervosa and bulimia nervosa, individuals place significant importance on their weight and body shape in their self-evaluations (APA, 2000). While sociocultural factors have been implicated in the development of body image disturbances and body satisfaction, it is clear from numerous studies that body dissatisfaction and poor body image are strongly related to eating disorder behavior (see Cash & Brown, 1987; Cash & Deagle, 1997). This finding has been replicated in samples of adult women, college students, adolescent females, preadolescent females, and both clinical and nonclinical populations (Cash & Smolak, 2011). In addition to being strongly associated with each other, there is evidence to suggest that poor body image and body dissatisfaction may be precursors to disordered eating behaviors, implying a causal pathway (e.g., Thompson, Coovert, Richards, Johnson, & Cattarin, 1995).

14.2 Empirical Research on Body Regard/Body Image in Both NSSI and ED

14.2.1 Body Regard in Eating Disorders

The study of body image disturbance is important for two reasons: (1) body image disturbance is widespread in almost all populations of females in Westernized countries, and (2) it is significantly related to numerous other psychological issues. Many studies conducted during the past 2 decades assessing large samples of females have found high rates of body image disturbance. These high percentages have been found in samples of adolescents (e.g., Nuemark-Sztainer, Paxton, Hannan, Haines, & Story, 2006) and young adult women (48 %; Cash & Henry, 1995). In a national survey of 4,000 adult women, 55 % indicated that they were dissatisfied with their overall appearance. About 89 % of the women surveyed reported wanting to lose weight (Garner, 1997). While the study of body image disturbance has focused on populations of adolescents and young adult women, the study of middle-aged women has been receiving increasing attention. A review of studies investigating the occurrence of body dissatisfaction in women over the age of 40 found rates comparable to younger women, indicating the tendency for body dissatisfaction to be continuous and stable across the life span (Slevec & Tiggemann, 2011).

The high prevalence of body image disturbance is alarming chiefly due to the established relationship between body dissatisfaction and eating pathology. Body dissatisfaction has been identified through repeated empirical studies as one of the most consistent, robust risk factors for the development of eating disorders (Slevec & Tiggemann, 2011). Stice and Shaw (2002) identified two mechanisms through which body dissatisfaction is thought to contribute to the development of eating disorders. The first pathway occurs when body dissatisfaction leads individuals to engage in dieting behavior, which is also a risk factor for eating disorders. The second pathway occurs when body dissatisfaction causes negative affect, which an individual may then try to manage through binge eating. One longitudinal study followed college women for several years beginning with their first year in school. Those who had body dissatisfaction at the beginning of the study showed more eating disorder symptoms 3 years later than those who had healthy body attitudes (Cooley & Toray, 2001).

While disturbances in body image and high concerns about shape and weight are central to the psychopathology of eating disorders, body image disturbance also commonly occurs in nonclinical samples of women (Farrell, Shafran, & Lee, 2006). These disturbances can still bring considerable distress and have been referred to as "normative discontent" (Rodin, Silberstein, & Streigel-Moore, 1984). A survey from 2004 found that one in four women reported engaging in unhealthy or abnormal eating behaviors or weight-control practices (Forman-Hoffman, 2004). A prospective study of over 1,000 adolescent females found that body dissatisfaction was a predictor of eating and weight-control pathology, low self-esteem, stress, and depression (Johnson & Wardle, 2005). Taken together, these results indicate that body dissatisfaction is a driving force in the development and maintenance of disordered eating behaviors.

14.2.2 Body Regard in NSSI

While not studied as extensively as with eating disorders, body image disturbances are also theorized to be particularly salient to understanding risk for NSSI. Research in this area began with exploring the possible relationship between body attitudes and experiences and suicidal behaviors. Orbach, Stein, Shani-Sela, and Har-Even (2001) theorized that having a fundamental hatred of the body facilitates acts of self-destruction. Specifically, they argued that when the body becomes a source of dissatisfaction, the natural self-preserving drive may be reduced such that an individual is less invested in protecting the body from harm. These negative perceptions and experiences of the body may take the form of rejecting one's body, feeling hate toward one's body, feeling detached, and feeling indifferent about body sensations. Orbach et al. also suggested that individuals having negative body experiences might also have a decreased sensitivity to pain and other unpleasant body sensations, making it more likely that they might attack their own body via self-injurious acts.

Building upon Orbach's ideas, Muehlenkamp (2012) broadened the conceptualization of the body relationship to the multidimensional construct of body regard and posits that negative body regard is a necessary, but not sufficient, risk factor for NSSI. She argues that individuals with poor body regard are less connected to their bodily experiences and have negative perceptions of their attractiveness, which contributes to a devaluing of and detachment from the body. This devaluing and detachment interacts with emotional distress to increase the likelihood the individual will use the body as a target for the distress and engage in NSSI over alternative coping strategies. Much like Orbach et al. (2001), Muehlenkamp is arguing that a compromised relationship with one's body facilitates acts of NSSI particularly when the individual is experiencing significant emotional distress. From this theoretical perspective, body regard is viewed as being a mechanism that facilitates and maintains NSSI behavior rather than being a direct cause for it to occur (Muehlenkamp, 2012).

Recent studies have focused on the relationship between body regard and NSSI, lending support to Muehlenkamp's (2012) ideas. A handful of studies have offered consistent support that there is a strong association between negative experiences of the body (e.g., body-size distortion, lack of familiarity with the body, body dissatisfaction, negative body esteem, etc.) and NSSI behavior in both clinical and community samples of youth (Duggan, Toste, & Heath, 2013; Muehlenkamp, Swanson, & Brausch, 2005; Nelson & Muehlenkamp, 2012; Yates, Carlson, & Egeland, 2008). For example, a study of Canadian high school students examined differences in eating pathology and body dissatisfaction between students with and without a history of NSSI (Ross, Heath, & Toste, 2009). Students who reported NSSI ($n = 59$) were compared to a control group ($n = 57$), and results indicated that self-injurers reported a significantly greater desire for thinness, more bulimic behaviors, and greater body dissatisfaction than the control group. Another study of high school freshmen found that those with a history of NSSI and reported body dissatisfaction were up to three times more likely to continue to engage in NSSI. Adolescents who reported engaging in NSSI less than three times also reported more body dissatisfaction than those with no NSSI history (Brunner et al., 2007). Negative body esteem has also been found to positively correlate with the frequency of NSSI (Bjärehed & Lundh, 2008). In a study using a combined sample of community and inpatient adolescents, Muehlenkamp and Brausch (2012) found that when body regard was taken into account, the relationship between negative affect and NSSI became nonsignificant. Most recently, Muehlenkamp, Bagge, Tull, and Gratz (2013) tested the idea that body regard is essential for NSSI in the context of emotion dysregulation with a sample of college students, finding that emotion dysregulation was only associated with NSSI frequency when negative body regard was also present. These findings in particular suggest that body regard is a crucial feature contributing to acts of NSSI.

14.2.3 Body Regard in Both Eating Disorders and NSSI

Given that body eating disorders and NSSI represent intentional harm inflicted onto the body, it makes sense that a person's relationship with the body would be relevant to both and thus their co-occurrence. Studies do support the salience of bodily experiences to the co-occurrence of NSSI and eating disorders, above and beyond the association to either behavior alone. Research of inpatients with a diagnosed eating disorder consistently finds that individuals who also engage in NSSI report significantly higher levels of body dissatisfaction and body alienation compared to those without NSSI (Claes, Vandereycken, & Vertommen, 2003; Solano, Fernández-Aranda, Aitken, López, & Vallejo, 2005). In a study examining the impact of body image on NSSI frequency within a sample of inpatient females diagnosed with an eating disorder, Muehlenkamp, Claes, Smits, Peat, and Vandereycken (2011) found that body image retained a significant association to NSSI after other variables such as trauma history and psychiatric symptoms were accounted for. Studies with community samples have reported similar results. For example, Ross et al. (2009) found that high school students who engaged in NSSI reported higher levels of eating disorder symptoms compared to no-NSSI peers. Among college students, Muehlenkamp, Peat, Claes, and Smits (2012) found that body-related concerns were strongly associated to the presence of both NSSI and eating disorder behaviors relative to either one individually. Collectively, the current empirical data indicates that even among individuals already known to have a compromised relationship with their body (e.g., those diagnosed with an eating disorder), engagement in NSSI is linked to significant body disturbances greater than that associated with eating disorder behavior alone.

One theory that can help explain why body experiences would be salient to the co-occurrence of eating disorders and NSSI is self-objectification theory

(Fredrickson & Roberts, 1997). This theory states that when the body is chronically objectified by society and oneself, an individual is at increased risk for numerous negative outcomes, which include eating disorders and self-injury. It is posited that objectification of the body contributes to the tendency to evaluate oneself, including self-worth, from an outsider's perspective that is largely focused on attractiveness. This self-objectification contributes to feeling disconnected from the body and often contributes to experiences of body dissatisfaction (Moradi & Huang, 2008). Strong support has documented the relationship between self-objectification and eating disorder behavior (see Moradi & Huang, 2008 for a review). Research has also found evidence that self-objectification is relevant to understanding risk for NSSI among both females and males (Muehlenkamp et al., 2005; Nelson & Muehlenkamp, 2012). These emerging results emphasize the importance of how the experience of the body, and perceiving the body as an external object, may contribute to both disordered eating and NSSI. The implications of this research are that it becomes important to help clients both value and connect with their body in order to reduce engagement in these behaviors.

14.2.4 Specific Aspects of Body Experiences

14.2.4.1 Interoceptive Awareness

Within the eating disorder literature, interoceptive awareness is identified as a major deficit many individuals experience. Interoceptive awareness is typically conceived as being an individual's ability to discriminate between individual bodily sensations and emotions and accurately respond to them. It can also refer to the extent to which an individual is able to identify "the specific visceral sensations relating to hunger and satiety" (Pollatos et al., 2008, p. 382). Numerous studies have documented poor interoceptive awareness across all the types of eating disorders (Pollatos et al., 2008), and it is noteworthy that interoceptive awareness generally improves following treatment for an eating disorder. For example, one study that followed anorexia nervosa patients over time found that deficits in interoceptive awareness were good predictors of a patient's severity of symptoms 5–10 years later, with poorer awareness corresponding to greater severity (Bizeul, Sadowsky, & Rigaud, 2001). Another study found that individuals who had been hospitalized and treated for anorexia nervosa for 6 months showed significant improvements in interoceptive awareness along with body mass index, eating attitudes, and anxiety (Matsumoto et al., 2006).

Since the construct of interoceptive awareness tends to incorporate physiological and behavioral components of emotion regulation as well as biological indicators of satiety, researchers have conceptualized it into different components and studied each component separately. Merwin, Zucker, Lacy, and Elliott (2010) have divided interoceptive awareness into two components: clarity about emotions and willingness to have those internal experiences. In their study of 50 eating disorder patients, only nonacceptance of emotional states predicted dietary restraint, and lack of clarity was not related. Another set of researchers include the concept of interoceptive sensitivity (e.g., an individual's sensitivity to bodily signals) in their studies of interoceptive awareness. Interoceptive sensitivity is based on theories of emotion positing that humans first notice cues of emotion and then interpret them. In a study of 28 female patients with anorexia nervosa and 28 healthy controls, Pollatos et al. (2008) found that the eating disorder patients showed poorer interoceptive sensitivity and awareness compared to controls even when controlling for anxiety and depression. The authors conclude that patients with anorexia nervosa appear to have deficits in both interoceptive awareness and sensitivity, but awareness might be greatly influenced by difficulties in describing and regulating emotions. Results from these studies indicate that individuals with eating disorders seem to be resistant to accepting their own bodily and emotional responses, which is then related to their actual eating disorder behaviors. Indeed, more recent interventions for eating disorders include components of improving emotion regulation skills such as mindfulness and acceptance, which may help ameliorate some of the interoceptive deficits identified.

Interoceptive awareness has also been studied in the context of NSSI, most often as it overlaps with disordered eating behaviors. In a study by Favaro and Santonastaso (1998), patients with bulimia were divided into groups that engaged in NSSI or not. The groups that reported more NSSI had higher interoceptive awareness scores, indicating greater deficits, than the group that reported little to no NSSI. Interestingly, the group of bulimic patients who reported no NSSI had the best self-reported interoceptive awareness. The authors concluded that interoceptive awareness appeared to be a salient characteristic among the patients who reported self-injury. A more recent study examined differences in interoceptive awareness in a sample of 80 Japanese female eating disorder patients and divided them into groups who had and had not engaged in NSSI in the past month (Fujimori et al., 2011). These groups were both compared to a sample of healthy control subjects. Results indicated that the combined group (eating disorder + recent NSSI) reported both higher body dissatisfaction and poorer interoceptive awareness than the eating disorder only and control groups. Similar results were reported by Ross et al. (2009) in a sample of over 400 Canadian high school students. Among other factors, this study found significant differences in interoceptive awareness between groups of injuring and non-injuring adolescents across genders. Interoceptive awareness was also found to be related to lifetime frequency of NSSI, indicating that adolescents who habitually engage in NSSI are less skilled in identifying and labeling their emotions or other internal states.

A recent study also examined the importance of emotion regulation and interoceptive awareness in both NSSI and disordered eating by investigating these factors in a sample of college undergraduate women (Muehlenkamp et al., 2012). The sample was divided into three groups: one with only a history of NSSI, one with a history of disordered eating only, and one with both. Results supported the hypotheses that emotional dysregulation was associated with both NSSI and disordered eating and was most pronounced in the group who engaged in both behaviors. The combination group also had higher levels of depressive symptoms and interoceptive awareness deficits than the other groups. Collectively, the empirical evidence points to the pattern of the combination of eating disorders and NSSI being related to an inability to detect internal cues associated with emotions as well as hunger and satiety. These studies provide one lens through which to view the experience of the body in NSSI and eating disorders, suggesting that the lack of awareness of both physical and emotional states is related to the severity, frequency, and factors associated with recovery for NSSI and eating disorders. Treatments that focus on enhancing interoceptive awareness will be important to consider when working with patients who present with both an eating disorder and NSSI.

14.2.4.2 Experience of Pain

Related to interoceptive awareness is the experience of pain in both NSSI and eating disorders. Individuals who are not in tune with internal body states and/or emotional experiences may also be less likely to experience external body states such as pain during acts of self-injury or restricting, purging, and/or bingeing. Indeed, this very pattern has been well documented in studies of eating disorder patients. Patients with anorexia, bulimia, and binge-eating disorder have all been found to have a higher pain threshold, which has been tested on various parts of the body and with different methods (see Papezova, Yamamotova, & Uher, 2005). Pain insensitivity has been found to be greater in bulimia, and the insensitivity continues after recovery from the disorder. The fact that pain insensitivity persists beyond recovery indicates that either an individual habituates to pain, or it serves as a trait marker for individuals who are predisposed to developing bulimia. Papezova et al. (2005) found that pain insensitivity was highest in individuals with bingeing-purging symptomatology compared to restricting. Furthermore, the authors found that lack of familiarity with one's body, or feeling alienated from one's body, was positively associated with pain threshold. One theory as to why eating disorder patients experience pain insensitivity is that they may also be experiencing dissociative symptoms. The authors concluded that while dissociative experiences (as measured by feelings of alienation) may be related to pain threshold in eating disorders, its contribution may be small.

It has also been suggested that one reason why individuals are able to engage in intentionally self-damaging acts of NSSI is because of pain insensitivity or diminished pain perception. Numerous studies of NSSI appear to support these claims. For example, studies have found that individuals with borderline personality disorder who also engage in NSSI have reduced pain perception (e.g., Niedtfeld et al., 2010) as do community samples of individuals with NSSI history (e.g., Hooley, Ho, Slater, & Lockshin, 2010). Other research has found that adolescents who engage in NSSI are likely to report not experiencing pain during NSSI (Stanley et al., 2010). In a study of eating disorder patients, those who also had a recent history of NSSI were assessed on their pain experience during NSSI (Claes, Vandereycken, & Vertommen, 2006). While the presence or absence of pain was not related to one type of eating disorder or another, the longer the duration of the patients' NSSI, the less pain was reported. Among the patients who reported experiencing no pain during NSSI, their levels of dissociation and traumatic experiences were higher than the patients who did report pain during NSSI. These results align nicely with the research on interoceptive awareness in that dissociation may be a factor in both a reduced awareness of the body's internal and emotional states and ability to feel pain.

Just as the research on interoceptive awareness included emotion regulation as a contributing factor to both disordered eating and NSSI, some research on pain perception in NSSI also includes emotion regulation as a factor that may potentially explain diminished pain perception in NSSI. Franklin, Aaron, Arthur, Shorkey, and Prinstein (2012) compared individuals with and without NSSI history on pain perception and emotion dysregulation. All participants completed a cold pressor task during which their hand was immersed in ice water and they indicated when they first felt pain (pain threshold) and when the pain became unbearable and they pulled their hand out (pain tolerance). Results of this study showed that the NSSI group demonstrated both increased pain tolerance and threshold and rated pain to a lesser intensity than the no-NSSI group. Significant correlations were also found between pain tolerance and emotion dysregulation even in the control group, although the correlations were stronger within the NSSI group. Overall, this study suggests that reduced pain perception is related to emotion dysregulation, which is in turn associated with NSSI, and may provide one explanation for how individuals with NSSI experience a higher pain threshold and tolerance.

14.2.4.3 Exercise

One final aspect to consider in the experience of the body as it relates to both disordered eating and NSSI is exercise. Overexercise can be a clinical symptom of both anorexia and bulimia (APA, 2000) and has been studied in the contexts of both eating disorders and self-harm behaviors. Disordered eating has also been reported by up to 58 % of female collegiate athletes, with up to 54 % of these women also reporting weight dissatisfaction (Stirling & Kerr, 2012). Up to 20 % of high school female athletes have been found to engage in disordered eating behaviors such as restricting and vomiting, especially during their competitive seasons. In a qualitative study of 17 female collegiate athletes, one theme that emerged was the enjoyment of hunger pains and being able to tolerate pain associated with the sport as being related to an increased vulnerability to disordered eating. Some women described the sensation of pain as rewarding their efforts to either lose weight or improve their physical skills through exercise.

The research on the role of exercise and pain in NSSI is quite limited. One relevant study examined overexercise as a potential risk factor for suicidal behavior in individuals with disordered eating. In a series of studies, Smith et al. (2013) found that overexercise was the only disordered eating behavior that was significantly related to suicidal behavior after taking into account many other factors. Another key result from these studies is that pain insensitivity and the acquired capability for suicide (habituation to painful and provocative events) helped to explain the relationship between overexercise and suicidal behaviors. In other words, overexercise was related to pain insensitivity and acquired capability, which were then related to suicidal behaviors. These relationships were found in various populations including individuals meeting criteria for bulimia and nonclinical college students. It seems reasonable to conclude that overexercise and pain insensitivity would function similarly in NSSI, with overexercise being related to increased pain threshold, thus contributing to NSSI behavior. More research is needed in this area to make any firm conclusions.

14.3 Treatment

Addressing aspects of body disregard/dissatisfaction, or distortion, as part of eating disorder treatment is an established standard of care. However, in existing NSSI treatment models, experiences of the body are not frequently included or identified as a target for treatment (Klonsky, Muehlenkamp, Lewis, & Walsh, 2011; Walsh, 2012). Treatments for NSSI typically emphasize emotion regulation, cognitive restructuring, interpersonal skills and relationships, as well as problem-solving and coping skill development. While these are all important components of treatment for NSSI, the empirical literature summarized in this chapter provides evidence that body regard should also be considered, if not definitely incorporated, into such treatments (Muehlenkamp, 2012). Addressing elements of body regard in treatment also appears to be essential when working with a patient presenting with both NSSI and eating disorder behaviors, given the research reviewed.

It could be argued that some of the methods used to target and treat NSSI and eating disorder behaviors may in fact improve body regard as a by-product of the skills taught. Within treatments such as dialectical behavior therapy (DBT; Linehan, 1993), individuals are taught skills that help them focus on bodily experiences to soothe the mind and reduce distress (e.g., mindfulness, emotional awareness, detection of early physiological cues to emotional arousal). Additionally, these treatments provide strategies for emphasizing body care, such as self-soothing and creating alternative sensations. One such activity that has budding research support is yoga. A study by Impett, Daubenmier, and Hirschman (2006) found that participating in hatha yoga for 2 months resulted in increased body awareness and regard and improvements in positive affect and life satisfaction. Yoga is an athletic activity that incorporates some aspects of the mindfulness and emotion regulation techniques used in treatments for NSSI and eating disorders. Thus, one aspect of treatments such as DBT that makes it effective may be because they teach skills to reduce body disregard and inadvertently promote body care and valuing (Muehlenkamp, 2012).

Other treatments take a cognitive approach to targeting NSSI and use challenge techniques that emphasize the negative consequences of the NSSI to the body through scarring and disfigurement. The cognitive challenges may also directly focus on changing beliefs of self-denigration which may indirectly enhance body regard since the body is an integral part of the overall self-concept. Newman (2009) provided examples of common core beliefs in individuals with NSSI which include hating the body, perceiving it as an enemy, and being body alienated. Other cognitive therapies use acceptance-based techniques in treatment with the intent of developing an acceptance or caring stance toward the body that could help prevent engagement in NSSI (Muehlenkamp, 2012).

Walsh (2012) has also made recommendations for working on body regard when treating self-injuring clients. He suggests that there are six dimensions of body regard with potential relevance to NSSI, including attractiveness, effectiveness, health, sexual behavior, sexual characteristics, and body integrity. For many individuals in treatment for NSSI, just asking about the body across these dimensions in relation to NSSI may open new avenues for discussion and provide hope that these "new" areas signify an effective approach to therapy compared to prior experiences. Assessing these different dimensions of body regard also helps the therapist and client identify specific domains to target that may be directly related to NSSI for each individual client, as well as identify aspects of the body that are viewed more positively. One could also infer that a client's level of body regard may be a relevant indicator of prognosis. For example, a client with higher levels of body regard may have a more positive prognosis and require a shorter treatment for ceasing NSSI because his or her level of body care and respect is close to being healthy. Thus, assessment of body attitudes is likely important to treatment conceptualization, and integrating body regard into treatment for NSSI may be warranted. Some specific treatment suggestions for merging body-related work into existing therapeutic approaches appear in the following section.

Behavioral interventions are one type of treatment technique that can be useful with NSSI and eating disorders because they provide problem-solving and action-oriented strategies that these individuals tend to be lacking in the midst of distress (Newman, 2009). Providing clients with experiential activities that can promote positive body experiences and simultaneously challenge the negative attitudes held about the body holds promise for reducing NSSI and eating disorder behaviors by improving body regard. Clinicians can design behavioral activities that help build positive body experiences, such as taking a bath, doing yoga, dancing, or trying a new haircut, in consultation with the client and their preferences. Activities that incorporate self-soothing and physically pleasant sensations, such as using fragrant lotion on the body or receiving a massage, can also be implemented both in and out of session. The use of alternate or replacement behaviors for the NSSI (or a binge/purging behavior) is also a common technique and may include activities that help improve a client's connection to the body or enhance perceptions of the body. Examples of replacement behaviors include mindful breathing exercises or other mindfulness-based activities such as washing the dishes, styling one's hair, squeezing a stress ball, or lifting weights. Mindful breathing helps calm emotional arousal while also focusing the individual on rhythmic breathing patterns, increasing body awareness. Other mindful activities help individuals focus on one thing at time while providing physical relief and promoting healthy interaction with the body (Muehlenkamp, 2012).

Having clients schedule exercise into their routine may also be beneficial in improving their perceptions of body effectiveness and reducing NSSI. Substituting exercise for NSSI has been successful in reducing self-injury in at least one case study (Wallenstein & Nock, 2007). Engaging in sport activities and exercising, along with removing NSSI instruments, have been found to be helpful ways to resist NSSI urges. It's possible that exercise works to prevent NSSI because it leads to a reduction in psychological tension and stress, it releases mood-enhancing endorphins, and/or it increases the sense of body regard. While exercise seems to be beneficial for some individuals who engage in NSSI, exercise should be monitored closely and with caution in clients who also present with symptoms of eating disorders, particularly if they have a history of or are currently engaging in overexercise.

Treatment techniques from cognitive therapy also lend themselves well to body work when treating NSSI and eating disorders. Cognitive interventions can smoothly transition from identifying automatic thoughts about NSSI or the disordered eating behavior to negative thoughts and beliefs underlying body disregard. Once identified, distorted and maladaptive thoughts about the body can be challenged, and self-criticism toward the body can be addressed and reduced. Clinicians can also work with clients to cognitively process the experiential techniques described in the preceding paragraphs to further develop positive body thoughts. It may also be useful to teach clients positive body self-talk or designing body-neutral replacement thoughts to help challenge negative attitudes and beliefs. For example, a clinician may reframe a statement such as "my body is worthless" to "my body allows me to hug those I care about" or "my body deserves respect just like I do." Techniques from dialectical behavior therapy may also be helpful, such as radical acceptance of the body, noting pros and cons of the body, and including body-related elements in developing self-respect as clients build more accepting and tolerant attitudes toward the body.

Lastly, teaching clients basic and advanced emotion regulation skills will likely help clients become more attuned to their body as well as adaptively manage their emotional distress. Lack of awareness of both physical and emotional states in individuals with NSSI or eating disorders highlights the need to teach emotion regulation skills. In clients with eating disorders, NSSI may be another method used for tension release, and thus finding alternate ways to cope with strong negative emotions is key for both behaviors. Having clients engage in mindfulness practices where they observe their body in various settings (calming sitting, while walking, in a certain pose, etc.) is an important step to helping clients identify emotions. Clients can learn about their body cues associated with emotional experiences so that they are better able to detect aversive signals before becoming overwhelmed. The ability to detect physiological signals can only improve if one is able to attend to the body, and if clients are able to, it will likely reduce body detachment or indifference. Once clients begin to see how the body plays a vital role in helping to understand themselves and their internal experiences, it is plausible that the client may develop a healthier relationship with the body and may relinquish some of the body disregard associated with NSSI and eating disorder behaviors.

Conclusion

Because the body is the central object in NSSI and a key diagnostic feature of eating disorders, it makes intuitive sense that a person may require some level of body disregard to intentionally harm it. Theoretical arguments and emerging empirical data support the importance of negative body regard to both NSSI and eating disorders and that it likely facilitates NSSI through various mechanisms such as decreasing pain sensitivity and reducing awareness of internal physiological and/or emotional states. While the research is in the early stages, it strongly suggests that body regard is salient to both the initiation and maintenance of NSSI as well as why NSSI co-occurs with eating disorders at such high rates. Consequently, treatments for the co-occurrence of these behaviors would likely benefit from including body regard as an explicit focus of the treatment. Finding ways to enhance an individual's connection to and valuing of the body is likely to facilitate bodily self-care in the same way disconnection from the body may facilitate self-destruction. Thus, adopting treatment techniques that aid an individual's ability to become in tune with bodily experiences such as yoga or mindfulness, along with cognitive strategies to ameliorate distorted body-related cognitions and body dissatisfaction, is highly recommended. Research on whether treatment for the co-occurrence of NSSI and eating disorder behaviors is enhanced by adding body-relevant interventions or whether decreases in NSSI coincide with increases in body regard is greatly needed.

References

American Psychiatric Association (APA). (2000). *Diagnostic and statistical manual of mental disorders* (4th ed. text rev.). Washington, DC: American Psychiatric Association.

Bergstrom, R. L., & Neighbors, C. (2006). Body image disturbance and the social norms approach: An integrative review of the literature. *Journal of Social and Clinical Psychology, 25*, 975–1000.

Bizeul, C., Sadowsky, N., & Rigaud, D. (2001). The prognostic value of initial EDI scores in anorexia nervosa patients: A prospective follow-up study of 5-10 years. *European Psychiatry, 16*, 232–238.

Bjärehed, J., & Lundh, L. G. (2008). Deliberate self-harm in 14-year-old adolescents: How frequent is it, and How is it associated with psychopathology, relationship variables, and styles of emotional regulation? *Cognitive Behaviour Therapy, 37*, 26–37.

Brunner, R., Parzer, P., Haffner, J., Steen, R., Roos, J., Klett, M., et al. (2007). Prevalence and psychological correlates of occasional and repetitive deliberate self-harm in adolescents. *Archives of Pediatric Adolescent & Medicine, 161*, 641–649.

Cash, T. F. (2004). Body image: Past, present, and future. *Body Image, 1*, 1–5.

Cash, T. F., & Brown, T. A. (1987). Body image in anorexia nervosa and bulimia nervosa: A review of the literature. *Behavior Modification, 11*, 487–521.

Cash, T. F., & Deagle, E. A. (1997). The nature and extent of body-image disturbances in anorexia nervosa and bulimia nervosa: A meta-analysis. *International Journal of Eating Disorders, 22*, 107–125.

Cash, T. F., & Henry, P. E. (1995). Women's body images: The results of a national survey in the USA. *Sex Roles, 33*, 19–28.

Cash, T. F., & Smolak, L. (Eds.). (2011). *Body image: A handbook of science, practice, and prevention*. New York, NY: Guilford.

Claes, L., Vandereycken, W., & Vertommen, H. (2003). Eating-disordered patients with and without self-injurious behaviours: A comparison of psychopathological features. *European Eating Disorders Review, 11*, 379–396.

Claes, L., Vandereycken, W., & Vertommen, H. (2006). Pain experience related to self-injury in eating disorder patients. *Eating Behaviors, 7*, 204–213.

Cooley, E., & Toray, T. (2001). Body image and personality predictors of eating disorder symptoms during the college years. *International Journal of Eating Disorders, 30*, 28–36.

Duggan, J. M., Toste, J. R., & Heath, N. L. (2013). An examination of the relationship between body image factors and non-suicidal self-injury in young adults: The mediating influence of emotion dysregulation. *Psychiatry Research, 206*, 256–264.

Farrell, C., Shafran, R., & Lee, M. (2006). Empirically evaluated treatments for body image disturbance: A review. *European Eating Disorders Review, 14*, 289–300.

Favaro, A., & Santonastaso, P. (1998). Impulsive and compulsive self-injurious behavior in bulimia nervosa: Prevalence and psychological correlates. *The Journal of Nervous and Mental Disease, 186*, 157–165.

Forman-Hoffman, V. L. (2004). High prevalence of abnormal eating and weight control practices among U.S. high-school students. *Eating Behaviours, 5*, 325–336.

Franklin, J. C., Aaron, R. V., Arthur, M. S., Shorkey, S. P., & Prinstein, M. J. (2012). Nonsuicidal self-injury and diminished pain perception: The role of emotion dysregulation. *Comprehensive Psychiatry, 53*, 691–700.

Fredrickson, B. L., & Roberts, T. A. (1997). Objectification theory: An explanation for women's lived experience and mental health risks. *Psychology of Women Quarterly, 21*, 173–206.

Fujimori, A., Wada, Y., Yamashita, T., Choi, H., Nishizawa, S., Yamamoto, H., et al. (2011). Parental bonding in patients with eating disorders and self-injurious behavior. *Psychiatry and Clinical Neurosciences, 65*, 272–279.

Garner, D. M. (1997). The 1997 body image survey results. *Psychology Today, 30*, 30–84.

Grogan, S. (1999). *Body image: Understanding body dissatisfaction in men, women, and children*. London: Routledge.

Hooley, J. M., Ho, D. T., Slater, J., & Lockshin, A. (2010). Pain perception and nonsuicidal self-injury: A laboratory investigation. *Personality Disorders, 1*, 170–179.

Impett, E. A., Daubenmier, J. J., & Hirschman, A. L. (2006). Minding the body: Yoga, embodiment, and well-being. *Sexuality Research & Social Policy, 3*, 39–48.

Johnson, F., & Wardle, J. (2005). Dietary restraint, body dissatisfaction, and psychological distress: A prospective analysis. *Journal of Abnormal Psychology, 114*, 119–125.

Klonsky, E. D., Muehlenkamp, J. J., Lewis, S., & Walsh, B. W. (2011). *Advances in psychotherapy: Nonsuicidal self-injury*. Cambridge, MA: Hogrefe.

Linehan, M. M. (1993). *Cognitive-behavioral treatment of borderline personality disorder*. New York, NY: Guilford.

Matsumoto, R., Kitabayashi, Y., Narumoto, J., Wada, Y., Okamoto, A., Ushijima, Y., et al. (2006). Regional cerebral blood flow changes associated with interoceptive awareness in the recovery process of anorexia nervosa. *Progress in Neuro-Psychopharmacology and Biological Psychiatry, 30*, 1265–1270.

Merwin, R. M., Zucker, N. L., Lacy, J. L., & Elliott, C. A. (2010). Interoceptive awareness in eating disorders: Distinguishing lack of clarity from non-acceptance of internal experience. *Cognition and Emotion, 24*, 892–902.

Moradi, B., & Huang, Y. P. (2008). Objectification theory and psychology of women: A decade of advances and future directions. *Psychology of Women Quarterly, 32*, 377–398.

Muehlenkamp, J. J. (2012). Body regard in nonsuicidal self-injury: Theoretical explanations and treatment directions. *Journal of Cognitive Psychotherapy, 26*, 331–347.

Muehlenkamp, J. J., Bagge, C. L., Tull, M. T., & Gratz, K. L. (2013). Body regard as a moderator of the relation between emotion dysregulation and non-suicidal self-injury. *Suicide and Life-Threatening Behaviors*. doi:10.1111/sltb.12032.

Muehlenkamp, J. J., & Brausch, A. M. (2012). Body image as a mediator of non-suicidal self-injury in adolescents. *Journal of Adolescence, 35*, 1–9.

Muehlenkamp, J. J., Claes, L., Smits, D., Peat, C. M., & Vandereycken, W. (2011). Non-suicidal self-injury in eating disordered patients: A test of a conceptual model. *Psychiatry Research, 188*, 102–108.

Muehlenkamp, J. J., Peat, C. M., Claes, L., & Smits, D. (2012). Self-injury and disordered eating: Expressing emotion dysregulation through the body. *Suicide and Life-Threatening Behavior, 42*, 416–425.

Muehlenkamp, J. J., Swanson, J. D., & Brausch, A. M. (2005). Self-objectification, risk taking, and self-harm in college women. *Psychology of Women Quarterly, 29*, 24–32.

Nelson, A., & Muehlenkamp, J. J. (2012). Body attitudes and objectification in non-suicidal self-injury: Comparing males and females. *Archives of Suicide Research, 16*, 1–12.

Newman, C. F. (2009). Cognitive therapy for nonsuicidal self-injury. In M. K. Nock (Ed.), *Understanding self-injury: Origins, assessment and treatment*. Washington, DC: American Psychological Association.

Niedtfeld, I., Schulze, L., Kirsch, P., Herpertz, S. C., Bohus, M., & Schmahl, C. (2010). Affect regulation and pain in borderline personality disorder: A possible link to the understanding of self-injury. *Biological Psychiatry, 68*, 383–391.

Nuemark-Sztainer, D., Paxton, S. J., Hannan, P. J., Haines, J., & Story, M. (2006). Does body satisfaction matter? Five-year longitudinal associations between body satisfaction and health behaviors in adolescent females and males. *Journal of Adolescent Health, 39*, 244–251.

Orbach, I., Stein, D., Shani-Sela, M., & Har-Even, D. (2001). Body attitudes and body experiences in suicidal adolescents. *Suicide and Life-Threatening Behavior, 31*, 237–249.

Papezova, H., Yamamotova, A., & Uher, R. (2005). Elevated pain threshold in eating disorders: Physiological and psychological factors. *Journal of Psychiatric Research, 39*, 431–438.

Pollatos, O., Kurz, A., Albrecht, J., Schreder, T., Kleeman, A. M., Schopf, V., et al. (2008). Reduced perception of bodily signals in anorexia nervosa. *Eating Behaviors, 9*, 381–388.

Rodin, J., Silberstein, L., & Streigel-Moore, R. (1984). Women and weight: A normative discontent. *Nebraska Symposium on Motivation, 32*, 267–307.

Ross, S., Heath, N. L., & Toste, J. R. (2009). Non-suicidal self-injury and eating pathology in high school students. *The American Journal of Orthopsychiatry, 79*, 83–92.

Slevec, J. H., & Tiggemann, M. (2011). Predictors of body dissatisfaction and disordered eating in middle-aged women. *Clinical Psychology Review, 31*, 515–524.

Smith, A. R., Fink, E. L., Anestis, M. D., Ribeiro, M. D., Gordon, J. D., Davis, K. H., et al. (2013). Exercise caution: Over-exercise is associated with suicidality among individuals with disordered eating. *Psychiatry Research, 206*(2–3), 246–255. doi:10.1016/j.psychres.2012.11.004.

Solano, R., Fernández-Aranda, F., Aitken, A., López, C., & Vallejo, J. (2005). Self-injurious behaviour in people with eating disorders. *European Eating Disorders Review, 13*, 3–10.

Stanley, B., Sher, L., Wilson, S., Ekman, R., Huang, Y. Y., & Mann, J. J. (2010). Non-suicidal self-injurious behavior, endogenous opioids and monoamine neurotransmitters. *Journal of Affective Disorders, 124*, 134–140.

Stice, E., & Shaw, H. E. (2002). Role of body dissatisfaction in the onset and maintenance of eating pathology: A synthesis of research findings. *Journal of Psychosomatic Research, 53*, 985–993.

Stirling, A., & Kerr, G. (2012). Perceived vulnerabilities of female athletes to the development of disordered eating behaviours. *European Journal of Sport Science, 12*, 262–273.

Thompson, J. K., Coovert, M. D., Richards, K. J., Johnson, S., & Cattarin, J. (1995). Development of body image, eating disturbance and general psychological functioning in female adolescents: Covariance structure modeling and longitudinal investigations. *International Journal of Eating Disorders, 18*, 221–236.

Wallenstein, M. B., & Nock, M. K. (2007). Physical exercise for the treatment of nonsuicidal self-injury: Evidence from a single-case study. *The American Journal of Psychiatry, 164*, 350–351.

Walsh, B. W. (2012). *Treating self-injury: A practical guide* (2nd ed.). New York, NY: Guilford.

Yates, T. M., Carlson, E. A., & Egeland, B. (2008). A prospective study of child maltreatment and self-injurious behaviour in a community sample. *Developmental and Psychopathology, 20*, 651–671.

15 Peer Influences on Non-suicidal Self-Injury and Disordered Eating

Lori M. Hilt and Emily H. Hamm

Abstract

In this chapter, we review models of peer influence and discuss the role of peer relationships in the onset and maintenance of disordered eating and non-suicidal self-injury (NSSI) during adolescence. Evidence suggests that unhealthy dieting and NSSI may be engaged in as a direct response to criticism from peers. This type of peer victimization may also increase negative affect, making emotion regulation more challenging which could increase self-harm. In addition to peer victimization, self-harm may develop through modeling, reinforcement, attempts to gain popularity, or other social mechanisms. Homophily effects are well documented, but additional longitudinal research is needed to better understand the mechanisms of peer influence on self-harm. Future research is also needed to address whether the co-occurrence of disordered eating and NSSI may be due to shared mechanisms of peer influence. The protective effects of peer relationships are also discussed along with clinical implications including strategies for prevention and intervention.

15.1 Introduction

In a recent episode of the popular television show *Glee*, a cheerleader attempted to convince a new rising star in the glee club that she was gaining weight and suggested she deal with it by purging, resulting in the development of a serious eating disorder. Although real-life peer influence on health-risk behaviors is likely less obvious and malicious, this plot line illustrates the potential power of peer influence in the development of self-harm.

L.M. Hilt (✉) • E.H. Hamm
Department of Psychology, Lawrence University, Appleton, WI, USA
e-mail: lori.m.hilt@lawrence.edu

L. Claes and J.J. Muehlenkamp (eds.), *Non-Suicidal Self-Injury in Eating Disorders*,
DOI 10.1007/978-3-642-40107-7_15,

Empirical evidence suggests that health-risk behaviors including non-suicidal self-injury (NSSI; deliberate destruction of one's body tissue without suicidal intent) and disordered eating (e.g., extreme dieting, fasting, and bingeing) are related to peer relationships. For example, NSSI is more common among young adolescent girls with a best friend who has engaged in NSSI (Prinstein et al., 2010), and body image and weight loss behaviors are more similar among friends within a clique than among peers in different cliques (Paxton, Schutz, Wertheim, & Muir, 1999), suggesting possible contagion of self-harm behaviors among peers. Furthermore, research on NSSI and disordered eating has suggested that these self-harm behaviors may be interpersonally motivated. In the context of NSSI, adolescents have reported that although they often engage in the behavior to regulate their emotions, they also self-injure in order to regulate their social environment. For example, in a study of over 100 adolescent psychiatric inpatients, 24 % endorsed a social reinforcement function for their past-year NSSI (Nock & Prinstein, 2004). Reasons for self-injuring included avoiding being with others (negative reinforcement) and attempting to change others' behavior (positive reinforcement). Within the context of disordered eating, some adolescents have reported engaging in extreme dieting behaviors in order to obtain acceptance or increase likability among peers (e.g., Gerner & Wilson, 2005; Oliver & Thelan, 1996).

The specific processes by which peers may influence NSSI and disordered eating behaviors are not well understood. In this chapter, we review general models of peer influence. We also review the literature on peer influence and self-harm behaviors to explore the question of whether peer relationships influence the onset and maintenance of NSSI and disordered eating. Extensive research suggests that peers can influence each other in both adaptive and maladaptive ways [for a review, see Brown, Bakken, Ameringer, and Mahon (2008)]. Thus, we consider how peers may both increase risk for self-harm and how they may buffer at-risk peers from developing self-harming behaviors. We also explore the question of *how* peers influence these behaviors and argue there may be common mechanisms of influence for NSSI and disordered eating that may be able to explain their co-occurrence and be addressed through prevention efforts.

Although social influence has been studied across the lifespan, much of the work on peer influence and health-risk behavior has focused on adolescence. During adolescence, peers become an increasingly important source of social support and influence as youth develop autonomy from parents (Furman & Buhrmester, 1992). Onset of self-harm behaviors peaks during adolescence (Rodham & Hawton, 2009), making this an opportune time to study mechanisms of risk and resilience. The literature reviewed in this chapter thus focuses primarily on adolescence.

15.2 General Models of Peer Influence

Adolescents interact with peers in a variety of contexts including schools, community groups, and social media networks. Peer influence has typically been examined empirically in the context of dyadic relationships or, in some cases, larger social networks such as school cliques. Occasionally, inpatient settings have also been used to study peer influences on self-harm (e.g., Rosen & Walsh, 1989). Multiple modes of peer influence have been documented to understand a variety of behaviors. A large literature on peer victimization suggests that both direct (e.g., teasing or name calling) and indirect (e.g., rumor spreading, social exclusion) forms of victimization may have deleterious effects on victims, including self-harm. A separate literature has explored why peers with similar behavior tend to affiliate and how behaviors may spread among peers (i.e., homophily). Finally, another literature has focused on the protective effects of high-quality peer relationships. Consideration of each of these models may offer ideas about the role of peers in the development and maintenance of self-harm.

15.2.1 Peer Victimization

Peer victimization is a multifaceted and pervasive problem that encompasses many potentially harmful behaviors perpetrated by youth and aimed at other youth (Hawker & Boulton, 2000). It may include name calling, social exclusion, teasing, and other forms of bullying. Many researchers divide peer victimization into two broad categories: *overt*, involving direct, openly aggressive name calling or physical/emotional aggression, and *relational*, including more indirect, covert behaviors such as rumor spreading, damaging reputations through gossip, and social exclusion (Crick & Grotpeter, 1996). These experiences are often assessed using self-report questionnaires such as the Revised Peer Experiences Questionnaire (RPEQ; Prinstein, Boergers, & Vernberg, 2001) which asks participants to indicate how often they have been the target of various peer victimization behaviors over the past year. Peer victimization is associated with multiple negative outcomes, especially in the social, psychological, and school adjustment domains (Hawker & Boulton, 2000). Research indicates that disordered eating and NSSI are two specific outcomes related to peer victimization in youth (e.g., Fairburn et al., 1998; Heilbron & Prinstein, 2010).

Peer Victimization and Disordered Eating. Teasing and disparaging comments from peers, both forms of overt victimization, are commonly associated with disordered eating and dieting behaviors in adolescence. Appearance-related teasing, in particular, is highly prevalent and salient throughout childhood and adolescence and commonly involves remarks about weight (Cash, 1995). In one study, over 20 % of both male and female adolescents reported being recipients of weight-related teasing at least a few times a year (Haines, Neumark-Sztainer, Eisenberg, & Hannan, 2006). One study found that teasing was associated with body/appearance dissatisfaction, which then statistically predicted adolescent girls' restrictive eating practices (Cattarin & Thompson, 1994). Another study reported a similar relationship between teasing and risk for developing bulimia or binge eating disorder (Fairburn et al., 1998).

Weight-related teasing is often measured using the Perceptions of Teasing Scale (POTS; Thompson, Cattarin, Fowler, & Fisher, 1995), a self-report questionnaire eliciting experiences of weight-related teasing (e.g., "People made fun of you because you were heavy") and competency teasing (e.g., "People made fun of you by repeating something you said because they thought it was dumb"). One large study of nearly 900 adolescent girls used a three-question adaptation of the POTS focusing only on weight, body shape, and appearance teasing to determine the influence of teasing, among other types of peer influence, on eating attitudes and behaviors (Lieberman, Gauvin, Bukowski, & White, 2001). Participants reported whether or not they had found the teasing distressing. Peers also nominated students in the grade who were recipients of non-weight-related relational aggression (e.g., "someone who is ignored by others") as well as weight- and/or appearance-related teasing. Results indicated that weight-related teasing was predictive of adolescents' dieting behaviors. Participants upset by the teasing were more likely to endorse more dieting restraint than participants who were teased but not upset. In addition, researchers found that adolescents' peer-reported overweight teasing predicted bulimic behavior. These findings suggest that adolescents' development of disordered eating behaviors may partially be in response to weight-related criticism from peers.

Peer Victimization and NSSI. Weight-related teasing and other forms of peer victimization are also related to NSSI. A study of 94 young adolescent girls used the weight-related items from the POTS along with the overt and relational subscales of the RPEQ to form a single indicator of peer victimization (Hilt, Cha, & Nolen-Hoeksema, 2008). Hilt and colleagues found that girls experiencing greater levels of peer victimization were more likely to self-injure for interpersonal reasons. Furthermore, perceived quality of peer relationships moderated this association such that victimized girls who reported lower quality peer communication were at greater risk for interpersonally motivated NSSI. Limitations of this study were that it was cross sectional and only examined girls. In a 2-year prospective study of nearly 500 young adolescent boys and girls, participants nominated peers who were targets of overt and/or covert victimization, and adolescents self-reported engagement in NSSI (Heilbron & Prinstein, 2010). Results revealed a different pattern for boys and girls in predicting baseline NSSI. Self-injuring boys (7.1 %) were more frequently identified by peers as receiving overt victimization than were boys who did not self-injure. Conversely, self-injuring girls (5.7 %) were less frequently nominated as victims of overt victimization than non-injuring girls. Peer victimization did not predict engagement in NSSI prospectively. The cross-sectional results for girls are not consistent with the results of the earlier study by Hilt and colleagues, but the studies differed considerably in measures and informants. Taken together, there is concurrent evidence that peer victimization is associated with NSSI for young adolescent girls and boys.

Although adolescents report engaging in NSSI for both intra- and interpersonal reasons, the most commonly reported reason is to regulate negative affect (Nock & Prinstein, 2004). Peer victimization is associated with increases in negative affect

(Hawker & Boulton, 2000), which could help explain the relationship between peer victimization and NSSI. One study tested this idea among a group of 99 psychiatrically hospitalized adolescent girls (Adrian, Zeman, Erdley, Lisa, & Sim, 2011). Adolescents completed questionnaires assessing relational and overt victimization along with negative friendship interactions. They also reported on their engagement in NSSI. Emotion dysregulation was assessed by questionnaires and a coded emotional reflection writing task. Results suggested that peer victimization and relational problems were indirectly related to the frequency and severity of NSSI via emotion dysregulation (Adrian et al., 2011). We explored a similar idea in our work with young adolescent girls recruited from the community (Hamm & Hilt, 2013). Adolescents reported on their experience as victims of relational peer aggression, their engagement in NSSI, and their use of rumination, a maladaptive emotion-regulation strategy that involves passively brooding about negative emotions. We found evidence for the indirect effect of relational victimization on NSSI via rumination. Both our study and the one by Adrian and colleagues were cross sectional, limiting interpretations regarding the causal nature of this relationship. However, they suggest a possible mechanism in the link between peer victimization and self-injury among both clinical and community samples.

Mechanisms of Influence. While no peer victimization studies we are aware of have examined disordered eating and NSSI together, similar mechanisms may be influencing these outcomes. Peer victimization appears to increase body image disturbance and negative affect while decreasing self-esteem (e.g., Hawker & Boulton, 2000; Lieberman et al., 2001). Hence, engaging in disordered eating, like NSSI, may be an attempt at regulating distressing emotions. In addition to mediation models, peer victimization could act as a stressor or moderator that interacts with other risk factors for self-harm such as self-criticism or abuse history. To our knowledge, these models have not been tested in the context of disordered eating and NSSI.

Peer victimization may be a more important predictor of self-harm behavior for adolescent girls compared to boys. Karen Rudolph has found that, relative to boys, girls place greater importance on peer relationships, experience more peer-related stress, and are more emotionally reactive to peer-related stress (e.g., Rudolph, 2002; Rudolph & Conley, 2005; Rudolph & Hammen, 1999). These differences might help explain why eating disorders and (to a lesser degree) NSSI occur more often among girls than boys.

In sum, peer victimization has been associated with self-harm behaviors, including disordered eating and NSSI. Much of the work on disordered eating has focused on weight-related teasing, while the work on NSSI has included both overt and relational forms of victimization. Self-harm behaviors may be a direct response to peer victimization. For example, an adolescent criticized for being overweight may adopt unhealthy eating behaviors in an attempt to lose weight, or a youth rejected by peers may self-injure in an attempt to gain social support. Additionally, peer victimization may increase negative affect or dysregulated emotion, leading to self-harm as a way to regulate. Preliminary evidence for these relationships is based predominantly on cross-sectional research, precluding an understanding of causal factors. This body of work has not examined onset versus maintenance of self-harm and has focused mostly on self-report. Thus, an important step for future research is to carefully examine these relationships prospectively using multiple methods and multi-informant measures of constructs. Additionally, future work should clarify the role of gender in the relationship between peer victimization and self-harm.

Considering this research from a clinical perspective, clinicians may want to assess for and consider the role of peer victimization in the client's self-harm. If a clinician learns that peer victimization is a factor maintaining an adolescent's self-harm, she/he may want to use psychoeducation to make this process transparent for the adolescent. Depending on the nature of the adolescent's peer network, social skills training may help the adolescent to build more positive peer relationships. It may also be important to help the adolescent build self-esteem and self-acceptance if peer criticism is a factor in self-harm behavior. Finally, as with any treatment for self-harm, it is important to teach adolescents adaptive coping strategies for dealing with negative affect.

15.2.2 Homophily

Much of the peer influence literature focuses on the idea that peers who affiliate tend to share similar attributes, and this homophily may be due to selection (i.e., birds of a feather flock together) and/or socialization (e.g., contagion via modeling) effects (Kandel, 1978). Selection involves similar peers (e.g., two adolescents who engage in NSSI) seeking each other out for friendship, while socialization involves peers who are initially dissimilar on some trait or behavior influencing each other (e.g., one adolescent with disordered eating influencing her friend to adopt similar behaviors). Both processes may also work in conjunction. For example, self-harming adolescents may select each other and then reinforce each other's behavior so that the self-harm within the group escalates in severity and frequency over time.

Socialization processes are of particular interest when trying to understand self-harm, and studying them requires a prospective design to examine temporal changes. Unfortunately, many studies involve cross-sectional designs, limiting conclusions regarding the causes of homophily which could be due to selection and/or socialization (Kandel, 1978). Furthermore, different mechanisms of socialization or contagion have also been suggested, including conformity, peer pressure, modeling, and reinforcement (Prinstein & Dodge, 2008). Some research has also focused on the role of popularity or social status and susceptibility to peer influence (e.g., Cohen & Prinstein, 2006). Although much of the research on the socialization of self-harm behaviors has focused on substance use, there is also evidence for socialization of disordered eating behavior (e.g., Paxton et al., 1999) and NSSI (e.g., Rosen & Walsh, 1989).

Much of the research on homophily has focused on either popularity or peer group affiliation. Popularity, the degree to which one is liked, accepted, or admired by peers, encompasses the unilateral attitude of a group towards an individual (e.g., Bukowski, Hoza, & Boivin, 1993). Popularity is equivalent to youth's sociometric status. Literature on popularity and related social processes distinguish between performing a behavior to secure or maintain popularity, performing a behavior in response to peer pressure (which is considered direct and overt), and general conformity to a group norm. In addition to popularity, research on peer groups' effects on health-risk behaviors, including disordered eating and NSSI, could be useful in identifying specific friend groups to target with prevention efforts at schools. Research suggests that health-risk behaviors are related to the peer groups students are affiliated with (La Greca, Prinstein, & Fetter, 2001).

Homophily and Disordered Eating. Research has demonstrated that appearance and attractiveness are often key components in peers' evaluation and acceptance. Indeed, children's overweight appearance has been associated with being less liked by peers (e.g., Lerner & Lerner, 1977). Youth are aware of this bias: Multiple studies have found that individuals perceive they will be better liked by friends or peers if thinner (e.g., Gerner & Wilson, 2005; Paxton et al., 1999). For example, in a study of 200 middle school students, the extent to which participants believed being thinner corresponded to being more liked by peers was the best predictor of disordered eating symptoms for girls and the second best predictor for boys (second to body- or eating-related teasing; Meyer & Gast, 2008). A prospective study of adolescent girls found that perceptions of peer pressure to be thin predicted the onset of binge eating and purging (Stice, 1998). These findings suggest that the perceived benefit of increased popularity and/or the perceived pressure from peers to conform to a thin ideal may be one factor contributing to the initiation and maintenance of disordered eating.

In the large study of adolescent girls conducted by Lieberman et al. (2001; detailed previously in the peer victimization section), researchers assessed several additional constructs to predict disordered eating, including popularity (measured by peer nomination) and self-reports of peer modeling, social reinforcement, and beliefs about the importance of appearance for popularity. Findings indicated that disordered eating was associated with being popular, the belief that weight and appearance are important for popularity, peer pressure in the form of modeling (e.g., having friends who are on a diet), and social reinforcement (e.g., having friends who have shown you how to lose weight). Although the data are cross sectional, precluding causal interpretations, these associations lend further evidence that disordered eating behavior may be reinforced by peers' favor.

Studies involving peer groups (i.e., cliques or social networks) have found that adolescents' friend groups can predict unhealthy eating behaviors (Mackey & La Greca, 2007). For example, studies with college students have shown that dietary restraint and binge eating symptoms converge over time among women who live together (Crandall, 1988; Meyer & Waller, 2001). Studies of young adolescent girls (in seventh and tenth grades) using social network analysis have shown that members of cliques are more similar than nonmembers on dietary restraint, extreme weight loss behaviors, and binge eating (Hutchinson & Rapee, 2007; Paxton et al., 1999). Furthermore, an individual's dieting and extreme weight loss behaviors can be predicted from her friends' scores on these measures (Hutchinson & Rapee, 2007). Some possible mechanisms of influence were explored in a study of almost 350 high school girls (Shroff & Thompson, 2006). Results suggested that internalization of media messages, thin-ideal appearance comparison, and peer suppression of feelings were statistical mediators of the association between peer relationship variables and adolescent disordered eating. This study was limited in that it relied only on self-report questionnaires, where adolescents reported on their perceptions of their peers' behavior and their own behavior. Future research could be enhanced by examining mechanisms of peer influence using friend-reported behaviors and a longitudinal design, as this cross-sectional study could not establish causal relationships between variables.

Although these studies of peer groups point to strong effects of homophily, they have generally been unable to tease apart selection and socialization effects due to their cross-sectional design.

Homophily and NSSI. Studies of youth with NSSI also suggest possible selection and socialization effects for their self-harm behaviors. For example, 82 % of an adolescent inpatient sample of self-injurers reported that friends outside of the hospital had self-injured within the past year (Nock & Prinstein, 2005). In another study, 38 % of adolescents with a history of NSSI reported getting the idea to self-injure from peers (Diliberto & Nock, 2008). Among a small sample of college students with a history of NSSI, 59 % reported that a friend first engaged in NSSI (Heath, Ross, Toste, Charlebois, & Nedecheva, 2009). These retrospective studies of adolescent and college student self-injurers suggest a possible socialization effect for NSSI, i.e., adolescents may be initiating NSSI after becoming friends with a peer already self-injuring.

Studies of NSSI in intensive treatment settings further point to socialization effects, because adolescents do not choose their peers in these situations, ruling out the likelihood of selection effects (Prinstein, Guerry, Browne, & Rancourt, 2009). For example, in a study of 12 adolescents in daily treatment together for 10 months, incidents of NSSI were often shared (i.e., if one adolescent self-injured, one or more were likely to also self-injure that same day or the next day; Rosen & Walsh, 1989). In another study of 12 adolescents studied during their stay at a psychiatric inpatient facility, deliberate self-harm (mostly NSSI in the form of cutting) was found to cluster among youth (Tiaminen, Kallio-Soukainen, Nokso-Koivisto, Kaljonen, & Kelenius, 1998). Two of the participants in this study who completed a follow-up interview indicated they had not self-injured prior to this hospitalization, suggesting a contagion.

Another larger study of adolescents recruited during their stay at a psychiatric treatment facility points to possible selection and socialization effects. Prinstein et al. (2010) sampled over 100 adolescents who reported on their frequency of NSSI and their perceptions of their close friends' health-risk behaviors (e.g., self-injury ideation) at three times during an 18-month interval. Baseline NSSI frequency was associated with perceptions of close friends' self-injurious thoughts and behaviors, suggestive of a possible selection effect. Increases in NSSI frequency from baseline to 18 months were also associated with perceptions regarding friends, suggestive of a possible socialization effect, which held controlling for depressive symptoms. Because friends' behaviors were not directly measured, it is possible that findings were biased by adolescents' perceptions (Prinstein et al., 2010); however, this longitudinal study adds additional preliminary evidence for socialization of NSSI.

Although longitudinal research on self-harm behavior is generally lacking, there is some further evidence of socialization effects for NSSI. Prinstein et al. (2010) also examined peer influences on NSSI in a large community sample of adolescents followed for one year. Nearly 400 sixth through eighth grade students identified their best friend and reported on their frequency of NSSI behavior at baseline and one year later. Adolescents' NSSI behavior at Time 2 was associated with having a best friend who engaged in NSSI at baseline, suggesting a socialization effect. Furthermore, this effect was stronger for girls and sixth grade students. Because this study relied on friends' reports of their own behavior and controlled for baseline depressive symptoms, socialization effects are likely valid.

Additional evidence for homophily of NSSI comes from research on peer cultures that may support or promote self-injurious behavior. For example, some research suggests that being a member of Goth subculture, which is often characterized as a subgenre of punk distinguished by its dark clothing and makeup, may increase an adolescent's likelihood of self-injuring (Young, Sweeting, & West, 2006). Young and colleagues' large study of older adolescents in Scotland asked participants to report on their identification with various youth subcultures. Participants also completed a clinical interview to assess psychological symptoms and self-injurious behaviors. After controlling for likely correlates (i.e., gender, depression, and substance use), identifying as Goth either currently or in the past predicted past self-harm (both NSSI and suicidal behavior). The association between self-injury and Goth subculture may be a product of ideals or norms held by the subculture, selection effects, or both. That is, self-harm may be viewed by those involved as a distinguishing feature of Goth subculture, which may facilitate experimentation with NSSI; or youth who self-injure may be drawn to a peer crowd that is concerned with darker themes, including injury and death. However, it should be noted that this study has been criticized as a mischaracterization of the subculture as a whole and that it does not make clear distinctions among body modification, non-suicidal self-injury, and suicidal behaviors (e.g., Phillipov, 2006).

Research points to the likely involvement of both selection and socialization effects in adolescent NSSI, though specific mechanisms of peer influence have not been systematically investigated. One study of Internet message boards offers some possible suggestions (Whitlock, Powers, & Eckenrode, 2006). Whitlock and colleagues found that participants in these online forums are often seeking social support, suggestive of a motivation for selection effects among virtual peer cultures. Additionally, participants posted suggestions (i.e., how-to) related to self-injury which may offer one mechanism of socialization. It is also noteworthy that some of the posts involved encouragement of treatment seeking, suggesting possible positive socialization effects.

Mechanisms of Peer Influence on Self-Harm. Although both disordered eating and NSSI are maladaptive behaviors that may be engaged in for social functions, it appears that disordered eating is more likely to be engaged in specifically for obtaining higher social status (i.e., being perceived as more popular). Adolescents may believe that their body shape is related to their social status, and research suggests there is some truth to this belief, which may directly reinforce disordered eating behavior. For example, as a slightly overweight adolescent begins purging or fasting, she/he may get more attention and acceptance from peers (i.e., increased status), directly reinforcing the disordered eating behaviors. To date, there is no documented evidence that NSSI increases social status, though it may elevate status within specific peer groups (e.g., Goth subculture; Young et al., 2006).

Though functions of these two types of maladaptive behavior may differ regarding popularity, they may share some similar functions related to social status. For example, beliefs about peers' perceptions of behavior are associated with engagement in maladaptive behaviors. In a study of adolescent girls, unhealthy eating behaviors and body dissatisfaction were correlated with perceptions regarding friend concern with appearance and thinness (Schutz & Paxton, 2007). Similarly, the perception of self-injury as beneficial or a symbol of strength by a friend or larger social group may be correlated with engaging in NSSI. Future research should focus on possible mechanisms of social status and NSSI.

Another possible shared mechanism of influence is increased attention from peers that may reinforce the self-harm. Research on NSSI has shown that a small percentage of self-injurers engage in NSSI in order to get attention from others (e.g., Nock & Prinstein, 2004, 2005). Even though this desire may not be a motivating force for many who self-injure, it is likely that increased attention from peers could reinforce this behavior. One prospective study of NSSI found that adolescents who self-injured perceived increases in social support from their fathers over the next year (Hilt, Nock, Lloyd-Richardson, & Prinstein, 2008). This study did not examine peer support; however, concerned friends could unintentionally reinforce self-harm behavior. This dynamic could equally apply to disordered eating which may also be reinforced more directly by increased popularity.

One important factor to consider in research on peer influence and self-harm is susceptibility to peer influence, i.e., what are the moderators of peer influence on self-harm? Research has found that youth who are low in self-confidence or high in social anxiety may be more susceptible to peer influence because of a desire to fit in (e.g., Cohen & Prinstein, 2006). Relatedly, adolescents lower in social status and higher in psychological problems including depressive symptoms and substance abuse have been found to be more susceptible to peer influence (Allen, Porter, & MacFarland, 2006). As mentioned in the peer victimization section, girls place more importance on the value of peer relationships in adolescence (Rudolph & Conley, 2005), suggesting they could be more susceptible to socialization. Some support for this comes from the Prinstein et al. (2010) community study of NSSI, where socialization effects were stronger for girls. Many studies of peer influence on disordered eating have only sampled girls (e.g., Hutchinson & Rapee, 2007; Paxton et al., 1999), so it is unclear whether similar effects would be evident among boys.

However, one study of adolescent girls and boys found that both girls' and boys' body shapes and dieting were associated with their peer status (Wang, Houshyar, & Prinstein, 2006). Multiple studies suggest that younger adolescents may be more susceptible to influence than older adolescents. For example, Pike (1995) only found homophily for binge eating among younger high school students (ninth and tenth graders). Prinstein et al. (2010) only found a contagion effect of NSSI among younger middle school students (sixth graders). Research on peer influence suggests that conformity may peak around ninth grade (Berndt, 1979; Steinberg, 2005), which generally corresponds to peaks in self-harm behavior (Muehlenkamp, Claes, Havertape, & Plener, 2012). These moderators suggest important targets for prevention efforts related to self-harm.

Another factor to consider is the role of peer influence in the onset versus maintenance of self-harm. Most studies of socialization examine whether self-harm either begins or increases over time as a function of having self-harming peers. Even though self-harm may be socially learned, functions for self-harm may shift to emotion regulation once the behavior has been initiated. Conversely, self-harm that begins with emotion-regulation motivations (i.e., to reduce negative affect) could then be maintained via peer reinforcement.

Clinically, it may be especially helpful to educate adolescents about contagion and other socialization processes that may be involved in his/her self-harm behaviors. Because friendships and peer status are often highly valued by adolescents, it may be more helpful to set "ground rules" for friendships than ask adolescents to avoid spending any time with self-harming friends. For example, adolescents could be asked to minimize discussions about self-harm with friends and learn strategies for doing this to avoid reinforcement. It would also be helpful to encourage adolescents to identify positive and supporting relationships and/or help them cultivate such relationships.

15.2.3 Protective Factors

Although the vast majority of research on peer influence and self-harm focuses on the deleterious effects of peer relationships, these relationships can also offer protection for adolescents. Protective factors may include such things as feeling connected to peers. Additionally, adaptive behavior may be socialized among peers [see Brown et al. (2008)], providing modeling of healthy attitudes and coping behavior.

High-quality peer relationships may provide social support and positive influences that can protect adolescents from self-harm. Research has found that the presence of at least one mutual friend is associated with better psychological outcomes [for a review, see Vitaro, Boivin, and Bukowski (2008)]. Some studies have found that a close friend can buffer youth with risk factors from experiencing poor outcomes. For example, one study showed that children victimized by their peers were less likely to show increases in internalizing and externalizing symptoms if they had a best friend (Hodges, Boivin, Vitaro, & Bukowski, 1999).

Research on peer support and self-harm behavior has predominately focused on risk, suggesting that poor perceived social support from peers is associated with self-harm, such as NSSI (e.g., Hilt, Cha, & Nolen-Hoeksema, 2008). The flip side of the coin suggests that perceived social support is associated with an absence of self-harm and perceived social support may help buffer against risk factors (e.g., Stice, Presnell, & Spangler, 2002).

Peer-Related Protective Factors and Disordered Eating. Shisslak and Crago (2001) reviewed protective factors in the development of disordered eating, many of which involve peer influence. Some of the protective factors hypothesized include a social network that supports a diverse range of physical weights and appearances, social support, and maintaining close relationships with peers relatively unconcerned with weight. In one small study of 30 high school girls, semi-structured interviews including both open- and closed-answered questions about weight and dieting behaviors were transcribed and coded by emerging themes (Wertheim, Paxton, Schutz, & Muir, 1997). Several participants reported witnessing peers or trying themselves to talk their friends out of unhealthy eating behaviors, including purging and unhealthy dieting. Hence, friends may be in a unique position to normalize healthy eating and to correct peers' potentially detrimental weight control behaviors.

Peer-Related Protective Factors and Self-Injury. Little research has examined the potential protective effect of peers on NSSI. One study referenced in the homophily section involving NSSI (Whitlock et al., 2006) has illuminated online message boards as a possible avenue for peer support. Out of the 3,219 individual posts examined over a 2-month period, researchers found that the most common type of exchange on the self-injury message boards was one poster offering informal support to another, which accounted for about 28 % of posts. Adolescents who struggle with social situations and lack peer support, or who do not disclose their self-injury to friends, may be using connections on an online forum for encouragement or help in diminishing or stopping their NSSI. Future research should attempt to ascertain the effects of message board viewing and participation on NSSI, as these descriptive data suggest that adolescents wishing to stop self-injuring may already be successfully utilizing online peer support. However, the possibility that some posters on message boards may inadvertently or deliberately encourage others' self-injury through triggering or competitive postings should also be examined.

Peer Support and Self-Harm. Association with peers who provide social support and model healthy behavior may be an effective prevention strategy against the development of self-harm. Caution may be warranted, however, in assuming that increased social support following engagement in self-harm is necessarily beneficial (Hilt, Nock et al., 2008). After peers notice or learn of self-harm in one of their friends, they may increase their attention to this individual, suggesting a fine line between the positive effects of this social support and accidental reinforcement of self-harm. Thus, although social support may buffer individuals at-risk for self-harm from developing it, the timing of social support could be an important factor to consider.

15.3 Further Implications for Prevention and Intervention

Given the findings related to the role of peer victimization and other mechanisms of peer influence in the development of both disordered eating and NSSI, it is important to consider the role of peers in the prevention and treatment of self-harm. Peer victimization may be best addressed at the level of the school system. This could involve promoting acceptance of peers for reasons unrelated to appearance and focusing on efforts to decrease teasing (Lieberman et al., 2001). Although some school-wide prevention programs aimed at reducing peer victimization exist (e.g., Olweus Bully Prevention Program; Olweus, 1994), few have been rigorously tested with randomized designs. Those that have been tested generally show mixed results, with many failing to reduce peer victimization (Vreeman & Carroll, 2007).

Intervening with the aim of preventing socialization may be even more challenging. Contagion of self-harming behaviors could be dealt with by isolating individuals whose self-harm tends to be imitated by peers (Rosen & Walsh, 1989), but this may only be feasible within clinical settings. Much of the work on preventing socially influenced self-harm has focused on drugs and alcohol using resistance training (e.g., Donaldson, Graham, Piccinin, & Hansen, 1995), which may not be directly relevant to disordered eating and NSSI, which are less likely to be directly offered or suggested compared to substances. One way to use research findings on socialization for preventive applications would be to focus efforts on youth who are most susceptible to peer influence, i.e., younger adolescents, girls, and perhaps those who already have other risk factors for the development of self-harm. One focus of prevention programs could be to help youth cultivate peer relationships that promote healthy attitudes and behaviors.

Regarding implications for treatment, research on group treatment for adolescents suggests a cautionary tale when dealing with socially influenced behaviors. Although it is cost-effective to treat problem behaviors in a group setting, some research has found iatrogenic effects for group treatment with adolescents in particular (Dishion, McCord, & Poulin, 1999). Dishion and colleagues found that group treatment for substance use and delinquency resulted in increases in these behaviors. They suggested that adolescents socially reinforce negative behaviors in peer group settings. Efficacious group treatments exist for bulimia (e.g., group cognitive-behavioral therapy) and NSSI (to an extent, e.g., dialectical-behavior therapy skills group), but they have been almost exclusively tested with adults [for reviews, see Robins and Chapman (2004); Wilson, Grilo, and Vitousek (2007)]. One controlled study examined dialectical-behavior therapy for suicidal adolescents and did not report any iatrogenic effects from the group skills training, which also included adolescents' parents (Rathus & Miller, 2002). Given the potential for socialization of self-harm among peers, any group treatment for adolescent self-harm must take care in how discussion of self-harm is handled within the group to avoid potential contagion or reinforcement.

15.4 Future Research

Throughout this chapter, we have suggested several areas in need of future research. One limitation among the current body of research is an overreliance on cross-sectional studies. These are helpful in identifying peer-related correlates of self-harm behavior, but longitudinal work is needed to examine mechanisms of influence. One important question that has not been addressed empirically, to our knowledge, is whether the co-occurrence of NSSI and disordered eating could be at least partially due to shared mechanisms of peer influence. Research examining peer victimization as a predictor of disordered eating and NSSI in separate studies suggests this could be one potential shared mechanism, either directly or indirectly via emotion dysregulation. Of particular interest is whether the same type of peer victimization (e.g., teasing about weight or appearance) would predict the co-occurrence of NSSI and disordered eating. Additionally, it appears that both disordered eating and NSSI may be socialized within peer groups. Observationally, the peak age of onset for disordered eating, NSSI, and susceptibility to peer influence is remarkably similar, suggesting a possible relationship. Other factors (e.g., increased stress, development of regulatory capacities) could explain the phenomenon, however, underscoring the importance of empirical investigation.

Most of the studies reviewed in this chapter relied on self-report of eating pathology and NSSI (along with other constructs). There are high rates of disordered eating and NSSI among community samples, making the ability to generalize to this population a benefit. A drawback is that we know considerably less about the contribution of peer influence to serious, clinical levels of self-harm which might be better assessed using a clinical interview. Future research that follows adolescents with socially influenced self-harm to examine how the behavior progresses would be helpful in understanding the long-term impact of peer-influenced self-harm. Finally, it is worth mentioning that peer influence processes are complex and transactional (Brown et al., 2008). Furthermore, they are only one of many hypothesized factors involved in the development of NSSI and disordered eating. Research that carefully measures peer influence processes along with other factors related to self-harm will be necessary to fully understand the relative contributions. In addition to research on better understanding the peer influence mechanisms on disordered eating and NSSI, research on prevention via these mechanisms is greatly needed.

References

Adrian, M., Zeman, J., Erdley, C. A., Lisa, L., & Sim, L. (2011). Emotional dysregulation and interpersonal difficulties as risk factors for nonsuicidal self-injury in adolescent girls. *Journal of Abnormal Child Psychology, 39*, 389–400.

Allen, J. B., Porter, M. R., & MacFarland, F. C. (2006). Leaders and followers in adolescent close friendships: Susceptibility to peer influence as a predictor of risky behavior, friendship instability, and depression. *Development and Psychopathology, 18*, 155–172.

Berndt, T. J. (1979). Developmental changes in conformity to parents and peers. *Developmental Psychology, 15*, 608–616.

Brown, B. B., Bakken, J. P., Ameringer, S. W., & Mahon, S. D. (2008). A comprehensive conceptualization of the peer influence process in adolescence. In M. J. Prinstein & K. A. Dodge (Eds.), *Understanding peer influence in children and adolescents* (pp. 17–44). New York: Guilford Press.

Bukowski, W. M., Hoza, B., & Boivin, M. (1993). Popularity, friendship, and emotional adjustment during early adolescence. *New Directions for Child Development, 60*, 23–37.

Cash, T. F. (1995). Developmental teasing about physical appearance: Retrospective descriptions and relationships with body image. *Social Behavior and Personality, 23*, 123–129.

Cattarin, J., & Thompson, J. K. (1994). A three year longitudinal study of body image and eating disturbance in adolescent females. *Eating Disorders, 2*, 114–125.

Cohen, G. L., & Prinstein, M. J. (2006). Peer contagion of aggression and health risk behavior among adolescent males: An experimental investigation of effects on public conduct and private attitudes. *Child Development, 77*, 967–983.

Crandall, C. S. (1988). Social contagion of binge eating. *Journal of Personality and Social Psychology, 55*, 588–598.

Crick, N. R., & Grotpeter, J. K. (1996). Children's maltreatment by peers: Victims of relational aggression. *Development and Psychopathology, 8*, 367–380.

Diliberto, T. L., & Nock, M. K. (2008). An exploratory study of correlates, onset, and offset of non-suicidal self-injury. *Archives of Suicide Research, 12*, 219–231.

Dishion, T. J., McCord, J., & Poulin, F. (1999). When interventions harm: Peer groups and problem behavior. *American Psychologist, 54*, 755–764.

Donaldson, S. I., Graham, J. W., Piccinin, A. M., & Hansen, W. B. (1995). Resistance skills training and onset of alcohol use: Evidence for beneficial and potentially harmful effects in public schools and private Catholic schools. *Health Psychology, 14*, 291–300.

Fairburn, C. G., Doll, H. A., Welch, S. L., Hay, P. J., Davies, B. A., & O'Connor, M. E. (1998). Risk factors for binge eating disorder: A community-based, case–control study. *Archives of General Psychiatry, 55*, 425–432.

Furman, W., & Buhrmester, D. (1992). Age and sex differences in perceptionsof networks of personal relationships. *Child Development, 63*, 103–115.

Gerner, B., & Wilson, P. D. (2005). The relationship between friendship factors and adolescent girls' body image concern, body dissatisfaction, and restrained eating. *International Journal of Eating Disorders, 37*, 313–320.

Haines, J., Neumark-Sztainer, D., Eisenberg, M. E., & Hannan, P. J. (2006). Weight teasing and disordered eating behaviors in adolescents: Longitudinal findings from Project EAT (Eating Among Teens). *Pediatrics, 117*, 209–215.

Hamm, E. H., & Hilt, L. M. (2013). *Nonsuicidal self-injury, relational victimization, and rumination: A mediation model.* Poster session presented at the biennial meeting of the Society for Research in Child Development, Seattle, WA.

Hawker, D. S. J., & Boulton, M. J. (2000). Twenty years' research on peer victimization and psychosocial maladjustment: A meta-analytic review of cross-sectional studies. *Journal of Clinical Psychology and Psychiatry, 41*, 441–455.

Heath, N. L., Ross, S., Toste, J. R., Charlebois, A., & Nedecheva, T. (2009). Retrospective analysis of social factors and nonsuicidal self-injury among young adults. *Canadian Journal of Behavioural Sciences, 41*, 180–186.

Heilbron, N., & Prinstein, M. J. (2010). Adolescent peer victimization, peer status, suicidal ideation, and nonsuicidal self-injury: Examining concurrent and longitudinal associations. *Merrill-Palmer Quarterly, 56*, 388–419.

Hilt, L. M., Cha, C. B., & Nolen-Hoeksema, S. (2008). Nonsuicidal self-injury in young adolescent girls: Moderators of the distress-function relationship. *Journal of Consulting and Clinical Psychology, 76*, 63–71.

Hilt, L. M., Nock, M. K., Lloyd-Richardson, E. E., & Prinstein, M. J. (2008). Longitudinal study of an interpersonal model of non-suicidal self-injury among young adolescents. *Journal of Early Adolescence, 28*, 455–469.

Hodges, E., Boivin, M., Vitaro, F., & Bukowski, W. M. (1999). The power of friendship: Protecting against an escalating cycle of peer victimization. *Developmental Psychology, 35*, 94–101.

Hutchinson, D. M., & Rapee, R. M. (2007). Do friends share similar body image and eating problems? The role of social networks and peer influences in early adolescence. *Behaviour Research and Therapy, 45*, 1557–1577.

Kandel, D. B. (1978). Homophily, selection, and socialization in adolescent friendships. *American Journal of Sociology, 84*, 427–436.

La Greca, A. M., Prinstein, M. J., & Fetter, M. D. (2001). Adolescent peer crowd affiliation: Linkages with health-risk behaviors and close friendships. *Journal of Pediatric Psychology, 26*, 131–143.

Lerner, R. M., & Lerner, J. V. (1977). The effects of age, sex, and physical attractiveness on child-peer relations, academic performance, and elementary school adjustment. *Developmental Psychology, 13*, 585–590.

Lieberman, M., Gauvin, L., Bukowski, W. M., & White, D. R. (2001). Interpersonal influence and disordered eating behaviors in adolescent girls: The role of peer modeling, social reinforcement and body-related teasing. *Eating Behaviors, 2*, 215–236.

Mackey, E. R., & La Greca, A. M. (2007). Adolescents' eating, exercise, and weight control behaviors: Does peer crowd affiliation play a role? *Journal of Pediatric Psychology, 32*, 13–23.

Meyer, T. A., & Gast, J. (2008). The effects of peer influence on disordered eating behaviour. *Journal of School Nursing, 24*, 36–42.

Meyer, C., & Waller, G. (2001). Social convergence of disturbed eating attitudes in young adult women. *Journal of Nervous and Mental Disease, 189*, 114–119.

Muehlenkamp, J. J., Claes, L., Havertape, L., & Plener, P. (2012). International prevalence of adolescent non-suicidal self-injury and deliberate self-harm. *Child and Adolescent Psychiatry and Mental Health, 6*, 10.

Nock, M. K., & Prinstein, M. J. (2004). A functional approach to the assessment of self-mutilative behavior in adolescents. *Journal of Consulting and Clinical Psychology, 72*, 885–890.

Nock, M. K., & Prinstein, M. J. (2005). Contextual features and behavioral functions of self-mutilation among adolescents. *Journal of Abnormal Psychology, 114*, 140–146.

Oliver, K. K., & Thelan, M. H. (1996). Children's perceptions of peer influence on eating concerns. *Behavior Therapy, 27*, 25–39.

Olweus, D. (1994). Bullying at school: Basic facts and effects of a school based intervention program. *Journal of Child Psychology and Psychiatry, 35*, 1171–1190.

Paxton, S. J., Schutz, H. K., Wertheim, E. H., & Muir, S. L. (1999). Friendship clique and peer influences on body image concerns, dietary restraint, extreme weight-loss behaviors, and binge eating in adolescent girls. *Journal of Abnormal Psychology, 108*, 255–266.

Phillipov, M. M. (2006). Self-harm in Goth youth subculture: Study merely reinforces popular stereotypes. *British Medical Journal, 332*, 1215–1216.

Pike, K. M. (1995). Bulimic symptomatology in high school girls. *Psychology of Women Quarterly, 19*, 373–396.

Prinstein, M. J., Boergers, J., & Vernberg, E. M. (2001). Overt and relational aggression in adolescents: Social-psychological functioning of aggressors and victims. *Journal of Clinical Child Psychology, 30*, 477–489.

Prinstein, J. J., & Dodge, K. A. (2008). Current issues in peer influence research. In M. J. Prinstein & K. A. Dodge (Eds.), *Understanding peer influence in children and adolescents* (pp. 3–13). New York: Guilford Press.

Prinstein, M. J., Guerry, J. D., Browne, C. B., & Rancourt, D. (2009). Interpersonal models of nonsuicidal self-injury. In M. K. Nock (Ed.), *Understanding nonsuicidal self-injury: Origins, assessment, and treatment* (pp. 79–98). Washington, DC: American Psychological Association.

Prinstein, M. J., Heilbron, N., Guerry, J. D., Franklin, J. C., Rancourt, D., Simon, V., et al. (2010). Peer influence and nonsuicidal self-injury: Longitudinal results in community and clinically-referred adolescent samples. *Journal of Abnormal Child Psychology, 38*, 669–682.

Rathus, J. H., & Miller, A. L. (2002). Dialectical behavior therapy adapted for suicidal adolescents. *Suicide and Life-Threatening Behavior, 32*, 146–157.

Robins, C. J., & Chapman, A. L. (2004). Dialectical behavior therapy: Current status, recent developments and future directions. *Journal of Personality Disorders, 18*, 73–89.

Rodham, K., & Hawton, K. (2009). Epidemiology and phenomenology of nonsuicidal self-injury. In M. K. Nock (Ed.), *Understanding nonsuicidal self-injury* (pp. 37–62). Washington, DC: American Psychological Association.

Rosen, P. M., & Walsh, B. W. (1989). Patterns of contagion in self-mutilation epidemics. *The American Journal of Psychiatry, 146*, 656–658.

Rudolph, K. D. (2002). Gender differences in emotional responses to interpersonal stress during adolescence. *Journal of Adolescent Health, 30*, 3–13.

Rudolph, K. D., & Conley, C. S. (2005). The socioemotional costs and benefits of social-evaluative concern: Do girls care too much? *Journal of Personality, 73*, 115–138.

Rudolph, K. D., & Hammen, C. (1999). Age and gender as determinants of stress exposure, generation, and reactions in youngsters: A transactional perspective. *Child Development, 70*, 660–677.

Schutz, H., & Paxton, S. (2007). Friendship quality, body dissatisfaction, dieting and disordered eating in adolescent girls. *British Journal of Clinical Psychology, 46*, 67–83.

Shisslak, C. M., & Crago, M. (2001). Risk and protective factors in the development of eating disorders. In J. K. Thompson & L. Smolak (Eds.), *Body image, eating disorders, and obesity in youth: Assessment, prevention, and treatment* (pp. 103–125). Washington, DC: American Psychological Association.

Shroff, H., & Thompson, J. K. (2006). Peer influences, body image dissatisfaction, eating dysfunction and self-esteem in adolescent girls. *Journal of Health Psychology, 11*, 533–551.

Steinberg, L. (2005). Cognitive and affective development in adolescence. *Trends in Cognitive Sciences, 9*, 69–74.

Stice, E. (1998). Modeling of eating pathology and social reinforcement of the think ideal predict onset of bulimic symptoms. *Behaviour Research and Therapy, 36*, 931–944.

Stice, E., Presnell, K., & Spangler, D. (2002). Risk factors for binge eating onset in adolescent girls: A 2-year prospective investigation. *Health Psychology, 21*, 131–138.

Thompson, J. K., Cattarin, J., Fowler, H., & Fisher, E. (1995). The Perception of Teasing Scale (POTS): A revision and extension of the Physical Appearance Related Teasing Scale (PARTS). *Journal of Personality Assessment, 65*, 146–157.

Tiaminen, T. J., Kallio-Soukainen, K., Nokso-Koivisto, H., Kaljonen, A., & Kelenius, H. (1998). Contagion of deliberate self-harm among adolescent inpatients. *Journal of the American Academy of Child and Adolescent Psychiatry, 37*, 211–217.

Vitaro, F., Boivin, M., & Bukowski, W. M. (2008). The role of friendship in child and adolescent psychosocial development. In M. J. Prinstein & K. A. Dodge (Eds.), *Understanding peer influence in children and adolescents* (pp. 568–585). New York: Guilford Press.

Vreeman, R. C., & Carroll, A. E. (2007). A systematic review of school-based interventions to prevent bullying. *Archives of Pediatric and Adolescent Medicine, 161*, 77–88.

Wang, S. S., Houshyar, S., & Prinstein, M. J. (2006). Adolescent girls' and boys' weight-related health behaviors and cognitions: Associations with reputation- and preference-based peer status. *Health Psychology, 25*, 658–663.

Wertheim, E. H., Paxton, S. J., Schutz, H. K., & Muir, S. L. (1997). Why do adolescent girls watch their weight? An interview study examining sociocultural pressures to be thin. *Journal of Psychosomatic Research, 42*, 345–355.

Whitlock, J. L., Powers, J. P., & Eckenrode, J. E. (2006). The virtual cutting edge: Adolescent self-injury and the Internet. *Developmental Psychology, 42*, 407–417.

Wilson, G. T., Grilo, C. M., & Vitousek, K. M. (2007). Psychological treatment of eating disorders. *American Psychologist, 62*, 199–216.

Young, R., Sweeting, H., & West, P. (2006). Prevalence of deliberate self-harm and attempted suicide within contemporary Goth youth subculture: Longitudinal cohort study. *British Medical Journal, 332*, 1058–1061.

Non-suicidal Self-Injury, Eating Disorders, and the Internet

16

Stephen P. Lewis and Alexis E. Arbuthnott

Abstract

Online communities and material regarding non-suicidal self-injury (NSSI) and eating disorders (ED) are abundant and easily accessible on the Internet. Internet platforms (e.g., social networks, message boards, blogs, video-, and photo-sharing sites) offer individuals who engage in these behaviors opportunities to interact with others with similar experiences (i.e., who have self-injured or who have ED difficulties). Researchers have found that although online activities can be positive in a number of ways (e.g., providing support to otherwise isolated individuals), they may be detrimental in others (e.g., contributing to continued and unhealthy self-destructive behaviors). In this chapter, we review extant literature on the potential benefits and risks of online activities related to NSSI and EDs, discuss avenues for future research, and present implications and guidelines for clinicians. We end with a case vignette illustrating the clinical guidelines presented.

16.1 Overview

The Internet has emerged as a highly salient part of many individuals' lives as a means to retrieve information and connect with others; research suggests that this may be especially the case for individuals who experience mental health difficulties (e.g., emotional difficulties), isolation, and stigmatization (Berger, Wagner, & Baker, 2005; McKenna, Green, & Gleason, 2002; Whitlock, Powers, & Eckenrode, 2006). As these issues are often central in the context of non-suicidal self-injury [NSSI; see Klonsky, Muehlenkamp, Lewis, and Walsh (2011)] and eating disorders [ED; see Fairburn and Harrison (2003); Treasure, Claudino, and Zucker (2010)], it is perhaps not surprising that there has been a proliferation of online NSSI and ED

S.P. Lewis (✉) • A.E. Arbuthnott
University of Guelph, Guelph, ON, Canada
e-mail: stephen.lewis@uoguelph.ca

L. Claes and J.J. Muehlenkamp (eds.), *Non-Suicidal Self-Injury in Eating Disorders*,
DOI 10.1007/978-3-642-40107-7_16,

content and communication on the Internet [for reviews, see Lewis, Heath, Michal, and Duggan (2012); Rouleau and von Ranson (2011)]. Accordingly, researchers have recognized the need to understand the scope and nature of online activities associated with NSSI and EDs as well as the potential impact these may have on those involved. It is important for researchers and clinicians to be knowledgeable within these areas of research. This is conducive to advancing empirical work in these growing fields and addressing these activities in clinical contexts.

16.2 Non-suicidal Self-Injury and the Internet

Growing attention has focused on the scope and nature of online activity regarding non-suicidal self-injury (NSSI). In 2010, the International Society for the Study of Self-injury (ISSS) recognized the importance of research in this area. By 2011, there were over 400 news stories published globally regarding online NSSI activity, most of which focused on the impact this may have on those who access it (Google, 2011; Sornberger, Joly, Heath, & Lewis, 2012). This trend continued well into 2012 with major social networking sites (e.g., Tumblr, Instagram, Pinterest) banning what they referred to as "pro self-harm" material (Google, 2012). With this widespread public attention, research in this area has increased. Indeed, the Internet has emerged as a highly accessible and often preferred vehicle for individuals to communicate about non-suicidal self-injury [for a review, see Lewis, Heath, Michal et al. (2012)].

To date, researchers have examined online NSSI activity on (a) personally made Web sites where individuals chronicle their NSSI experiences, (b) video-sharing Web sites (e.g., YouTube), (c) major social networks (e.g., MySpace, Facebook), (d) discussion forums, and (e) question-and-answer Web sites (which allow users to post and respond to questions on almost any topic). Given the high rates of NSSI, its numerous consequences, and the salience of the Internet as a means to communicate about NSSI, researchers and clinicians need to be aware about the potential benefits and risks associated with such e-activity.

16.2.1 Potential Benefits of Online Non-suicidal Self-Injury Activity

16.2.1.1 Support and Validation

It has been suggested that many individuals who self-injure and who go online to communicate about NSSI feel isolated and stigmatized in their daily offline lives [see Lewis, Heath, Michal et al. (2012)]. Thus, for many individuals, the Internet may offer an anonymous means by which to communicate with others—typically others who also self-injure (Lewis, Heath, St. Denis, & Noble, 2011; Whitlock et al., 2006). To this end, the most widely cited benefit associated with online NSSI activity involves the aspect of social support (Baker & Fortune, 2008; Jones et al., 2011; Lewis et al., 2011; Lewis, Heath, Sornberger, & Arbuthnott, 2012; Murray & Fox, 2006; Rodham, Gavin, & Miles, 2007; Whitlock et al., 2006). Accordingly, individuals not only receive support from others but they also provide it (Lewis & Baker, 2011; Lewis et al., 2011; Rodham et al., 2007; Niwa & Mandrusiak, 2012; Smithson et al., 2011; Whitlock et al., 2006). Related to this, many youth and young adults who self-injure and who communicate about NSSI via the Internet also do so to obtain validation about their experiences (e.g., to gain a sense that they are not alone) (Baker & Fortune, 2008; Lewis, Heath, Michal et al., 2012; Lewis, Rosenrot, & Messner, 2012; Niwa & Mandrusiak, 2012; Rodham et al., 2007).

16.2.1.2 Non-suicidal Self-Injury Reductions

Reported to a lesser extent is that communicating about NSSI online may, at least in part, associate with reductions in NSSI frequency (Johnson, Zastawny, & Kulpa, 2010; Murray & Fox, 2006; Baker & Lewis, 2013; Lewis, Heath, Sornberger et al., 2012). Preliminary support for this comes from two research approaches. In the first, brief surveys have been administered to members of NSSI e-communities in which respondents indicate that pursuant to joining the e-community, they have self-injured less often (Johnson et al., 2010; Murray & Fox, 2006). In the second, researchers have content-analyzed individuals' online posts within NSSI e-communities; findings from these studies indicate that some individuals upload messages that they have self-injured less often as a result of communicating with others about NSSI online or by accessing online NSSI material (Baker & Lewis, 2013; Lewis, Heath, Sornberger et al., 2012). Notwithstanding these reports, the extent to which online NSSI communication associates with NSSI reductions is unclear, and inferences about this should be made cautiously. Not only are these reports scant, the degree to which online NSSI activity actually yields NSSI reductions is uncertain, as are the forms of online activity that may associate with these reductions and the mechanisms involved in this process.

16.2.2 Risks of Online Non-suicidal Self-Injury Activity

16.2.2.1 Normalization and Reinforcement

The most frequently reported risk associated with online NSSI activity pertains to NSSI becoming normalized and reinforced; that is, through continued online activity, the risk for continued NSSI behavior is exacerbated (Duggan, Heath, Lewis, & Baxter, 2011; Lewis & Baker, 2011; Lewis et al., 2011; Lewis, Heath, Sornberger et al., 2012; Rodham et al., 2007; Whitlock et al., 2006). As described next, online activity may normalize and reinforce NSSI in a number of ways.

Sharing NSSI Experiences. On a variety of online platforms, individuals share their NSSI experiences with others. As noted earlier, this may allow individuals to obtain needed support and validation (see Lewis, Heath, Michal et al., 2012). However, in many cases, individuals describe their NSSI experiences in ways which focus on distress and emotional pain (Lewis, Heath, Sornberger et al., 2012; Niwa & Mandrusiak, 2012); consequently, these messages tend to have melancholic and hopeless themes (Lewis & Baker, 2011; Lewis et al., 2011;

Lewis, Heath, Michal et al., 2012; Lewis, Heath, Sornberger et al., 2012). It is also not uncommon for NSSI to be presented as a viable and at times justifiable response to manage emotional pain (Lewis & Baker, 2011). To this end, the aspect of NSSI recovery and the presentation of hopeful messages about the prospect of recovery are seldom presented (Lewis, Heath, Sornberger et al., 2012). In many instances, recovery is presented as either impossible or extremely difficult, and NSSI is presented as uncontrollable and impossible to resist (Baker & Lewis, 2013; Lewis & Baker, 2011; St. Denis, Lewis, Rodham, & Gavin, 2012). Taken together, it has been suggested that if these messages resonate with the individual accessing them and they are repeatedly accessed, they may reinforce NSSI as a normative response to assuage emotional distress and pain and that little can be done to stop self-injuring; in turn, this may lead to continued NSSI and reticence to seek help or make efforts to stop NSSI (e.g., Lewis & Baker, 2011; Lewis, Heath, Michal et al., 2012).

Shared NSSI Strategies. Across numerous message boards (Whitlock et al., 2006) and personal NSSI Web sites (Lewis & Baker, 2011) researchers have found that individuals who self-injure share potentially detrimental NSSI strategies with others who self-injure. Examples include posting NSSI methods (e.g., new ways to cut or burn skin) as well as ways to hide NSSI from others (e.g., suggesting locations on the body to injure which may not be visible to others) (Lewis & Baker, 2011; Whitlock et al., 2006); shared less frequently are first-aid tips, which offer suggestions and tips for individuals to use before self-injuring (e.g., disinfecting a razor) and after (e.g., cleaning and caring for a resultant injury) (Lewis & Baker, 2011). By disseminating these strategies to those who self-injure, it may work to reinforce NSSI by virtue of increasing people's capabilities to self-injure and promoting the notion that NSSI should be hidden from others (Lewis & Baker, 2011; Whitlock et al., 2006).

16.2.2.2 Triggering Non-suicidal Self-Injury Urges

Another concern identified by researchers is the aspect of triggering (Lewis & Baker, 2011; Lewis et al., 2011). Triggering refers to the notion that certain forms of online material are especially upsetting for those who access it. In turn, this produces heightened NSSI urges, which ultimately exacerbates NSSI risk. Accordingly, it is not uncommon for NSSI Web sites and e-communities to carry trigger warnings, which serve to caution others that by accessing additional NSSI content (within the Web site or e-community) individuals may be triggered to self-injure. Concerns over triggering seem to be particularly salient for more graphic NSSI material, such as photographs (Baker & Lewis, 2013; Lewis & Baker, 2011; Duggan et al., 2011), videos (Duggan et al., 2011; Lewis et al., 2011; Lewis, Heath, Sornberger et al., 2012), and vivid text descriptions of NSSI enactment (Lewis & Baker, 2011; Whitlock et al., 2006).

Despite the large number of trigger warnings posted online and widespread assumption that NSSI e-material triggers NSSI, the degree to which this transpires is not well documented (see Lewis, Heath, Michal et al., 2012). In a study exploring the nature of personal NSSI Web sites (which allow individuals to keep a log of their experiences with NSSI), a small number of Web sites provided direct testimony from site owners that they had self-injured after accessing what they referred to as triggering NSSI images and text on other Web sites (Lewis & Baker, 2011). In another study investigating viewers' responses to NSSI videos on YouTube (as indexed by video comments), a small percentage of individuals provided testimony that the graphic content of NSSI videos triggered the viewer (who posted the comment) to self-injure (Lewis, Heath, Sornberger et al., 2012). Interestingly, not all individuals seem to be impacted by graphic NSSI imagery in the same way. A recent study examining people's comments about NSSI photographs in an online forum found that some individuals were triggered by the content, whereas others indicated that by virtue of viewing the images, they had a reduced urge to self-injure (Baker & Lewis, 2013). In sum, it seems that (at least some) individuals are differentially impacted by potentially triggering NSSI material when online; this underscores the need for more empirical work in this area.

16.2.2.3 Pro Self-Injury Content

As noted earlier, several major social networks have made efforts to ban what they refer to as *pro self-harm* content, a broad referent referring to material actively promoting NSSI, suicide, and eating disorder behavior. Unlike the scope and nature of pro-eating disorder content on the Internet (discussed in the next section), pro-NSSI content is not well studied. Only a handful of studies have reported exclusively pro-NSSI content, which involves statements and online content (e.g., imagery, video), which promotes and/or justifies NSSI as a viable response to distress (Lewis & Baker, 2011; Lewis et al., 2011; Whitlock et al., 2006). As such, the existence of pro-NSSI content, including possible pro-NSSI Web sites and e-communities, merits further empirical exploration.

16.3 Eating Disorders and the Internet

Individuals with EDs frequently use the Internet to discuss ED activities (e.g., Wilson, Peebles, Hardy, & Litt, 2006). ED Web sites are often classified as either pro-ED (e.g., pro-anorexia [*pro-ana*], pro-bulimia [*pro-mia*]) or pro-recovery. Pro-ED Web sites focus on individuals who wish to begin or maintain eating disorder behaviors; these Web sites sometimes promote ED behaviors as a lifestyle choice rather than an illness and often provide dieting tips, techniques for engaging in destructive behaviors, and *thinspiration* (i.e., words or images meant to inspire ED behaviors such as fasting) with the intention of reinforcing and maintaining ED behaviors (Borzekowski, Schenk, Wilson, & Peebles, 2010; Chesley, Alberts, Klein, & Kreipe, 2003). Many Web sites do not explicitly describe themselves as pro-ED (i.e., they do not describe EDs as a lifestyle choice), but still have some of the same pro-ED content and level of harm as self-proclaimed pro-ED Web sites (Borzekowski et al., 2010). In contrast, pro-recovery Web sites focus on individuals who wish to recover, are in the process of recovering, or have already recovered from an eating disorder (Wilson et al., 2006). Pro-recovery Web sites describe eating disorders as destructive illnesses, promote support and understanding for individuals with eating disorders, discourage the use of potentially triggering material (e.g., posting weights, sharing ED tips and techniques), and provide information on recovery (Chesley et al., 2003). While some pro-ED Web sites share features of pro-recovery Web sites (e.g., providing recovery links), they assume that the individual is choosing to actively participate in the ED (Dias, 2003).

Although both pro-ED and pro-recovery Web sites are frequently visited by individuals with EDs (e.g., Peebles et al., 2012; Chesley et al., 2003; Wilson et al., 2006), Web sites with pro-ED content may be more prevalent online (Borzekowski et al., 2010). Pro-ED search terms are entered into Google's search engine more than 13 million times annually, with *pro-ana* being the most frequently used search term (Lewis & Arbuthnott, 2012). It is thus not surprising that the majority of the research on ED material online has focused on pro-ED Web sites over pro-recovery Web sites. Despite the fundamental differences between pro-ED and pro-recovery Web sites, they appear to share similar benefits and risks and are discussed together below.

16.3.1 Potential Benefits of Online Eating Disorder Activity

16.3.1.1 Support and Validation

Increased Support Online. Online ED Web sites frequently offer opportunities for interactions (e.g., through forums, chat rooms, blog comments) between individuals with EDs (Borzekowski et al., 2010). Individuals with EDs are socially stigmatized and may feel poorly understood within their offline relationships. Online ED communities may offer these individuals the opportunity to share experiences and gain mutual support in an accepting environment and thus may be beneficial to individuals with EDs who visit these e-communities (Cspike & Horne, 2007; Mulveen & Hepworth, 2006; Ransom, La Guardia, Woody, & Boyd, 2010; Tierney, 2008).

Unlike offline support groups, where only those individuals directly involved in a conversation typically benefit from the interaction, a large number of individuals may benefit from e-communities. Within online ED forums, *posters* (i.e., individuals who post a thread in the forum), *feedback givers* (i.e., those who give feedback to the poster), and *silent browsers* (i.e., individuals who read content posted by others without actively participating in the e-community) may all benefit through the personal disclosures, emotional support (e.g., empathy giving, feelings of not being alone, feelings that others understand), and informational support (e.g., recovery resources, education about EDs) shared in the forum threads (Flynn & Stana, 2012). When surveyed, members of a pro-ED forum reported getting more support from other members regarding general life stressors as compared to eating concerns; more support for both types of concerns was perceived in the e-community than offline (Ransom et al., 2010). Furthermore, the ability to use the Internet at any time, from anywhere, enhances the value of the Internet as a medium of support for individuals with EDs (Tierney, 2008; Wesemann & Grunwald, 2008); on one bulimia forum, 43 % of new threads were created between 11 P.M. and 5 A.M.—a time period in which offline support is likely to be unavailable (Wesemann & Grunwald, 2008).

Content of Online Support. Several studies have analyzed the content of ED e-communities (e.g., Fox, Ward, & O'Rourke, 2005; Juarascio, Shoaib, & Timko, 2010; Mulveen & Hepworth, 2006; Wesemann & Grunwald, 2008). A study of excerpts from pro-ED e-communities found that while users supported each other in losing weight, little attention was paid to the manner in which the weight was lost (i.e., whether ED behaviors were used); users also displayed a high degree of responsibility when extreme weight loss occurred by encouraging one another toward health (Mulveen & Hepworth, 2006). Similarly, a study of public pro-ED groups on Facebook and MySpace social networking sites found that while both social support and eating disorder specific content were present, interactions were primarily focused on social support and contained less specific ED content than expected; furthermore, negative reactions from members toward overly eating disorder specific content were common (Juarascio et al., 2010). Thus, content on the pro-ED e-communities may reflect the ambivalence that an individual with an ED may experience prior to being ready to begin a recovery process; these e-communities allow users a safe place to process this ambivalence (Mulveen & Hepworth, 2006).

Pro-recovery forums were found to have similar content to pro-ED forums (Riley, Rodham, & Gavin, 2009; Wesemann & Grunwald, 2008). A content analysis of forum threads in a pro-recovery bulimia forum was found to most frequently contain problem-oriented threads (i.e., alternatives to ED behaviors; food, calories, or weight; emotional experiences; recovery information and offline supports), followed by communication-oriented threads (i.e., topics unrelated to the ED, including communication of a personal and private nature directed at specific members), and a small number of meta-communication threads (i.e., communication on the forum as the topic of discussion) (Wesemann & Grunwald, 2008). Thus, similar to pro-ED Web sites, pro-recovery Web sites may also provide a space for individuals with EDs not just to communicate with one another but also to process their ED and negotiate their self-images with others also attempting to recover from EDs (Wesemann & Grunwald, 2008).

16.3.2 Risks Associated with Online Eating Disorder Activity

16.3.2.1 Reinforcement of Eating Disorder Behaviors

Eating disorder Web sites have been criticized for reinforcing and maintaining ED behaviors [for a review, see Rouleau and von Ranson (2011)]. Some content and patterns of social interaction found on ED Web sites and e-communities are associated with ED behaviors (e.g., Blair, Kelly, Serder, & Mazzeo, 2012; Harper,

Sperry, & Thompson, 2008; Jett, LaPorte, & Wanchisn, 2010; Juarez, Soto, & Pritchard, 2012; Peebles et al., 2012; Wilson et al., 2006) and may promote an eating disorder identity (e.g., Gavin, Rodham, & Poyer, 2008; Haas, Irr, Jennings, & Wagner, 2010; Riley et al., 2009), as outlined below.

Eating Disorder Content. Eating disorder Web sites may be harmful when viewers learn about and copy dangerous behaviors (Borzekowski et al., 2010; Cspike & Horne, 2007); thus, similar to online NSSI activity, there is concern that certain forms of online ED material (e.g., providing tips and strategies) may contribute to the reinforcement of ED behavior. Among adolescent patients with eating disorders, 96 and 46.4 % who viewed pro-ED Web sites and pro-recovery Web sites, respectively, reported learning new techniques to lose weight or purge (Wilson et al., 2006). Similarly, after exposure to pro-ED Web sites, female college students without a history of EDs reported using techniques on the pro-ED Web sites to reduce their caloric intake over the following week (Jett et al., 2010). The most harmful Web sites tend to have warnings about distressing material, attempt to deter *wannabes* (i.e., individuals who are dabbling in ED behaviors), and give tips and techniques for engaging in multiple forms of extreme ED behaviors—many of which could lead to immediate and life-threatening problems (Borzekowski et al., 2010). Within pro-ED e-communities, ED symptoms or problems may be reframed as signs of success (Gavin et al., 2008).

Associations with Eating Disorder Behaviors. Pro-ED Internet activity has been associated with eating disorder behaviors (e.g., Blair et al., 2012; Harper et al., 2008; Jett et al., 2010; Juarez et al., 2012; Peebles et al., 2012; Wilson et al., 2006), increases in negative affect (Bardone-Cone & Cass, 2006, 2007; Theis, Wolf, & Kordy, 2011), and reductions in self-esteem (Theis et al., 2011). One study comparing the viewing of a pro-ED Web site and a control Web site found that women reported a decreased caloric intake after viewing the pro-ED Web sites (Jett et al., 2010). Similarly, another study found that a greater intention to exercise and perceptions of being at a heavier weight were reported after the pro-ED Web site was viewed relative to when a control Web site was viewed (Bardone-Cone & Cass, 2006, 2007). Adolescents with EDs and who accessed pro-ED Web sites had a longer duration of illness (Wilson et al., 2006). Using both pro-ED and pro-recovery Web sites was associated with a greater number of hospitalizations (Wilson et al., 2006). There seems to be a relation between increased viewing of ED Web site and more ED pathology; specifically, women who visited pro-ED Web sites daily for at least 12 months reported greater eating pathology and impairment, more extreme weight loss behaviors, and more harmful post-Web site usage activities (Peebles et al., 2012).

Competition and Thinspiration. Competition between individuals with EDs, and self-comparisons to thinspiration, may further reinforce ED behaviors (Cspike & Horne, 2007; Rouleau & von Ranson, 2011). Some pro-ED Web sites allow users to post photos of themselves and receive validation from the e-community

(Fox et al., 2005). Thinspiration allows users to compare their own image to those images already validated by others (Rouleau & von Ranson, 2011). The majority (i.e., 59 %) of pro-ED Web site users reported visiting pro-ED Web sites in order to obtain thinspiration (Cspike & Horne, 2007). Indeed, the most dangerous pro-ED Web sites are found through the search terms related to *thinspiration* and *thinspo*, relative to other pro-ED search terms (Lewis & Arbuthnott, 2012). Less harmful pro-ED Web sites may still provide dieting tips but may also provide information related to recovery (Borzekowski et al., 2010; Lewis & Arbuthnott, 2012).

Eating Disorder Identities. Eating disorder Web sites may also reinforce ED identities that work to maintain ED behaviors (e.g., Gavin et al., 2008; Haas et al., 2010; Riley et al., 2009). Disclosures of ED behaviors and pro-ED thoughts, as well as the group bond created by sharing a secret pro-ED identity, may contribute to the strengthening of personal (Gavin et al., 2008; Haas et al., 2010) and collective (Haas et al., 2010; Whitehead, 2010) ED identities. Two themes have been identified for managing a pro-anorexia identity online: maintaining a sense of the pro-anorexic self as abnormal (i.e., different from others) and keeping the ED identity a secret (Gavin et al., 2008). These are reinforced on pro-anorexia e-communities by co-constructing anorexic identities through disclosures of loyalty to anorexia and associated behaviors, self-loathing and self-deprecation, advice giving (e.g., tips and techniques to lose weight, managing offline social situations), and group encouragement and cohesion (Gavin et al., 2008; Haas et al., 2010).

The organization of an in-group (i.e., members of the e-community) and out-group (e.g., *wannabes*) may reinforce a collective eating disorder identity and may influence members to make claims proving that they belong to the e-community (Fox et al., 2005; Haas et al., 2010; Riley et al., 2009; Whitehead, 2010). Staged photographs and signatures containing weights (e.g., highest weight, lowest weight, current weight, and goal weights) are commonly used to support an ED identity (Fox et al., 2005). In both pro-anorexia forums (Boero & Pascoe, 2012; Riley et al., 2009) and pro-recovery forums (Riley et al., 2009), body talk (i.e., physical descriptions, descriptions of doing something with the body, bodily experiences) has been used to provide evidence toward ED identity claims (e.g., as a pro-anorexic, as recovering) and the right to participate in the e-community. Discourse analysis suggests that while both pro-anorexia and pro-recovery Web sites contained communication related to a thin-ideal and claims to group membership, only the pro-anorexia Web sites reframed health concerns as markers of eating disorder success as a means to establish a pro-ED identity (Riley et al., 2009).

16.3.2.2 Thwarting Recovery

Pro-ED Web sites often operate under the presumption that the individuals using these Web sites do so with the intention of maintaining their ED behaviors (e.g., Rouleau & von Ranson, 2011). The emergence of pro-ED on the Internet has been speculated to reflect the desire of those who suffer from EDs to be in control of their ED behaviors (Fox et al., 2005). Labeling the ED as a lifestyle choice or way of life, and the eating disorder as a personal friend or enemy (e.g., *ana* or *mia*), empowers the individuals who use these e-communities to perceive themselves as choosing the ED behaviors, rather than suffering from a mental illness (Mulveen & Hepworth, 2006). When this perception is challenged, those who identify themselves as pro-ED may actively protect their pro-ED self-identity. For example, when pro-anorexia users were exposed to pro-recovery comments, they became more likely to continue posting pro-ED photos on Flicker (Yom-Tov, Fernandez-Luque, Weber, & Crains, 2012). The sharing of tips and techniques around concealment of the eating disorder is common on pro-ED Web sites (e.g., Borzekowski et al., 2010) and may further influence individuals with EDs to avoid seeking treatment (Rouleau & von Ranson, 2011).

The perception that *outsiders* (e.g., doctors, family, friends) fail to understand the role of the ED in a pro-ED individual's life is frequently discussed on ED e-communities (Fox et al., 2005). This distrust in medical authority and advice may contribute to the pro-ED e-community's rejection of the ED as a mental illness, and the subsequent normalization and acceptance of the community's understandings and practices (Mulveen & Hepworth, 2006). In this regard, pro-recovery Web sites tend to differ from pro-ED Web sites. Although medical and psychological language in reference to ED behaviors and functions is absent on the pro-ED Web sites, it is central to communications on pro-recovery Web sites (Riley et al., 2009).

16.4 Implications for Researchers

16.4.1 Online Non-suicidal Self-Injury Activity

With growing research suggesting that online NSSI activity may affect those involved, it will be essential to formally investigate the impact of online NSSI activity. In particular, efforts are needed to examine whether online NSSI activity impacts NSSI thoughts and behavior and which processes are involved (e.g., how and why NSSI may be reinforced in some cases). The impact this has on NSSI intervention may also merit empirical consideration; for instance, if some forms of NSSI e-activity reinforce NSSI, this may limit the effectiveness of certain treatments. Related to this, the notion of triggering warrants further research—especially in light of recent findings that individuals may be affected by NSSI images in different ways (Baker & Lewis, 2013).

It will also be important for researchers to explore the motivations for online NSSI activity more formally. Although some motives for online NSSI activity can be inferred from the literature (e.g., to get social support), this has not been formally studied, and it cannot be assumed that all potential motives have been elucidated. A clear understanding of what contributes to these activities is critical in terms of gaining further insight into why these activities are repeated in some cases and how they may be addressed when the nature of the online activity is worrisome (e.g., reinforces NSSI).

Although a significant amount of research and public attention has focused on the risks of online NSSI activity, many researchers indicate that the Internet may carry significant promise as a means to reach those who self-injure and to address NSSI (Lewis & Baker, 2011; Lewis et al., 2011; Lewis, Heath, Michal et al., 2012; Lewis, Heath, Sornberger et al., 2012; Lewis, Rosenrot, & Messner, 2012; Whitlock et al., 2006; Whitlock, Lader, & Conterio, 2007). Indeed, researchers have reported that many young people who self-injure would prefer getting NSSI help and resources via the Internet (Hasking, Martin, & Berger, 2010). Thus, efforts are needed to identify novel ways to use e-technology to reach those who engage in online NSSI activity and to provide needed NSSI resources and help. Finally, as the nature of e-activity changes over time in popularity, scope, and nature, it will be imperative for researchers to keep pace with these changes.

16.4.2 Online Eating Disorder Activity

Several research directions have emerged from current knowledge of ED Web sites and e-communities. The role of these Web sites and ED e-communities in the development, maintenance, and cessation of an ED needs to be further elucidated with longitudinal data. A large amount of research has already been conducted examining the nature and content of ED Web sites (e.g., Fox et al., 2005; Juarascio et al., 2010; Mulveen & Hepworth, 2006; Wesemann & Grunwald, 2008), and this research has informed clinicians regarding the benefits and risks associated with ED e-communities. Less is known about the members' experiences of ED e-communities and the perceived functions that these communities serve for these members in all stages of the ED.

Given the known risks and benefits of ED e-communities and the similarities between pro-ED and pro-recovery e-communities (e.g., Riley et al., 2009; Wesemann & Grunwald, 2008), the use of online support groups within recovery programs needs to be carefully studied in future research. Similarly, although ED e-communities have been criticized for impeding the recovery process, research has found that the opposite may also be true; e-communities may offer users a safe place to process existing ambivalence regarding recovery and to receive support toward healthier behaviors (e.g., Wesemann & Grunwald, 2008). Thus, the influence of ED e-communities on the recovery process has yet to be determined.

16.5 Implications for Clinical Practice

Clinicians working with clients engaging in NSSI and/or who struggle with ED difficulties need to know whether their clients are also engaging in forms of online activity that may impact the course of treatment. To assist clinicians in these cases, we discuss aspects of assessment, formulation, and treatment below.

16.5.1 Initial Steps

Online activity may have a great deal of relevance to clients engaging in NSSI and/or who struggle with EDs. As noted above, the Internet may represent a salient and preferred mode of communication for many of these individuals (Cspike & Horne, 2007; Lewis, Heath, Michal et al., 2012; Lewis, Heath, Sornberger et al., 2012; Mulveen & Hepworth, 2006). At the same time, some clinicians may be less familiar with the scope and nature of online activities and terminology used to refer to these activities. For many clinicians, the Internet may be less salient in their daily lives (Whitlock et al., 2007). Thus, familiarization with the types of online activities individuals engage in when online may be helpful. Table 16.1 outlines some common online activities and describes related terms. Increased familiarity with these terms may assist in clinical assessment, as discussed next.

16.5.2 Assessment

Similar to assessment recommendations for NSSI (see Klonsky et al., 2011), a functional assessment may have utility as a means to assess online activities related to NSSI, EDs, or both. Indeed, this approach has been recommended in recently published guidelines to assess online NSSI activity (Lewis, Heath, Michal et al., 2012). Using a functional assessment, clinicians can work with clients with the goal of understanding the scope and nature of their clients' online activities (regarding NSSI, EDs, or both).

In the initial session, clinicians can orient their clients to the use of a functional log as a means of monitoring and tracking the online activities of their clients. It is recommended that clients be asked to try this between the first and second sessions. From here, clinicians will be able to further assess the client's online activities in a more detailed manner during the second session and then in subsequent meetings as needed. Among the types of data to record in the functional log are as follows (a) events/interactions, thoughts, and feelings that preceded the online activity; (b) the events/interactions online and the thoughts and feelings during the online activity; and the (c) events/interactions, thoughts, and feelings following the online activity. To understand the potential impact of a client's online activity over the course of treatment, a weekly log can be maintained by the client between sessions, which clinicians can review with clients during their meetings.

Once the initial assessment is complete, a broader assessment of the client's online activities can be conducted. Table 16.2 outlines a number of potentially useful questions that may facilitate this process. By conducting a more in-depth assessment, clinicians will be better able to identify the types of online activities engaged in by the client (e.g., types of interactions, types of Web sites accessed); in turn, this is conducive to determining if the client is accessing potentially problematic material (e.g., which may contribute to reinforcement of NSSI and/or EDs), material that is more adaptive and supportive in nature (e.g., which advocates for recovery and help-seeking), or in some cases, both.

Table 16.1 Internet factsheet: key terms and related activities

	Community Web sites	Social networking Web sites	Video-/photo-sharing Web sites
Terms	*Chat forum*: space dedicated to real-time chat among individuals who are accessing the Web site *Moderated*: content and membership on Web site are controlled and regulated by creator *Discussion forum* (*message board*): online space where users can openly exchange information and opinions regarding a common interest/theme *e-Communities*: electronic community/social network of users who share a common interest *Peer driven*: created and moderated by a nonprofessional *Professionally driven*: created and moderated by a mental health professional	• *Facebook* *Friends*: people you connect and share profile information with Post: public sharing of information on a wall Profile: user space containing personal information, online exchanges, and photos Wall: user profile space where friends can post and share information • *MySpace* *Blog*: a personal journal created by user • *Twitter* *Followers*: size of audience following individual's tweets/profile *Tweet*: real-time information sharing in 140 characters or less • *General* (*common terms found across all social networking Web sites*) *Group*: collection of individuals who keep in touch surrounding a particular theme *Instant chat/messaging* (*IM*): live, real-time chat that occurs in present time between members *Members*: individuals who join a group *Messages*: private exchange of material (e.g., messages, photos) *Public vs. private group*: membership required	*Account:* viewer to verify they are a mature audience (18 years and older) *Character*: videos containing live individual(s) *Comments*: public remarks/ observations posted by video viewers pertaining to a specific video *Noncharacter*: videos containing visual representations such as images, video stills, and/or text *Subscribe*: to receive updates when a specific video uploader posts new videos *Top favorite*: a user indicates a specific video is their preferred *Video uploader*: user who creates and shares videos *Video view count*: number of video views, also referred to as "hits"
Example	http://self-injury.net[a] http://www.psyke.org/[a] http://www.something-fishy.org[a]	http://www.facebook.com http://www.myspace.com http://www.twitter.com http://www.xanga.com (account needed to access groups)	http://www.youtube.com http://www.flickr.com

Reprinted and adapted with permission from: Lewis, S.P., Heath, N.L., Michal, N.J., & Duggan, J.M. (2012). Nonsuicidal self-injury and the Internet: What mental health professionals need to know. *Child and Adolescent Psychiatry and Mental Health*, *6*, 13: doi:10.1186/1753-2000-6-13

[a]Web sites are examples and are not suggested as recommendations

Table 16.2 Recommended questions about online NSSI/ED activity

I. Activity type
Review log: What type(s) of online activities do you use concerning NSSI/ED (informational, interactive, social networking, and video viewing/sharing/posting)?
If community
What are the resources available in the community/forum?
Is this Web site professionally or peer driven? Is the Web site moderated?
Is the Web site focused on recovery? Is it focused on continuing NSSI/ED?
What specific activities do you engage in on these Web sites (live chat, posting, information seeking)?
Social networking
What social networking Web sites are you affiliated with?
Do you have friendships/connections with people concerning about NSSI/ED?
If yes, what is the nature of the relationship(s)?
If yes, have these relationships extended outside of the activity?
Are you a member of any group related to NSSI/ED?
If yes, what are the themes surrounding that group (against, pro, neutral)?
If yes, is this group public or private?
If yes, is it moderated?
Are there any visual representations of NSSI or ED (e.g., thinspiration) in these groups?
What specific activities do you engage in on these Web sites (live chat, messaging, posting, information seeking)?
Video/picture sharing
What specific Web sites do you visit?
Do you create videos/photos related to NSSI?/ED?/Thinspiration?
If yes, discuss themes/content of videos created
If yes, are these videos character or noncharacter videos?
If yes, what purpose does creating these videos serve (e.g., creative outlet)?
What types of videos/photos do you watch?
Are these character or noncharacter videos?
What are the general themes in these videos (against NSSI, pro-NSSI, neutral)?
Do these videos present visual presentations of NSSI?/ED?/Thinspiration?
If yes, are these visual presentations accompanied by a warning?
Are these visual presentations of NSSI/ED triggering?
If yes, discuss nature, intensity, and degree of triggering material
What other specific activities do you engage in on these Web sites (messaging, commenting, following channels)?
II. Frequency
Review log: Discuss frequency of NSSI/ED online activities (explore usage, during week and weekend)
III. Functional assessment of NSSI/ED behaviors in relation to Internet activities
Review log: When/why did you first start engaging in NSSI/ED online activities? Explore first episode
Has your NSSI/Have your ED behaviors increased/decreased/remained the same since you began engaging in NSSI/ED online activities?

(continued)

Table 16.2 (continued)

What are events/interactions, thoughts, and feelings that preceded/occur during/follow the online activity?
Do you self-injure before/after engaging in NSSI online activities?
If yes, explore online activities that may confer/reduce NSSI risk

Note: Reprinted and adapted from: Lewis, S.P., Heath, N.L., Michal, N.J., & Duggan, J.M. (2012). Nonsuicidal self-injury and the Internet: What mental health professionals need to know. *Child and Adolescent Psychiatry and Mental Health*, *6*, 13: doi:10.1186/1753-2000-6-13

When conducting the functional assessment, it is recommended that clinicians not circumscribe the assessment to just the activity type (e.g., whether a client is visiting a message board or watching a YouTube video) since some clients may not accurately report what they do online or be cognizant of the impact their online activity may have on their thoughts, feelings, or behavior (i.e., NSSI or ED behavior). Thus, alongside what the client is doing online (i.e., the activity type), it is important to assess the frequency and duration of the client's online activity; this includes when the behaviors occur over the course of a day as this information helps to determine if the client's online activities are negatively affecting their daily lives (e.g., disrupting sleep, work, school) (Lewis, Heath, Michal et al., 2012).

Lastly, clinicians should carefully review the functional log in an effort to understand why certain online activities may be enacted by the client and to better understand how these online activities affect the client (i.e., positively and/or negative). Identification of possible antecedents to online activities and variables reinforcing them can shed insight into what might precede (and drive) potentially problematic online activity. In turn, this can inform a plan to address these activities. Although many clinicians may be primarily focused on identifying and curbing potentially problematic online activity, it is important to bear in mind that for many individuals, online activity related to NSSI and EDs provides needed support and validation (Cspike & Horne, 2007; Lewis, Heath, Michal et al., 2012). For this reason, practitioners should be cautious when making conclusions about what forms of online activity are detrimental to the client. If harmful online activities are identified, however, it is important to intervene and work with clients to change the nature of their online activities alongside intervention for their NSSI and/or ED.

16.5.3 Intervention

Promoting change in the context of people's online activities may be challenging, especially if clients do not view their online activity as problematic. As such, requests for clients to cease engaging in online activities related to NSSI and EDs are not recommended—in part because it is first important to identify the impact these activities have on the client using a functional assessment (discussed above) and doing so may result in the online activity becoming secretive. If there are risks associated with the client's e-activities and these become secretive, this may be counterproductive in the context of treatment and recovery.

Guidelines to address online NSSI activity in the context of clinical care have been offered (Lewis, Heath, Michal et al., 2012) and may have utility for problematic online ED activity as well. Recommendations suggest that as an initial step in addressing these online activities, clinicians determine the client's readiness for change. To do this, the stages of change model (Prochaska & Velicer, 1997) may be useful. Accordingly, motivational interviewing may be relevant and serve as a means to effectively manage a client's ambivalence toward online activity desistance and to increase desire to change his/her online behavior. Although no line of work has directly examined this therapeutic approach in the context of addressing online activity related to NSSI or ED behaviors, motivational interviewing has been used to increase motivation to change with clients who engage in NSSI (Kress & Hoffman, 2008), EDs (Macdonald, Hibbs, Corfield, & Treasure, 2012) and those with Internet addiction (Griffiths & Meredith, 2009).

When clients are open to adopting alternative activities in place of problematic online behavior, clinicians can use a number of strategies. Clinicians may opt to work with clients to develop a list of offline activities (e.g., exercise, communicating with friends or family) that can be used in place of problematic online activities. However, as indicated above, it may be unhelpful to attempt to discourage online activity altogether. As noted above, the Internet may be highly salient for many who engage in NSSI and/or ED behaviors (Lewis, Heath, Michal et al., 2012; Rouleau & von Ranson, 2011). As a result, replacing problematic online activities with more adaptive ones may be more effective. One part of this is directing clients to adaptive online activities. From here, the functional log can continue to be used as a means of understanding the impact of these newer and more adaptive online activities and to establish a new set of healthy online activities for clients. As identifying reputable Web sites to recommend to clients can be difficult, readers may find Table 16.3 helpful, which outlines and describes a number of recommended, supportive, recovery-focused, and monitored Web sites for both NSSI and EDs. Many of these Web sites can also be recommended to people in the lives of the client who can play a supportive role in recovery (e.g., family, romantic partners). As the course of treatment progresses, a brief check-in with respect to the client's online activities should occur as a part of assessing the client's overall functioning. If abrupt changes in the client's online activities are reported, it may be indicative of a change in their overall wellbeing.

16.6 Summary

With the influx in Internet use and social networking over the past several years, the aspects of online activity regarding NSSI and EDs have emerged as new and important areas of empirical focus. Research from these efforts have identified a number of similarities between online NSSI and online ED activities with respect to potential benefits (e.g., social support) and risks (e.g., reinforcement); however,

Table 16.3 Web sites providing quality NSSI and eating disorder resources

	Organization	Resource	Stakeholders
NSSI	Self-injury outreach and support (SIOS) http://www.sioutreach.org	Nonprofit outreach initiative providing information and resources about self-injury	Individuals who self-injure Mental health professionals Physicians School professionals Family Friends
	Cornell research program on self-injurious behavior http://www.crpsib.com	Summarizes research and provides resources related to understanding, identifying, treating, and preventing self-injury	Mental health professionals Physicians School professionals
	Self abuse finally ends (SAFE) http://www.selfinjury.com	Treatment center Web site providing information and resources about self-injury, with a focus on interventions for individuals who self-injure	Individuals who self-injure Mental health professionals Physicians School professionals Family Friends
Eating disorders	National eating disorders association (NEDA) http://www.nationaleatingdisorders.org	Nonprofit organization dedicated to the prevention and advocacy for eating disorders	Individuals with eating disorders Mental health professionals School professionals and coaches Family Friends
	Academy for eating disorders http://www.aedweb.org	Professional association committed to ED research, education, treatment, and prevention	Mental health professionals Physicians Researchers General public

there may also be unique benefits and risks associated with each (e.g., triggering in the context of online NSSI activity, thinspiration in the context of online ED activity). In light of the infancy of these fields, more research is needed to better understand the impact these online activities may have and how to effectively address the potential harm some activities might confer. Alongside empirical work, clinicians may need to consider these impacts in clinical contexts when working with clients who self-injure and/or who struggle with eating disorder difficulties.

16.7 Case Vignette

Now 17, Jessica has been self-injuring since she was 15. She cuts episodically but this becomes more frequent during times of stress. Jessica describes herself as "sensitive" and reports being emotionally reactive; she struggles managing her emotions. Jessica has low self-esteem and a poor body image. In the past, she has binged and purged though she does not meet diagnostic criteria for an eating disorder. After seeing several fresh cuts on her arm, Jessica's mother brought her to see a therapist.

As a part of the initial assessment, Jessica's therapist conducted a comprehensive assessment of Jessica's self-injury and other mental health difficulties. Jessica's therapist also explored her online activities. After asking several initial questions about her Internet behavior, Jessica's therapist introduced the use of a functional log. To help Jessica understand how to use the log, her therapist drew from an incident that Jessica mentioned when responding to the initial questions about her Internet activity. Specifically, Jessica reported that a few nights ago she was feeling very upset and alone. Everyone in her home had gone to bed. She decided to go online to visit a self-injury message board, which she has found supportive in the past. She said she goes there because they "get me. . .they know what it's like." On this particular night, Jessica started to read a new post from a member of the message board. The individual who posted the message had also posted a link to photos of his self-injury. Jessica clicked on the link and saw the images. She reported that this really upset her and "really made me want to cut."

By completing the log together, Jessica was able to make initial connections between how she felt prior to going online, what she accessed (i.e., the images), and how she felt after viewing this content. Although she recognized that seeing the images of self-injury increased her urge to hurt herself, she maintained that she had no intentions to stop visiting the message board because "it's not all bad like you think. . .it mostly helps." Her therapist validated Jessica's concern and acknowledged that if she finds the message board supportive, it is understandable that she would not want to stop visiting it. As homework, Jessica agreed that she would set aside time each day to complete the log between meetings with her therapist.

Over the next several sessions, Jessica completed the functional log and her therapist took time during each session to review it. These discussions helped Jessica to better understand that although she received needed support from most of her online activities, some of the content she accessed in the message board was upsetting and even "triggering." In turn, this contributed to a conversation about the advantages and disadvantages associated with certain forms of her Internet activity. Jessica's therapist used a number of motivational interviewing techniques over the next several sessions, which allowed Jessica to generate her own reasons for and against different types of online activities related to self-injury. As a result, Jessica noticed that she had more reasons to refrain from a number of her online activities (including visiting the abovementioned message board) than reasons for engaging in these activities. Jessica and her therapist also developed a list of healthy online activities that she could use when she felt alone and her therapist provided a list of several self-injury Web sites that might be helpful to use when she felt upset or had urges to self-injure; they also worked on and developed a number of offline strategies (e.g., calling a friend, relaxation techniques, painting) that Jessica could use during these times.

Over the course of therapy, Jessica visited the self-injury message board less often, and she and her therapist worked on a variety of coping strategies rooted in dialectical and cognitive behavior therapies to manage her self-injury. They also worked on her response to distress more generally and began to address her low self-esteem and poor body image. As therapy progressed, Jessica found that she self-injured less often; she also had no subsequent binge-purge episodes, especially as she began to feel better about herself and became more accepting of her body.

References

Baker, D., & Fortune, S. (2008). Understanding self-harm and suicide websites: A qualitative interview study of young adult website users. *Crisis, 39*, 118–122.

Baker, T. G., & Lewis, S. P. (2013). Responses to online photographs of non-suicidal self-injury: A thematic analysis. *Archives of Suicide Research, 17*, 223–235.

Bardone-Cone, A. M., & Cass, K. M. (2006). Investigating the impact of pro-anorexia websites: A pilot study. *European Eating Disorders Review, 14*, 256–262.

Bardone-Cone, A. M., & Cass, K. M. (2007). What does viewing a pro-anorexia website do? An experimental examination of website exposure and moderating effects. *International Journal of Eating Disorders, 40*, 537–548.

Berger, M., Wagner, T. H., & Baker, L. C. (2005). Internet use and stigmatized illness. *Social Science & Medicine, 61*, 1821–1827.

Blair, C. E., Kelly, N. R., Serder, K. L., & Mazzeo, S. E. (2012). Does the Internet function like a magazine? An exploration of image-focused media, eating pathology, and body dissatisfaction. *Eating Behaviors, 13*, 398–401.

Boero, N., & Pascoe, C. J. (2012). Pro-anorexia communities and online interactions: Bringing the pro-ana body online. *Body & Society, 18*, 27–57.

Borzekowski, D. L. G., Schenk, S., Wilson, J. L., & Peebles, R. (2010). e-Ana and e-Mia: A content analysis of pro-eating disorder websites. *American Journal of Public Health, 100*, 1526–1534.

Chesley, E. B., Alberts, J. D., Klein, J. D., & Kreipe, R. E. (2003). Pro or con? Anorexia nervosa and the Internet. *Journal of Adolescent Health, 32*, 123–124.

Cspike, E., & Horne, O. (2007). Pro-eating disorder websites: Users' opinions. *European Eating Disorder Review, 15*, 196–206.

Dias, K. (2003). The ana sanctuary: Women's pro-anorexia narratives in cyberspace. *Journal of International Women's Studies, 4*, 31–45.

Duggan, J. M., Heath, N. L., Lewis, S. P., & Baxter, A. (2011). An examination of the scope and nature of non-suicidal self-injury online activities: Implications for school mental health professionals. *School Mental Health, 4*, 56–67.

Fairburn, C. G., & Harrison, P. J. (2003). Eating disorders. *The Lancet, 361*, 407–416.

Flynn, M. A., & Stana, A. (2012). Social support in a men's online eating disorder forum. *International Journal of Men's Mental Health, 11*, 150–169.

Fox, N., Ward, K., & O'Rourke, A. (2005). Pro-anorexia, weight-loss drugs and the internet: An 'anti-recovery' explanatory model of anorexia. *Sociology of Health & Illness, 27*, 944–971.

Gavin, J., Rodham, K., & Poyer, H. (2008). The presentation of "pro-anorexia" in online group interactions. *Qualitative Health Research, 18*, 325–333.

Google News (2011, February 25). Health Section. Retrieved from http://www.news.google.com.

Google News (2012, February 28). Health Section. Retrieved from http://www.news.google.com.

Griffiths, M. D., & Meredith, A. (2009). Videogame addiction and treatment. *Journal of Contemporary Psychotherapy, 39*, 47–53.

Haas, S. M., Irr, M. E., Jennings, N. A., & Wagner, L. M. (2010). Communicating thin: A grounded model of online negative enabling support groups in the pro-anorexia movement. *New Media & Society, 13*, 40–57.

Harper, K., Sperry, S., & Thompson, J. K. (2008). Viewership of pro-eating disorder websites: Association with body image and eating disturbances. *International Journal of Eating Disorders, 41*, 92–95.

Hasking, P., Martin, G., & Berger, E. (2010, June). *How do we help those who self-injure? An examination of what young people think.* Paper presented at International Society for the Study of Self-injury Conference, Chicago, IL.

Jett, S., LaPorte, D. J., & Wanchisn, J. (2010). Impact of exposure to pro-eating disorder websites on eating behaviours in college women. *European Eating Disorder Review, 18*, 410–416.

Johnson, G. M., Zastawny, S., & Kulpa, A. (2010). E-message boards for those who self-injure: Implications for E-health. *International Journal of Mental Health and Addiction, 8*, 566–569.

Jones, R., Sharkey, S., Ford, T., Emmens, T., Hewis, E., Smithson, J., et al. (2011). Online discussion forums for young people who self-harm: User views. *The Psychiatrist, 35*, 364–368.

Juarascio, A. S., Shoaib, A., & Timko, C. A. (2010). Pro-eating disorder communities on social networking sites: A content analysis. *Eating Disorders, 18*, 393–407.

Juarez, L., Soto, E., & Pritchard, M. E. (2012). Drive for muscularity and drive for thinness: The impact of pro-anorexia websites. *Eating Disorders, 20*, 99–112.

Klonsky, E. D., Muehlenkamp, J. J., Lewis, S. P., & Walsh, B. (2011). *Non-suicidal self-injury.* Cambridge, MA: Hogrefe.

Kress, V. E., & Hoffman, R. (2008). Non-suicidal self-injury and motivational interviewing: Enhancing readiness for change. *Journal of Mental Health Counseling, 30*, 311–329.

Lewis, S. P., & Arbuthnott, A. E. (2012). Searching for thinspiration: The nature of Internet searches for pro-eating disorder websites. *Cyberpsychology, Behavior and Social Networking, 15*, 200–204.

Lewis, S. P., & Baker, T. G. (2011). The possible risks of self-injury web sites: A content analysis. *Archives of Suicide Research, 15*, 390–396.

Lewis, S. P., Heath, N. L., Michal, N. J., & Duggan, J. M. (2012). Non-suicidal self-injury, youth, and the Internet: What mental health professionals need to know. *Child and Adolescent Psychiatry and Mental Health, 6*, 13.

Lewis, S. P., Heath, N. L., Sornberger, M. J., & Arbuthnott, A. E. (2012). Helpful or harmful? An examination of viewer's responses to nonsuicidal self-injury videos on YouTube. *Journal of Adolescent Health, 51*, 380–385.

Lewis, S. P., Heath, N. L., St. Denis, J. M., & Noble, R. (2011). The scope of nonsuicidal self-injury on YouTube. *Pediatrics, 127*, e552–e557.

Lewis, S. P., Rosenrot, S. A., & Messner, M. A. (2012). Seeking validation in unlikely places: The nature of online questions about non-suicidal self-injury. *Archives of Suicide Research, 16*, 263–272.

Macdonald, P., Hibbs, R., Corfield, F., & Treasure, J. (2012). The use of motivational interviewing in eating disorders: A systematic review. *Psychiatry Research, 200*, 1–11.

McKenna, K. Y. A., Green, A., & Gleason, M. (2002). Relationship formation on the internet: What's the big attraction? *Journal of Social Issues, 58*, 9–31.

Mulveen, R., & Hepworth, J. (2006). An interpretative phenomenological analysis of participation in a pro-anorexia Internet site and its relationship with disordered eating. *Journal of Health Psychology, 11*, 283–296.

Murray, C. D., & Fox, J. (2006). Do Internet self-harm discussion groups alleviate or exacerbate self-harming behaviour? *Australian e-Journal for the Advancement of Mental Health, 5*(3), 1–9.

Niwa, K. D., & Mandrusiak, M. N. (2012). Self-injury groups on facebook. *Canadian Journal of Counselling and Psychotherapy, 46*, 1–20.

Peebles, R., Wilson, J. L., Litt, I. F., Hardy, K. K., Locks, J. D., Mann, J. R., et al. (2012). Disordered eating in a digital age: Eating behaviors, health, and quality of life in users of websites with pro-eating disorder content. *Journal of Medical Internet Research, 14*, e148.

Prochaska, J. O., & Velicer, W. F. (1997). The transtheoretical model of health behavior change. *American Journal of Health Promotion, 12*, 38–48.

Ransom, D. C., La Guardia, J. G., Woody, E. Z., & Boyd, J. L. (2010). Interpersonal interactions on online forums addressing eating concerns. *International Journal of Eating Disorders, 43*, 161–170.

Riley, S., Rodham, K., & Gavin, J. (2009). Doing weight: Pro-ana and recovery identities in cyberspace. *Journal of Community & Applied Social Psychology, 19*, 348–359.

Rodham, K., Gavin, J., & Miles, M. (2007). I hear, I listen and I care: A qualitative investigation into the function of a self-harm message board. *Suicide and Life-Threatening Behavior, 37*, 422–430.

Rouleau, C. R., & von Ranson, K. M. (2011). Potential risks of pro-eating disorder websites. *Clinical Psychology Review, 31*, 525–531.

Smithson, J., Sharkey, S., Hewis, E., Jones, R., Emmens, T., Ford, T., et al. (2011). Problem presentation and responses on an online forum for young people who self-harm. *Discourse Studies, 13*, 487–501.

Sornberger, M., Joly, M., Heath, N. L., & Lewis, S. P. (2012, June). *What hath research wrought: Evaluating knowledge transfer of NSSI via online news media.* Symposium: New Millenium Media & Non-suicidal Self-injury: Implications for Mental Health Professionals. Canadian Psychological Association Annual Convention, Halifax, NS.

St. Denis, J. M., Lewis, S. P., Rodham, K., & Gavin, J. (2012, July). *The first cut may not be the deepest: Descriptions of NSSI as an addiction.* Presented at the 7th Annual Meeting of the International Society for the Study of Self-injury (ISSS), Chapel Hill, NC.

Theis, F., Wolf, M., & Kordy, H. (2011, March). *Experimental examination of the exposure to pro-eating disorders and pro-recovery website contents.* Paper presented at the 2nd INTACT Symposium, Prague.

Tierney, S. (2008). The dangers and draw of online communication: Pro-anorexia websites and their implications for users, practitioners, and researchers. *Eating Disorders, 14*, 181–190.

Treasure, J., Claudino, M. A., & Zucker, N. (2010). Eating disorders. *The Lancet, 375*, 583–583.

Wesemann, D., & Grunwald, M. (2008). Online discussion groups for bulimia nervosa: An inductive approach to Internet-based communication between patients. *International Journal of Eating Disorders, 41*, 527–534.

Whitehead, K. (2010). "Hunger hurts but starving works": A case study of gendered practices in the online pro-eating-disorder community. *Canadian Journal of Sociology, 35*, 595–626.

Whitlock, J. L., Lader, W., & Conterio, K. (2007). The Internet and self-injury: What psychotherapists should know. *Journal of Clinical Psychology: In Session, 63*, 1135–1143.

Whitlock, J. L., Powers, J. P., & Eckenrode, J. E. (2006). The virtual cutting edge: Adolescent self-injury and the Internet. *Developmental Psychology, 42*, 407–417.

Wilson, J. L., Peebles, R., Hardy, K. K., & Litt, I. F. (2006). Surfing for thinness: A pilot study of pro-eating disorder web site usage in adolescents with eating disorders. *Pediatrics, 118*, e1635–e1643.

Yom-Tov, E., Fernandez-Luque, L., Weber, I., & Crains, S. P. (2012). Pro-anorexia and pro-recovery photo sharing: A tale of two warring tribes. *Journal of Medical Internet Research, 14*, e151.

Prevention and Postvention of NSSI and Disordered Eating

17

Lara J. Cox and Michael P. Levine

Abstract

Non-suicidal self-injury (NSSI) and eating disorders (EDs) are comorbid disorders with a number of common risk factors, including negative emotionality, negative body image, impulsivity, and emotional dysregulation. Existing work in the ED field draws upon the nonspecific vulnerability-stressor model and critical social perspectives to engage adolescents as well as prevention specialists in the prevention process. Although there is very little empirical research on the prevention of NSSI, there are guidelines in the areas of preventing ED, depression, and suicide. Postvention, or interventions that occur after a disorder has already developed, is a concept developed in the field of suicidology to provide aid to the family, friends, and school community of an individual who has completed suicide. As NSSI and EDs affect a living sufferer in addition to those around them, postvention is modified here to include identification, assessment, and referral of the affected individual, as well as programs to support families, friends, and schools. After reviewing the key concepts and existing prevention and postvention research, this chapter uses the mental health intervention spectrum model of prevention to propose an ecological prevention/postvention model with interventions at the level of the media, community, school system, family, student body, and affected individual.

L.J. Cox (✉)
Department of Psychiatry, New York University, New York, NY, USA
e-mail: lara.cox@nyumc.org

M.P. Levine
Department of Psychology, Kenyon College, Gambier, OH, USA

L. Claes and J.J. Muehlenkamp (eds.), *Non-Suicidal Self-Injury in Eating Disorders*, DOI 10.1007/978-3-642-40107-7_17, © Springer-Verlag Berlin Heidelberg 2014

17.1 Introduction

Non-suicidal self-injury (NSSI) is comorbid with a spectrum of problems related to negative body image, disordered eating, and clinically significant eating disorders (e.g., Hilt, Nock, Lloyd-Richardson, & Prinstein, 2008; Ross, Heath, & Toste, 2009). In fact, it appears that NSSI, negative body image, and disordered eating are elements in a larger spectrum of significant problems in self-care pertaining to "disembodiment" (Piran & Teall, 2012) and "body disregard" (Muehlenkamp, 2012).

It is unlikely that the prevalence of NSSI or eating disorders will be substantially reduced by applying a detect-then-treat model. Consequently, this chapter has four fundamental goals. First, it offers a conceptual and empirical foundation for prevention specialists seeking to reduce the incidence of NSSI and eating disorders among adolescents. Ages 13–20 are high-risk periods for the onset of eating disorders (Smolak & Levine, 1996) and NSSI tends to begin between the ages of 12 and 16 (Klonsky, 2011; Nock & Prinstein, 2004). The second goal is to present guidelines for developing integrated interventions at various points along the National Research Council/Institute of Medicine's spectrum of prevention (National Research Council, 2009). Third, as prevention shades into clinical intervention, this chapter addresses postvention for families, friends, and others seeking to understand and support those adolescents who are already showing signs of disordered eating and/or NSSI. A final goal is to develop further directions for the joint prevention of NSSI and disordered eating.

17.2 Assumptions Related to NSSI and Eating Disorders

In this chapter, NSSI is defined as the direct, deliberate self-infliction of pain and tissue damage in the absence of suicidal intent or psychosis, for purposes that are not socially sanctioned (see also Chap. 1, Claes & Muehlenkamp, 2013). Moreover, it is distinguished from stereotypic or self-stimulating behavior associated with mental retardation or developmental delay (Nock & Favazza, 2009; Svirko & Hawton, 2007). The most common forms of NSSI are cutting, burning, hitting, and biting (Nock & Prinstein, 2004).

It is very useful to conceptualize the well-known eating disorders as the extremes of a set of intertwined spectra or continua that are unhealthy but ordinary to the point of being normative and culturally syntonic (Levine & Smolak, 2006). The strands are (a) negative or distorted body image; (b) unhealthy forms of weight management; (c) valuing the self in terms of perceived weight and shape in relation to unrealistic standards of beauty, fitness, muscularity, and power; (d) irrational fear of fat feeding a drive for thinness and leanness; (d) harsh self-surveillance and self-criticism feeding and being fed by shame, anxiety, depression, and difficulties in self-regulation; and (e) binge eating. People who have eating concerns and behaviors that generate mild-to-moderate problems and who have moderate to high levels of (a) and (b), plus one of (c)–(e), do not have a recognized eating disorder such as anorexia nervosa (AN), bulimia nervosa (BN), or EDNOS.

However, their unhealthy attitudes and behaviors constitute disordered eating (Levine & Smolak, 2006, 2009; Levine, Piran, & Jasper, in press). Note that weight management behaviors such as diet pill or laxative abuse, exercising while injured, or binge eating followed by self-induced vomiting are not considered to be NSSI because pain or injury are typically neither immediate nor the conscious function of the behavior.

17.3 Definitions and Assumptions Relevant to Prevention and Postvention

17.3.1 Prevention

Prevention focuses on anticipating and forestalling illness or disorder. Thus, prevention involves protecting current states of health and reinforcing effective functioning (Levine & Smolak, 2006, 2009). It attempts to reduce the *incidence* of disorders by implementing and evaluating carefully planned interventions designed to reduce risk factors and to increase protective factors that promote health and strengthen resilience in the event of predictable challenges and unforeseen stressors.

This chapter uses the *"mental health intervention spectrum"* model of prevention. This is a continuum from health promotion → prevention (universal, selective, and indicated or "targeted") → treatment (case identification, intervention, and aftercare) (National Research Council, 2009). Identification, referral, and effective therapy and support are important components of an approach to building integrated systems for health promotion, prevention, and treatment (Levine, 1987; Lieberman, Toste, & Heath, 2009), as they help prevent further comorbidity, chronicity, and mortality (Levine & Smolak, 2006). However, using the National Research Council (2009) guidelines, these processes are considered "treatment," not prevention.

Health promotion seeks to influence the general public or a whole population in ways that strengthen physical and mental health. Promotion of mental health is designed to "enhance individuals' ability to achieve developmentally appropriate tasks [and] a positive sense of self-esteem, mastery, well-being, and social inclusion, and to strengthen their ability to cope with adversity" (National Research Council, 2009, p. 67).

Universal prevention programs seek to change and reinforce government policies, social institutions, and common cultural practices in order to improve the "public health" of extremely large groups of citizens.

Selective prevention also involves changes in public policy and group practices, but the primary audiences are large groups of people who are asymptomatic but considered at risk for biological, psychological, or sociocultural reasons. For example, selective prevention programs seeking to reduce the incidence of NSSI and disordered eating might focus on girls ages 10–14 who live in a society that defines women in terms of looks and passivity and who have a parent who suffers from severe depression. The typical multi-lesson eating disorders prevention curriculum for middle school girls would fall between universal and selective prevention on the mental health intervention continuum (Levine & Smolak, 2009).

Indicated/targeted prevention refers to programs for people who have been identified as being at high risk due to warning signs in the form of clear precursors or mild symptoms. Their at-risk status "indicates" a need for a preventive intervention. Ideally, determination of at-risk status for selective through indicated prevention programs is based on screening methods with well-documented sensitivity and specificity (Levine & Smolak, 2006).

17.3.2 Postvention

A concept relevant to prevention that is not fully included in the mental health intervention model is postvention. It is typically applied to those affected by a suicide and, in the case of completed suicide, it refers to activities aimed at preventing adverse outcomes, including suicidal behavior, among survivors (Aguirre & Slater, 2010). There has been very little work directed specifically at postvention for NSSI or an eating disorder, in which the "survivors" include not only family and friends but also the identified sufferer. Literature searches for postvention yield only one article for NSSI (Trepal, Wester, & MacDonald, 2006) and none for eating disorders.

In the present chapter, the concept of postvention has been adapted in two related ways. The first form of postvention, which lies between indicated prevention and treatment on the mental health intervention continuum, is designed to reduce the duration and severity of eating disordered behaviors and NSSI by identifying, building a caring relationship with, and helping individuals whose symptoms have reached a clinically significant level. The second form attempts to support individuals with newly identified NSSI and eating disorders, as well as people in their social systems, by decreasing stressors and increasing support and resilience in the contexts of families, peers, schools, and communities. A key factor in these interventions is specific, detailed response protocols designed in advance of an incident (Komar, 1994).

17.4 Common Risk Factors for Disordered Eating and NSSI

When seeking to prevent two intersecting disorders, a reasonable place to begin is identification of shared and modifiable risk factors. It is challenging to disentangle putative causal risk factors (Table 17.1) from correlates and consequences, from early manifestations or warning signs (Table 17.2), and from longitudinal predictors that turn out to be proxies for other, perhaps as yet unknown, causal variables (Smolak, 2012; Stice, 2002). With these caveats in mind, Table 17.1 presents risk factors that meet three criteria: they are shared by disordered eating and NSSI; a body of evidence strongly suggests that they are involved in the

Table 17.1 Shared risk factors for eating disorders and NSSI

Factor	Description and comment
Genetic vulnerability to anxiety and mood disorder	Nonspecific predisposition for some as yet undetermined combination or interrelationship of unstable serotonin systems, stress reactivity, temperamental fearfulness (related to negative affect, below)
Chronic family stress and dysfunction	High family conflict and stress + low levels of problem solving and support, insecure attachments, poor communication
Negative affect	A dispositional tendency to increased levels of stress, distress, dysphoria, tension, worry, despair, guilt, hopelessness, etc.
Intimidation, teasing, and/or harassment	Interpersonal experiences with peers, family members, coaches, physicians, etc., that leave the person feeling anxious, ashamed, out of control, and powerless
Body dissatisfaction (negative body image, appearance dissatisfaction)	Beliefs, perceptions, and feelings that one's body, and in particular one's weight and shape, is flawed because of its failure to live up to internalized standards of beauty and attractiveness
Low self-esteem and negative self-concept	Beliefs, perceptions, and feelings that one's self, including significant aspects of one's self in addition to one's physical appearance, is inferior, inadequate, too different, and/or unacceptable
Emotional dysregulation	Increased emotional intensity and reactivity, limited emotion regulation strategies, nonacceptance of one's emotions, alexithymia; may also include dissociation
Impulsivity	Self-reports of generalized tendency to act without thinking or contemplating risk, especially in the presence of intense emotions or external stressors (there is mixed evidence regarding behavioral indicators of impulsivity); risk factor for NSSI and bulimic syndromes

Based on research reviewed and conclusions drawn by Cox et al. (2012); Glenn and Klonsky (2010); Levine et al. (in press); Nock, Joiner, Gordon, Lloyd-Richardson, and Prinstein (2006); Smolak (2012); Stice (2002); Svirko and Hawton (2007), among others. Many of these risk factors are not specific to eating disorders or NSSI.

multiple pathways to the development of both disorders; and they have clear implications for prevention. This list is based largely on correlational work, as longitudinal data do not yet exist for all the factors. However, these are reliable correlates that are reasonable targets for prevention because they are both identifiable and modifiable.

In refining and applying the information in Table 17.1, three things are important. First, no one risk factor is necessary or sufficient, so prevention of NSSI and disordered eating needs to address a variety of risk factors. Second, all these factors are deeply embedded in multidimensional psychosocial contexts. Third, developmental determinants of some of these risk factors will need to be addressed.

Table 17.2 Warning signs for NSSI and disordered eating

Type of warning sign	NSSI warning signs	ED warning signs
Emotional	Inability to cope with strong emotions as evidenced by frequent outbursts of anger or tears	Moodiness and irritability Oversensitivity to criticism Guilt and shame about eating
	Frequent expressions of anxiety, depression, hopelessness, or self-denigrating comments	Chronic, unrelenting dissatisfaction with self, regardless of performance
Behavioral	Possession of implements potentially used to self-injure (razor blades, knives, shards of glass, lighters, etc.)	Possession of diet pills, laxatives, purgatives, and emetics; exercising regularly and intensively despite illness, injury, or dangerous weather
	Evidence of self-injury in schoolwork such as journals, art projects, or writing samples	Evidence of preoccupation with weight, shape, fat, and calories—in speech, schoolwork, art, etc.
	Secretive behavior such as spending unusual amounts of time in the restroom	Secretive vomiting; heading for the restroom immediately after eating
	Isolation or withdrawal	Isolation or withdrawal
	Friendship with peers engaging in NSSI	Friendship with peers engaging in "fat talk" and a "dieting culture"
	Visiting websites or message boards related to depression and NSSI	Visiting and championing pro-anorexia or pro-bulimia websites or message boards
Physical	Frequent or unexplained scars, cuts, burns, or bruises	Signs of starvation, cuts on the back of the fingers from inducing vomiting, swelling of glands under jaw from frequent vomiting
	Consistent use of inappropriate clothing for the weather (e.g., wearing long sleeves/pants in hot weather to cover injured areas)	Consistent use of inappropriate clothing for the weather or the event, to cover emaciation or to manage body image issues

Based on information found in Juhnke et al. (2011), Levine (1987), Levine and Smolak (2006), and Lieberman et al. (2009)

For example, negative affect, negative body image, and body disregard or disembodiment all play a role in both disordered eating and NSSI (Muehlenkamp, 2012; Piran & Teall, 2012; Smolak, 2012). A lot of evidence indicate that threats to one's sense of control, self-objectification, internalization of impossible ideals of thinness or muscularity, and perfectionist standards contribute to negative affect and negative body image. Consequently, prevention programs need to address factors, including mass media, that influence those variables during late childhood and early adolescence (Levine & Smolak, 2006, 2009; Smolak & Levine, 1996).

17.5 Models Guiding Prevention

17.5.1 Nonspecific Vulnerability-Stressor Model

It has long been known that the risk factors predisposing individuals to a broad range of psychopathology in adolescence and adulthood tend to overlap [see Chap. 7 in Levine and Smolak (2006)]. Examples of nonspecific risk factors are lack of coping skills and other behavioral competencies (e.g., goal setting, problem solving, communication), cumulative life stress, and lack of social support. To these can be added a number of the risk factors listed in Table 17.1. The likelihood and number of psychiatric comorbidities increase with exposure to greater numbers of risk factors (Mendes, Souza Crippa, Souza, & Loureiro, 2012).

This nonspecific relationship between stressors, vulnerabilities, and maladaptive behavior has several important implications (Levine et al., in press; Levine & Smolak, 2006; Whitlock & Knox, 2009). Prevention need not wait until all risk factors are clarified and organized into a dynamic model. According to the nonspecific vulnerability-stressor (NSVS) model, problems will be prevented and health and resilience facilitated when stakeholders in healthy development work together to eliminate or reduce stressors while strengthening the personal and interpersonal lives of adolescents. Stressors range from normative developmental challenges (e.g., issues of autonomy, relatedness, identity, sexuality) to common but frequent threats (e.g., sexual harassment, family conflicts such as divorce) to major losses and trauma (Levine & Smolak, 2006; Smolak & Levine, 1996; Whitlock & Knox, 2009).

Adolescents will benefit when those committed to prevention provide multiple, overlapping opportunities for the "5 *C*s" of youth development (Levine et al., in press): *C*ompetence (life skills), *C*onnection, *C*haracter (standing up for one's beliefs), *C*onfidence, and *C*aring. The five *C*s flourish when those engaged in prevention work together *and* with adolescents to make multiple environments (e.g., school, athletics, the arts, family) safer, more respectful, and more responsive. One important set of environments in this effort is found online (Whitlock & Knox, 2009). According to the NSVS model, prevention is expressly developmental, behavioral, and ecological (Levine & Smolak, 2006). In this regard the NSVS model emphasizes the transformation of policies, practices, norms, media messages, etc., at the population and community levels (Whitlock & Knox, 2009).

17.5.2 Critical Social Perspectives, Disembodiment, and Body Disregard

The adolescent's developing body resides at the nexus of biological, psychological, interpersonal, and sociocultural forces (Piran & Teall, 2012). Embodiment, which Muehlenkamp casts in terms of body regard, refers to a "connection to, ownership of, and understanding of the body (e.g., body integrity)" (2012, p. 332). To be "embodied" is to be present in and engaged with one's own feelings, desires, capacities, relationships, and cultural identities (Menzel & Levine, 2011). People who are more embodied are attuned to bodily needs and signals (e.g., hunger, satiety, pain, passion), respect and care for their body, accept and appreciate their appearance, and enjoy and cultivate a variety of physical experiences.

To be disembodied, then, is to experience one's body and its connection to action, relationships, and cultures as mysterious, untrustworthy, awkward, dangerous, belonging to others, out of control, and/or meaningless. To be disembodied is to live in—or avoid many forms of living because of the likelihood of—frequent experiences of shame, self-criticism, dissociation, and either stultifying self-consciousness or mindless impulsivity with respect to the body (Muehlenkamp, 2012). Both NSSI and disordered eating reflect and amplify disembodiment (Muehlenkamp, 2012; Piran and Teall, 2012). The experience of disembodiment increases receptivity to direct and modeled messages from family, peer groups, and mass media that the "body is an acceptable physical outlet upon which to manage aversive internal states" (Muehlenkamp, 2012, p. 334). Disembodiment can be expressed in a wide variety of ways. For example, research with adolescent girls indicates that having a negative body image increases risk for depression, binge eating, physical inactivity, and unhealthy weight management, including cigarette smoking and illegal drug use.

Piran (2001, 2010) and Piran and Teall (2012) have documented how adverse social experiences negatively affect the physical domain, the mental domain (e.g., identity, norms, values), and experiences of powerlessness in relation to the body as the site of subjectivity and control (or lack thereof). For many adolescent boys and girls, the result of normative cultural messages, gender roles, prejudice, and teasing is disconnection, dis(rupted) embodiment, and behavioral tendencies that represent and express body disregard (Muehlenkamp, 2012; Piran & Teall, 2012).

Disembodiment theories and the NSVS model are "Critical Social Perspectives" (Piran & Teall, 2012) that direct prevention to emphasize social changes and social justice (Levine et al., in press; Piran, 2001). These models also highlight relationship building as the foundation for empowering youth to engage in analysis of unhealthy sociocultural influences and to put the resulting knowledge, based on their lived experiences, to use in spearheading social transformations. Piran's (1999, 2001, 2010) quantitative and qualitative prevention studies have demonstrated that engagement in a program shaped by a critical social perspective helps adolescent girls shift the experience of their bodies from a self-conscious, private, and silent nexus of anxiety, shame, and helplessness to an individual and shared experience of "embodied self-care and agency in transforming their social environment" and themselves (Levine et al., in press).

17.6 Existing Prevention and Postvention Programs

17.6.1 Eating Disorders Prevention

The substantial developments over the past 15 years in the prevention of negative body image, disordered eating, and eating disorders have been evaluated in several meta-analytic reviews (e.g., Stice, Shaw, & Marti, 2007) and in many narrative literature reviews (e.g., Levine & Smolak, 2006, 2009; Piran, 2010). These reviews point to three guiding principles (adapted from Levine and McVey 2012).

17.6.1.1 Principle 1: A Critical Social Perspective

Eating disorder prevention will likely fail, and may well be harmful, if it concentrates on "those people" with "their clinical disorders." To reiterate, problems pertaining to body image and body management are embedded in cultural attitudes, norms, and practices. For example, negative body image, disordered eating, and eating disorders thrive in settings where the female body, the small male body, the fat body, the ethnic body, and so forth are subjected to objectification, teasing, intimidation, harassment, and social constraints (Levine & Smolak, 2006; Piran, 2001). Therefore, consciousness raising for adults and adolescents is an important element in establishing and applying a critical social perspective. Analysis and clarification of lived experiences become the basis for constructive action, such as improvements in school policies and practices, peer norms, and healthy attitudes modeled by teachers and other staff. Peer engagement in social and environmental transformations is consistent with the fundamental meaning of prevention and with the commitment that many schools and other organizations have to facilitating education and cultivating youth development through respect, tolerance, safety, citizenship, and leadership (Levine & McVey, 2012).

The relational component of the critical social perspective also means that prevention requires a careful assessment phase that necessarily involves many people, including adolescents. It is very important to engage a range of the stakeholders—males as well as females—in schools and other important environments for adolescents (see Chap. 15 in Levine & Smolak, 2006; Piran, 2001, 2010). Collaborative evaluation of specific contexts provides the data and working relationships for development of social, organizational, and physical–environmental changes.

17.6.1.2 Principle 2: An Ecological Perspective

Many different types of curricular prevention programs for adolescents have positive effects during and immediately after the program, only to have those effects dissipate with longer follow-up (Levine & Smolak, 2006). It is not surprising that individual changes within one context are insufficient. Children and adolescents receive multiple, overlapping, and unhealthy messages and incentives emanating from multiple social sources that support risk factors for negative body image and disordered eating (Levine & Smolak, 2006; Piran, 2010).

This problem is well known in the drug prevention field. A meta-analysis by Tobler et al (2000) of nearly 200 studies demonstrated that drug prevention programs that facilitate *systemic* changes clearly have the most positive, sustained results. Studies of eating disorders prevention for adolescent females (Piran, 2010) and prevention of steroid and supplement abuse for adolescent males (Goldberg et al., 2000) reinforce the critical importance of intervention at various levels in the ecology of adolescents. Changes in influences beyond the individual classroom have been accomplished in many ways: in-service training of staff; training of teachers, coaches, and peers in program delivery; inclusion of parents and grandparents in homework assignments and events; integrated lessons in a variety of subjects; coordinated changes in peer norms and school policies pertaining to teasing (as one example); student involvement in after-school programs such as live theater with dramatic but program-consistent content; and public service announcements devised and delivered by students. A proposal for an ecological, multisystems approach to prevention of NSSI and eating disorders is presented in Table 17.3. Here, two examples of successful applications are presented.

One encouraging example of an ecological approach that also embodies a critical social perspective is the *Full of Ourselves* curricular program for girls ages 12–14 (Steiner-Adair et al., 2002). Using some 70 activities, organized into eight units delivered across 2–4 months, this program brings young adolescent girls together to help them become more assertive and more supportive of each other while learning to detect and challenge unhealthy cultural messages concerning gender, beauty, weight- and shape-related prejudice, and eating. Participants are strongly encouraged to develop and express a multifaceted sense of self while working with other girls and adult mentors to be an active presence in reshaping cultural messages. An RCT with 6-month follow-up found that *Full of Ourselves* produced a sustained increase in body satisfaction, coupled with improved knowledge about weight-based prejudice, mass media, and healthy behavior (Steiner-Adair et al., 2002).

Another promising ecological approach is seen in the work of McVey and colleagues in Toronto (see Levine and McVey (2012), for a fuller description). Based on a program of risk factor and prevention research with middle school students that produced a curriculum for boys and girls and a template for a girls-only conscious-raising support group, McVey, Tweed, and Blackmore (2007) developed *Healthy Schools–Healthy Kids*. This 8-month school-based intervention integrated an improved curriculum with teacher and staff training, parent education, separate support groups for boys and girls, and promotion of positive messages via posters and public service announcements. In addition, all students saw and discussed a 50-min play devoted to understanding and resisting media and peer pressures. An RCT found that at 6-month follow-up, seventh grade girls and boys reported significantly less body dissatisfaction. Moreover, girls participating in the program also reduced their awareness and internalization of the slender beauty ideal. McVey and colleagues have continued to build an ecological approach, demonstrating, for example, the feasibility and utility of a web-based curriculum for teachers and public health staff who work with 9–12-year olds (Levine & McVey, 2012).

17.6.1.3 Principle 3: Multifaceted Competence Development

At the individuals-within-classrooms level of adolescent ecology, school-based programs that work best in preventing adolescent drug use are interactive and engaging, and they emphasize positive peer norms, resistance skills, media literacy, stress management, and other "life skills" or competencies (Botvin & Griffin, 2002; Tobler et al., 2000). In addition to *Full of Ourselves*, several different programs demonstrate the value of multifaceted competence development in preventing negative body image and disordered eating. *Athletes Targeting Healthy Exercise and Nutrition Alternatives* (ATHENA) is a universal-selective program for promoting health and preventing eating problems and unhealthy weight/shape management in female athletes, cheerleaders, and members of dance and drill teams (Elliot et al., 2006; Ranby et al., 2009). A manual is used to train coaches and peer leaders to model, teach, and reinforce clear expectations for healthy attitudes and behaviors; positive norms for self and others; media literacy skills; drug (e.g., steroids and diet pills) resistance behaviors; and goal setting and other life skills. Psychoeducation, behavioral instruction and rehearsal, individual demonstrations of competence, and positive norm development all take place during regular team practices.

A large-scale RCT of ATHENA showed that, at the end of the program, participants were significantly less likely to begin using diet pills, amphetamines, anabolic steroids, and muscle-building supplements; reported healthier eating and fewer injuries; and significantly reduced their intentions to diet for weight loss and to use self-induced vomiting and drugs for weight control (Elliot et al., 2006; Ranby et al., 2009). As predicted, ATHENA successfully increased four significant mediators: self-efficacy in controlling mood, the perception that few peers endorse and use body-shaping drugs, media literacy, and drug-resistance skills. The first three of these may have implications for preventing NSSI as well.

Media literacy is a collection of skills for resisting unhealthy messages and for generating alternative and much healthier messages for oneself and one's peers (Levine & Smolak, 2006). It is a critical component of the ATHENA program and its companion intervention, the *Athletes Training and Learning to Avoid Steroids* (ATLAS) program, which has been successful with male high school football players (Goldberg et al., 2000). Media literacy is also a promising component of universal-selective programs for preventing negative body image and disordered eating in young adolescents (see reviews by Levine et al., in press; Levine and Smolak, 2006).

Media literacy is one type of the cultural literacy that is a pillar of the critical social perspective (Piran, 2010). An extremely significant innovation in prevention is a form of cultural literacy known as dissonance-based intervention (DBI). DBI is a reliably effective targeted prevention program for young college women who are at risk due to high levels of weight preoccupation and negative body image (Stice, Rohde, & Shaw, 2013). Working in accordance with a detailed manual, group leaders use minimal persuasion (hence the potential for cognitive dissonance) to induce participants to write essays, conduct role plays, and engage in other cognitive–behavioral activities to analyze, resist, and dilute sociocultural pressures to internalize the slender beauty ideal. These counter-attitudinal actions, particularly in a group context, are designed to promote attitude change motivated by the need to reduce dissonance. An RCT found that adolescent girls with high levels of body concern who received the DBI in four weekly 1 h sessions showed greater decreases in body dissatisfaction at 2-year follow-up and in eating disorder symptoms at 3-year follow-up (Stice, Rohde, Shaw, & Gau, 2011).

17.6.2 Depression and Suicide Prevention

Very little has been written about the prevention of NSSI (see Sect. 17.6.3). Therefore, given the relationships between negative emotionality, mood disorders, and NSSI, it is useful to consider lessons from depression prevention when developing an NSSI prevention program. NSSI may be an earlier indicator of a shared diathesis with suicidality (Cox et al., 2012), so lessons from suicide prevention may also be applied.

Many interventions seeking to prevent depression in adolescents and young adults are universal-selective programs that feature some blend of cognitive–behavioral therapy (CBT), psychoeducation, and/or interpersonal psychotherapy (IPT). Typically, there are 8–12 hour-long sessions, delivered either by school staff or a mental health professional, or as computerized exercises available in the classroom or at home (Calear, Christensen, Mackinnon, Griffiths, & O'Kearney, 2009; Van Voorhees et al., 2009). Lessons focus on identifying and changing dysfunctional thoughts and beliefs, improving self-esteem and protective behaviors such as pleasurable activities and engagement with social supports, and teaching life skills such as communication, problem solving, relaxation, and coping (Calear et al., 2009; Gillham et al., 2012). A systematic review of RCTs for school-based depression prevention programs showed overall small effect sizes, both immediately post-intervention and with long-term follow-up (Corrieri et al., 2013). Nevertheless, an economics study using mathematical simulation (Mihalopoulos, Vos, Pirkis, & Carter, 2012) found that a theoretical school-based program for depression was highly cost-effective; the cost of $5,400 per disability-adjusted life year (DALY) was far below the threshold of $50,000 per DALY commonly considered good value for money.

Most of the broad variety of suicide prevention programs are universal, although these range from gatekeeper training programs to community-level developments such as public education campaigns and media guidelines. The US Air Force's (USAF) suicide prevention is of particular interest for prevention of EDs and NSSI because it is a comprehensive, top-down program that includes health promotion efforts, universal and indicated interventions, screening, and postvention strategies (Knox, Litts, Talcott, Feig, & Caine, 2003). Operating at all levels of the mental health promotion spectrum, the USAF effected changes at the system-wide level, including transformations in policy, education, officer training, and monitoring of groups and individuals. Access to mental health services was improved by increasing the number of mental health providers dedicated to prevention while integrating human service systems. Multiple universal prevention strategies were implemented simultaneously. Leaders were given training and education in suicide awareness and in guidelines for use of mental health services, and senior USAF leaders received annual messages and briefings on suicide and referral. Information on suicide was also integrated into the mandatory curriculum for officer training. With regard to selective and indicated prevention, commanders were given a behavioral health survey to assess the well-being of their units. Training on risk factors, intervention skills, and referral procedures was provided to enlisted personnel at two levels: every member was given training in nonsupervisory "buddy care," while selected unit gatekeepers received additional training in leadership and supervision. Finally, a critical incident stress management team was created to respond to traumatic events, including completed suicides, and to provide postvention services.

The USAF's comprehensive program resulted in a 33 % reduction in completed suicides in the 6 years following its implementation (Knox et al., 2003). The social norm for help seeking was also changed, from being viewed as a sign of weakness to a statement of strength and responsibility. However, although this program is effective, it does not address certain issues relevant to adolescents. For example, reliance on an ingrained hierarchy of authority may be counterproductive in working with adolescents, who may resist or only temporarily adopt interventions perceived as coming only from adults. In addition, the USAF program does not address social media, a rapidly growing arena for problems involving youth.

A systematic review of school-based suicide prevention programs found that, although not all studies assessed number of self-reported suicide attempts, those that did found decreased rates among those exposed to the intervention (Cusimano & Sameem, 2011). Therefore, several school-based suicide prevention programs will be reviewed. The Signs of Suicide suicide prevention program, which can be administered in a single session, is a school-based universal strategy that helps adolescents help each other (Aseltine & DeMartino, 2004). It consists of a video and discussion guide that raise awareness of suicide and related issues, teach students to recognize signs of depression and suicide in themselves or others, and provide specific action steps for responding based on the ACT model. The first step is to *A*cknowledge the signs of suicide displayed by an individual and take the adolescent seriously. The second is to let the adolescent know that you *C*are and want to help. Last, the helping student should *T*ell a responsible adult. The Signs of Suicide program also involves a brief self-screening for depression and the provision of information about appropriate resources. In an RCT, adolescents who received the Signs of Suicide program were 40 % less likely to report a suicide attempt over 3-month follow-up than those who did not (Aseltine & DeMartino, 2004).

Part of the USAF program is gatekeeper training, which is designed to prepare individuals who may come into contact with a suicidal person to identify the warning signs for suicide, to reach out to the person, and to help the person to access care. When this concept is applied to adolescents, potential gatekeepers include teachers and other school staff, clergy, medical professionals, police, social service workers, parents, and anyone who works closely with youth. Young people may also be trained as gatekeepers. Training involves education about suicide and its warning signs, the idea that suicide is preventable, and guidance similar to the ACT template (Tompkins, Witt, & Abraibesh, 2010). Gatekeeper training usually consists of a single 1–2 h session, though it may also involve a refresher session several months later. A review of gatekeeper training studies found increased levels of self-reported knowledge, self-efficacy, and knowledge of services among individuals trained as gatekeepers. Moreover gatekeeper training programs decreased rates of suicidal acts by 16–73 % among the target populations, though only one study reviewed was specific to adolescents (Isaac et al., 2009).

The Sources of Strength program integrates the gatekeeper model with a youth-led messaging campaign to change norms and behaviors pertaining to suicide and help seeking (Wyman et al., 2010). The goals of Sources of Strength support the five *C*s of youth development. Specifically, to increase youth–adult communication ties, students are encouraged to name and engage trusted adults. To reduce implicit suicide acceptability, students are guided to create and reinforce the expectation that friends ask adults for help for suicidal friends. Similarly, students are helped to identify, develop, and use interpersonal and formal coping resources.

Implementation of the Sources of Strength program begins with selection of peer leaders from diverse social cliques, including those considered high risk. At each school, two to three adult advisors receive 4–6 h of training, while peer leaders receive 4 h of interactive training on resilience, how to increase resources for themselves and other students, and how to model engagement of "trusted adults" to help depressed or suicidal peers. Peer leaders also disseminate messages about sources of strength, including compassion, through presentations, public service announcements, and by video or text on social networking sites. This program's focus on peer leaders, trusted adults, and help-seeking skills is extremely important. On measures of suicide perceptions and norms, social connectedness, and peer leader behaviors, the program produced effect sizes ranging from 0.21 to 0.75 (Wyman et al., 2010).

17.6.3 NSSI Prevention

While many chapters and articles offer recommendations for preventing NSSI (e.g., Juhnke, Granello, & Granello, 2011; Lieberman et al., 2009; Whitlock & Knox, 2009), extensive literature search reveals only one empirically tested program. The Signs of Self-Injury (SOSI) program (Muehlenkamp, Walsh, & McDade, 2010), adapted from the Signs of Suicide program (Aseltine & DeMartino, 2004), is a school-based program designed to increase knowledge and decrease acts of NSSI. The SOSI program also attempts to increase help-seeking behaviors by improving attitudes about helping and by increasing individuals' perceived capacity to respond effectively to those engaging in NSSI and to refer them to help. Along with information about NSSI and the ACT model, the SOSI video includes practice vignettes, an example of an initial, constructive meeting between a counselor and student, and an interview with an older adolescent discussing her recovery from NSSI. The video is followed by a moderated class discussion. In a quasi-experimental study, adolescents participating in the SOSI program showed significant improvements in knowledge about NSSI and less discomfort with or avoidance of NSSI in peers, along with a significant increase in desire to approach and help. There was a clear but nonsignificant trend towards fewer past-month acts of NSSI at 5 weeks post-intervention (Muehlenkamp et al., 2010). Though larger scale evaluation is needed, the SOSI program is a potentially effective option for school-based NSSI prevention.

17.6.4 NSSI and Eating Disorders Postvention

To date there is no literature addressing postvention of eating disorders, and the only article describing a postvention plan for NSSI focuses on the family of the affected individual (Trepal et al., 2006). Thus, this section presents five fundamental and interrelated principles that need to be embraced by family members, friends, teammates, and others who care about and are affected by an adolescent suffering from NSSI or an eating disorder. First, these problems need to be taken as seriously as if one discovered that the adolescent had type I diabetes or asthma.

Second, NSSI and eating disorders are complex because they negatively affect physical health, cognition, emotions, and relationships. No one is helped by beliefs and proclamations that "it's just a diet gone wrong" or "she's just trying to get attention so she can compete with her sister" or "he just doesn't want to be teased anymore." These two principles emphasize the importance of helping loved ones and friends become educated and to be aware of understandable but misguided interpretations and statements they can avoid making to the person and to each other. Organizations such as Self-Injury Outreach and Support (SiOS; http://www.sioutreach.org), the National Eating Disorders Association (NEDA; http://www.nationaleatingdisorders.org), and the National Association of Anorexia Nervosa and Associated Disorders (ANAD; http://www.anad.org) offer free or low-cost information packets for parents, schools, and friends.

Third, shame and the attribution of blame are unproductive and potentially harmful to everyone involved. No one causes these behaviors, *and* everyone has a responsibility to participate in the person's process of recovery. Fourth, problems such as NSSI and eating disorders exact a frightful toll, not only on the adolescent but also on family, friends, and, in some instances, school staff. Adolescents with NSSI or eating disorders may appear in control at times, and sometimes they act in ways that are deceptive, mean, and manipulative—though they do not intend to hurt others or "drag them down." And yet the disorder itself, the secrecy and half-truths, the shame and anxiety, the vacillations between self-control and loss of control—all this constitutes severe, prolonged stress, especially for the family (Goddard, Raenker, & Treasure, 2012). Finally, while acknowledging the significant negative impact of NSSI on the family and peers, it is important to keep in mind that each person, including postvention personnel, will likely have "a unique and valid perspective" (Trepal et al., 2006, p. 343), ranging from fear and avoidant isolation to nonchalance to over-involvement or anger due to a sense of continuing crisis. Thinking and talking in terms of what is "typical" is unhelpful for all concerned.

When the disorder is identified, the process of working with the school and medical personnel to find, engage, participate in, and pay for high-quality clinical services is likely to add to the family's challenges. Most clinicians working with adolescents who have problems such as eating disorders and/or NSSI expect to collaborate with the family in helping both the adolescent and the family (Goddard et al., 2012; Hill et al., 2013; Levine et al., in press). Family members can benefit considerably from training in regulating and expressing their own emotions, effective listening and communicating when anxious or frustrated, and the distinction between direction and guidance (Goddard et al., 2012; Hill et al., 2013).

Along the same lines, supporting a person during the exciting peaks, the discouraging valleys, and the frustrating or boring plateaus of treatment, progress, relapse, and recovery is at best challenging and at worst extremely stressful. Participants in the process need support themselves, and some will need treatment for long-standing conditions (e.g., depression, substance abuse, marital conflict) that make it hard for family or friends to be there for the recovering person. Programs that treat adolescents usually work with families to improve their ability to support the adolescent through stages of change and recovery while supporting each other as individuals and as a family (Levine et al., in press; Vale, Nixon, & Kucharski, 2009). Some eating disorder programs in major cities and/or embedded in large hospitals are able to offer, as part of an array of services, free, open weekly support groups for families, friends, and anyone whose life is touched by a person with an eating disorder. These groups, many of which are facilitated by mental health professionals, provide information about the disorder and treatment, validation of the stressful nature of caregiving, and models of coping and hope.

Much has been written about identification, assessment, and treatment of individuals engaging in NSSI (e.g., Nixon & Heath, 2009; Nock, 2009). In contrast, there is little specific guidance for postvention (see brief mention by Lieberman et al., 2009; see also Trepal et al., 2006, and there are no outcome studies. Thus, the following describes potentially valuable recommendations for active, programmatic postvention for the family of an adolescent engaging in NSSI.

Postvention efforts should include the family, as some family members are likely to have strong and potentially unhelpful emotional reactions, such as shame, high levels of anxiety, and anger (Trepal et al., 2006). Family difficulties in managing these reactions may cause an inconsistent, confusing, and exhausting mix, across people or across time for a given person, of withdrawal from the person who is self-injuring and angry and intrusive attempts to control that individual. This may intensify family conflict, cause triangulation, or decrease communication, all of which may inadvertently worsen NSSI and significantly increase family distress. Consequently, families should be educated about the functional nature of NSSI, the differences between it and suicide, and ways to address understandable but potentially problematic emotional and behavioral reactions to NSSI.

This psychoeducation is an integral part of the training and support each member receives in order to feel that he or she is contributing to the well-being and progress of the affected individual and the family. As is the case with eating disorders, this education includes a no-fault model in which the individual is separated from her or his symptoms and neither the individual nor the family is blamed for the behavior. Based on studies of psychoeducation for families of people with other severe mental health problems, it is likely that families of those with NSSI will also benefit from learning about the course of NSSI, its prognosis, and treatment options including medication (Trepal et al., 2006). The family system/structure should also be assessed, and skills for decreasing or avoiding problematic communication and minimizing conflict may be taught to ensure that lines of supportive communication remain open while not impeding the individual's well-being.

In the school setting, a Crisis Response Team model similar to that often applied in postvention for suicide has been suggested (Lieberman et al., 2009). Teachers and staff should be trained about the warning signs for NSSI, suggestions for reaching out, and the protocol for response and referral. A school-based mental health professional, counselor, or nurse should be designated as the point person for NSSI referral issues and should create a "circle of care" involving the adolescent, the person making the referral, the school administration, family, and community mental health agencies. Affected peers should be identified and assessed for distress and risk factors. With regard to public discussion, large-scale assemblies or PA system announcements about NSSI should be avoided. The media and authority figures should also avoid presenting simplistic explanations for NSSI, including that it is intended to be manipulative (similar to recommendations found in O'Carroll and Potter, 1994, for suicide).

Conclusions and Future Directions

The success of various targeted interventions for older adolescents and young adults at risk for eating disorders, coupled with clinical experience in addressing NSSI, indicates that a medical model of detect-then-treat will indeed help high-risk adolescents (Lieberman et al., 2009; Stice et al., 2007, 2013). However, as detect-then-treat models intervene only after the development of the disorder, they can affect incidence only by reducing contagion and are therefore unlikely to have large effects on lifetime prevalence (Levine & Smolak, 2006). Given the nascent development of prevention for NSSI (Muehlenkamp et al., 2010; Whitlock & Knox, 2009) and the incomplete status of eating disorders prevention (Levine & McVey, 2012), at this time, no one knows how to prevent their comorbidity. It is known that prevention across the mental health intervention spectrum requires a "more ecological approach to prevention as the promotion of public health and well-being through policies and other interventions that target, not high-risk *individuals*, but rather institutions, communities, and other large groups" (Levine & Smolak, 2006, p. 363). Problems so clearly rooted in sociocultural factors require solutions drawn from a critical social perspective, social transformations, and social justice.

Table 17.3 summarizes and organizes ideas from the theory and research reviewed in this chapter (e.g., Knox et al., 2003; Piran, 1999, 2001) by proposing a continuum of multisystem, integrated interventions with adolescents. Table 17.3 also draws from drug prevention research (see Levine & Smolak, 2006, Chap. 10, for a review), proposals in the NSSI (Lieberman et al., 2009; Whitlock & Knox, 2009) and eating disorders fields (Levine & Smolak, 2006), and actual ecological programs currently under development, such as McVey's spectrum of mental health interventions for eating disorders in the province of Ontario, Canada (see review by Levine and McVey, 2012).

Table 17.3 Proposed ecological prevention and postvention model for NSSI and eating disorders

Level of intervention	Target	Proposed activity/program
Health *promotion* –> universal-selective *prevention*	School system	Health-promoting schools initiative, including participation from stakeholders such as students, teachers, parents, and other community members
		Anti-bullying policy, including special focus on social media, integrated with (a) policies concerning teasing/harassment related to weight, shape, gender, sexual orientation, and ethnicity; and (b) peer-led media contests and campaigns in school or in the community that promote tolerance and respect
	Media	Media guidelines for discussing NSSI and EDs, based on CDC guidelines for reporting on suicide (O'Carroll & Potter, 1994)
	Students	Media literacy and cultural literacy training across the curriculum, including responsible use of social media
		Curricula given in regular courses focused on life skills such as self-esteem, emotions and adaptive emotional regulation, healthy coping, communication, and problem solving; health courses may teach CBT skills for identifying and challenging dysfunctional thought and behavior patterns
	Community	Youth-led campaign to shift cultural norms about prejudice and intimidation and about help seeking among adolescents, including (a) media campaigns linked to media literacy education in school and (b) informing and educating civic organizations, business leaders, and medical and mental health professionals
Selective –> indicated *prevention*	School system	Annual school-wide screening for existing NSSI and disordered eating as well as known risk factors (e.g., depressive symptoms) integrated with (a) increased access to school-based mental health providers and (b) coordination with community mental health services focused on adolescents
		In-service gatekeeper training for teachers/staff on risk factors, warning signs of NSSI and EDs, application of the Acknowledge-Care-Tell (ACT) model, and guidelines for support of students receiving treatment

(continued)

Table 17.3 (continued)

Level of intervention	Target	Proposed activity/program
Selective –> indicated *prevention*	Health and fitness professionals	CME training for pediatricians and family physicians about NSSI and EDs; encourage screening at well-child visits for signs of NSSI and eating disorders (interview and physical exam)
		Continuing professional education and training for psychiatrists, psychologists, social workers, dietitians, nurses, athletic trainers, and fitness professionals in the community, focusing on different roles and skills involved in ACT and support vs. therapy
Selective –> indicated *prevention*	Parents and adult leaders (clergy, coaches, youth group leaders)	Education and gatekeeper training for adults active in parent–teacher associations, religious organizations, youth groups (scouts, equestrians, 4-H) in identifying risk factors, warning signs of NSSI and EDs, intervention skills using the ACT model, guidelines for use of mental health services, and providing support
		Ongoing contact via refresher courses, mailings, resource websites, and local mini-conferences (including awards for service) for leaders and adolescents (coupled with media attention to the issues)
	Students	Identification of diverse "youth leaders" and provision of special training on resilience factors, help seeking, and warning signs prior to youth conducting a mentored campaign (e.g., "I've Got Your Back"), including the use of social media, to promote positive messages and actions regarding helping peers
		Basic gatekeeper training for all students on risk factors, warning signs, and intervention and referral skills, using ACT model; creative and performance-based integration of this material into curriculum and into the arts (e.g., theater)
Targeted *prevention* –> *clinical intervention*	Students identified by screening, self-report, or peer/adult gatekeepers	School, with community advice and support, creates opportunity for on-campus or after-school prevention groups, including moderated online computer-assisted interventions; groups may teach CBT skills, acceptance-based emotional regulation, and mindfulness-based practices for improvement of body image and increased embodiment

(continued)

Table 17.3 (continued)

Level of intervention	Target	Proposed activity/program
Postvention	Affected individual	Assessment and referral to treatment by school-based mental health professional
		Creation of "circle of care" by trained point person, involving family, mental health providers, gatekeeper/referring individual (if applicable and appropriate)
		Follow-up in school setting to monitor progress and ensure adequate supports
	Family of affected individual	Psychoeducation about disordered eating and NSSI, including the no-fault model
		Assessment of family structure's functioning in providing necessary support, autonomy, etc.; focus on strengthening relationships between affected individual and family members as individuals and as a family
		Support and training for family members, including communication skills and conflict management
	School system	Creation of mental health team, including school-based mental health professional
		Specific protocol for assessment and referral of affected individual—and for smoothing student's return to school if inpatient, partial hospitalization, or intensive outpatient treatment is deemed to be necessary
		Specific protocol for identification and assessment of affected peers
		Specific policies to create guidelines for school-based communication about NSSI and EDs

Table 17.3 is intended to be an inspiration for further discussion, specific programming, and various types of formative and summative evaluations. One key to success in these daunting but important and exciting tasks is careful and creative planning by collaborative groups consisting of a variety of stakeholders (Piran, 2010). In this regard, prevention leaders can look for opportunities to synthesize multiple strategies (Levine & Smolak, 2006). For example, a peer-led and media-based education program for consciousness raising with adolescents and staff about risk factors for the spectrum of body disregard and about the nature and benefits of body regard (Muehlenkamp, 2012) can be combined with training in understanding and using media effects. The entire effort can then be used as community education and advocacy; the school's group could work with local media, service groups, and business organizations to publicize the program and honor the leaders and participants. This in turn could become the basis for

collaborative presentation of the program and materials at regional conferences or in statewide educator newsletters.

Finally, in thinking about collaboration, stakeholders, creativity, and multiple strategies, it is critically important to remember that adolescents themselves must be included in the design, implementation, evaluation, and refinement of prevention and postvention. A successful integrated program will not only produce the five *C*s of positive youth development, it will embody it.

References

Aguirre, R. T. P., & Slater, H. (2010). Suicide postvention as suicide prevention: Improvement and expansion in the United Sates. *Death Studies, 34*, 529–540.

Aseltine, R. H., Jr., & DeMartino, R. (2004). An outcome evaluation of the SOS Suicide Prevention Program. *American Journal of Public Health, 94*, 446–451.

Botvin, G. J., & Griffin, K. W. (2002). Preventing substance use and abuse. In K. M. Bear & G. G. Bear (Eds.), *Preventing school problems – Promoting school success: Strategies and programs that work* (pp. 259–298). Bethesda, MD: National Association of School Psychologists.

Calear, A. L., Christensen, H., Mackinnon, A., Griffiths, K. M., & O'Kearney, R. (2009). The YouthMood Project: A cluster randomized controlled trial of an online cognitive behavioral program with adolescents. *Journal of Consulting and Clinical Psychology, 77*, 1021–1032.

Claes, L., & Muehlenkamp, J. J. (2013). Non-suicidal self-injury and eating disorders: Dimensions of self-harm. In L. Claes & J. J. Muehlenkamp (Eds.), *Non-suicidal self-injury in eating disorders*. Heidelberg: Springer.

Corrieri, S., Heider, D., Conrad, I., Blume, A., Konig, H. H., & Riedel-Heller, S. G. (2013). School-based prevention programs for depression and anxiety in adolescence: A systematic review. *Health Promotion International*. Advance online publication. PMID 23376883.

Cox, L. J., Stanley, B. H., Melhem, N. M., Oquendo, M. A., Birmaher, B., Burke, A., Brent, D.A. (2012). A longitudinal study of nonsuicidal self-injury in offspring at high risk for mood disorder. *Journal of Clinical Psychiatry, 73*, 821–828.

Cusimano, M. D., & Sameem, M. (2011). The effectiveness of middle and high school-based suicide prevention programmes for adolescents: A systematic review. *Injury Prevention, 17*, 43–49.

Elliot, D. L., Moe, E. L., Goldberg, L., DeFrancesco, C. A., Durham, M. B., & Hix-Small, H. (2006). Definition and outcome of a curriculum to prevent disordered eating and body-shaping drug use. *Journal of School Health, 76*, 67–73.

Gillham, J. E., Reivich, K. J., Brunwasser, S. M., Freres, D. R., Chajon, N. D., Kash-Macdonald, V. M., Seligman, M. E. (2012). Evaluation of a group cognitive-behavioral depression prevention program for young adolescents: A randomized effectiveness trial. *Journal of Clinical Child and Adolescent Psychology, 41*, 621–639.

Glenn, C. R., & Klonsky, E. D. (2010). A multimethod analysis of impulsivity in nonsuicidal self-injury. *Personality Disorders: Theory, Research, and Treatment, 1*, 67–75.

Goddard, E., Raenker, S., & Treasure, J. (2012). Involving careers: A skills-based learning approach. In J. Alexander & J. Treasure (Eds.), *A collaborative approach to eating disorders* (pp. 149–162). London: Routledge.

Goldberg, L., MacKinnon, D. P., Elliot, D. L., Moe, E. L., Clarke, G., & Cheong, J. (2000). The Adolescents Training and Learning to Avoid Steroids program: Preventing drug use and promoting health behaviors. *Archives of Pediatric and Adolescent Medicine, 154*, 332–338.

Hill, L., Dagg, D., Levine, M. P., Smolak, L., Johnson, S., Stotz, S. A., & Little, N. (2013). *Family eating disorders manual: Guiding families through the maze of eating disorders*. Worthington, OH: Center for Balanced Living.

Hilt, L. M., Nock, M. K., Lloyd-Richardson, E. E., & Prinstein, M. J. (2008). Longitudinal study of nonsuicidal self-injury among young adolescents: Rates, correlates, and preliminary test of an interpersonal model. *Journal of Early Adolescence, 28*, 455–469.

Isaac, M., Elias, B., Katz, L. Y., Belik, S. L., Deane, F. P., Enns, M. W., & Swampy Cree Suicide Prevention Team (2009). Gatekeeper training as a preventative intervention for suicide: A systematic review. *Canadian Journal of Psychiatry, 54*, 260–268.

Juhnke, G. A., Granello, D. H., & Granello, P. F. (2011). Working with students who engage in nonsuicidal self-inflicted injury. In G. A. Juhnke, P. F. Granello, & D. H. Granello (Eds.), *Suicide, self-injury, and violence in the schools: Assessment, prevention, and intervention strategies* (pp. 85–108). Hoboken, NJ: Wiley

Klonsky, E. D. (2011). Non-suicidal self-injury in United States adults: Prevalence, sociodemographics, topography and functions. *Psychological Medicine, 41*, 1981–1986.

Knox, K. L., Litts, D. A., Talcott, G. W., Feig, J. C., & Caine, E. D. (2003). Risk of suicide and related adverse outcomes after exposure to a suicide prevention programme in the US Air Force: Cohort study. *British Medical Journal, 327*(7428), 1376.

Komar, A. A. (1994). Adolescent school crises: Structures, issues, and techniques for postventions. *International Journal of Adolescence and Youth, 5*, 35–46.

Levine, M. P. (1987). *How schools can help combat student eating disorders*. Washington, DC: National Education Association.

Levine, M. P., & McVey, G. L. (2012). Prevention, prevention science, and an ecological perspective: A framework for programs, research, and advocacy. In G. L. McVey, M. P. Levine, N. Piran, & H. B. Ferguson (Eds.), *Preventing eating-related and weight-related disorders: Collaborative research, advocacy, and policy change* (pp. 19–43). Toronto: Wilfred Laurier University Press.

Levine, M. P., Piran, N., & Jasper, K. J. (in press). Treatment and prevention of eating disorders in adolescence. In T. P. Gullotta & G. R. Adams (Eds.), *Handbook of adolescent behavioral problems: Evidence-based approaches to prevention and treatment* (2nd ed.). New York, NY: Kluwer.

Levine, M. P., & Smolak, L. (2006). *The prevention of eating problems and eating disorders: Theory, research, and practice*. Mahwah, NJ: Lawrence Erlbaum Associates.

Levine, M. P., & Smolak, L. (2009). Prevention of negative body image and disordered eating in children and adolescents: Recent developments and promising directions. In L. Smolak & J. K. Thompson (Eds.), *Body image, eating disorders, and obesity in youth* (2nd ed., pp. 215–239). Washington, DC: American Psychological Association.

Lieberman, R. A., Toste, J. R., & Heath, N. L. (2009). Nonsuicidal self-injury in the schools: Prevention and intervention. In M. K. Nixon & N. L. Heath (Eds.), *Self-injury in youth: The essential guide to assessment and intervention* (pp. 195–215). New York, NY: Routledge, Taylor & Francis Group.

McVey, G., Tweed, S., & Blackmore, E. (2007). Healthy Schools-Healthy Kids: A controlled evaluation of a comprehensive universal eating disorder prevention program. *Body Image, 4*, 115–136.

Mendes, A. V., Souza Crippa, J. A., Souza, R. M., & Loureiro, S. R. (2012). Risk factors for mental health problems in school-age children from a community sample. *Maternal and Child Health Journal*. Advance online publication. DOI 10.1007/s10995-012-1202-9.

Menzel, J. E., & Levine, M. P. (2011). Embodying experiences and the promotion of positive body image: The example of competitive athletics. In R. M. Calogero, S. Tantleff-Dunn, & J. K. Thompson (Eds.), *Self-objectification in women: Causes, consequences, and counteractions* (pp. 163–168). Washington, DC: American Psychological Association.

Mihalopoulos, C., Vos, T., Pirkis, J., & Carter, R. (2012). The population cost-effectiveness of interventions designed to prevent childhood depression. *Pediatrics, 129*, 723–730.

Muehlenkamp, J. J. (2012). Body regard in nonsuicidal self-injury: Theoretical explanations and treatment directions. *Journal of Cognitive Psychotherapy, 26*, 331–347.

Muehlenkamp, J. J., Walsh, B. W., & McDade, M. (2010). Preventing non-suicidal self-injury in adolescents: The Signs of Self-Injury Program. *Journal of Youth and Adolescence, 39*, 306–314.

National Research Council. (2009). *Preventing mental, emotional, and behavioral disorders among young people: Progress and possibilities*. Washington, DC: The National Academies Press.

Nixon, M. K., & Heath, N. L. (Eds.). (2009). *Self-injury in youth: The essential guide to assessment and intervention*. New York, NY: Routledge, Taylor & Francis Group.

Nock, M. K. (Ed.). (2009). *Understanding nonsuicidal self-injury: Origins, assessment, and treatment*. Washington, DC: American Psychological Association.

Nock, M. K., & Favazza, A. R. (2009). Nonsuicidal self-injury: Definition and classification. In M. K. Nock (Ed.), *Understanding nonsuicidal self-injury* (pp. 9–18). Washington, DC: American Psychological Association.

Nock, M. K., Joiner, T. E., Jr., Gordon, K. H., Lloyd-Richardson, E. E., & Prinstein, M. J. (2006). Non-suicidal self-injury among adolescents: Diagnostic correlates and relation to suicide attempts. *Psychiatry Research, 144*, 65–72.

Nock, M. K., & Prinstein, M. J. (2004). A functional approach to the assessment of self-mutilative behavior. *Journal of Consulting and Clinical Psychology, 72*, 885–890.

O'Carroll, P. W., & Potter, L. B. (1994). Suicide contagion and the reporting of suicide: Recommendations from a national workshop. United States Department of Health and Human Services. *Morbidity and Mortality Weekly Report – Recommendations and Reports, 43*(RR-6), 9–17.

Piran, N. (1999). Eating disorders: A trial of prevention in a high risk school setting. *Journal of Primary Prevention, 20*, 75–90.

Piran, N. (2001). Re-inhabiting the body from the inside out: Girls transform their school environment. In D. L. Tolman & M. Brydon-Miller (Eds.), *From subjects to subjectivities: A handbook of interpretative and participatory methods* (pp. 218–238). New York, NY: New York University Press.

Piran, N. (2010). A feminist perspective on risk factor research and on the prevention of eating disorders. *Eating Disorders: The Journal of Treatment & Prevention, 18*, 183–198.

Piran, N., & Teall, T. (2012). The developmental theory of embodiment. In G. McVey, M. P. Levine, N. Piran, & H. B. Ferguson (Eds.), *Preventing eating-related and weight-related disorders: Collaborative research, advocacy, and policy change* (pp. 169–198). Waterloo, OH: Wilfred Laurier Press.

Ranby, K. W., Aiken, L. S., Mackinnon, D. P., Elliot, D. L., Moe, E. L., McGinnis, W., & Goldberg, L. (2009). A mediation analysis of the ATHENA intervention for female athletes: Prevention of athletic-enhancing substance use and unhealthy weight loss behaviors. *Journal of Pediatric Psychology, 34*, 1069–1083.

Ross, S., Heath, N. L., & Toste, J. R. (2009). Non-suicidal self-injury and eating pathology in high school students. *American Journal of Orthopsychiatry, 79*, 83–92.

Smolak, L. (2012). Risk and protective factors in body image problems. In G. L. McVey, M. P. Levine, N. Piran, & H. B. Ferguson (Eds.), *Preventing eating-related and weight-related disorders: Collaborative research, advocacy, and policy change* (pp. 147–167). Waterloo, ON: Wilfred Laurier University Press.

Smolak, L., & Levine, M. P. (1996). Developmental transitions at middle school and college. In L. Smolak, M. P. Levine, & R. H. Striegel-Moore (Eds.), *The developmental psychopathology of eating disorders: Implications for research, prevention, and treatment* (pp. 207–233). Hillsdale, NJ: Erlbaum.

Steiner-Adair, C., Sjostrom, L., Franko, D. L., Pai, S., Tucker, R., Becker, A. E., & Herzog, D. B. (2002). Primary prevention of eating disorders in adolescent girls: Learning from practice. *International Journal of Eating Disorders, 32*, 401–411.

Stice, E. (2002). Risk and maintenance factors for eating pathology: A meta-analytic review. *Psychological Bulletin, 128*, 825–848.

Stice, E., Rohde, P., & Shaw, H. (2013). *The body project: A dissonance-based eating disorder prevention intervention* (updated edition) – *Facilitator Guide*. New York, NY: Oxford University Press.

Stice, E., Rohde, P., Shaw, H., & Gau, J. (2011). An effectiveness trial of a selected dissonance-based eating disorder prevention program for female high school students: Long-term effects. *Journal of Consulting and Clinical Psychology, 79*, 500–508.

Stice, E., Shaw, H., & Marti, C. N. (2007). A meta-analytic review of eating disorder prevention programs: Encouraging findings. *Annual Review of Clinical Psychology, 3*, 207–231.

Svirko, E., & Hawton, K. (2007). Self-injurious behavior and eating disorders: The extent and nature of the association. *Suicide and Life-Threatening Behavior, 37*, 409–421.

Tobler, N. S., Roona, M. R., Ochshorn, P., Marshall, D. G., Streke, A. V., & Stackpole, K. M. (2000). School-based adolescent prevention programs: 1998 meta-analysis. *Journal of Primary Prevention, 20*, 275–336.

Tompkins, T. L., Witt, J., & Abraibesh, N. (2010). Does a gatekeeper suicide prevention program work in a school setting? Evaluating training outcome and moderators of effectiveness. *Suicide and Life-Threatening Behavior, 40*, 506–515.

Trepal, H. C., Wester, K. L., & MacDonald, C. A. (2006). Self-injury and postvention: Responding to the family in crisis. *The Family Journal, 14*, 342–348.

Vale, H., Nixon, M. K., & Kucharski, A. (2009). Working with families and adolescents with NSSI. In M. K. Nixon (Ed.), *Self-injury in youth: The essential guide to assessment and intervention* (pp. 237–256). New York, NY: Routledge.

Van Voorhees, B. W., Fogel, J., Reinecke, M. A., Gladstone, T., Stuart, S., Gollan, J., & Bell, C. (2009). Randomized clinical trial of an Internet-based depression prevention program for adolescents (Project CATCH-IT) in primary care: 12-week outcomes. *Journal of Developmental and Behavioral Pediatrics, 30*, 23–37.

Whitlock, J., & Knox, K. L. (2009). Intervention and prevention in the community. In M. K. Nixon & N. L. Heath (Eds.), *Self-injury in youth: The essential guide to assessment and intervention* (pp. 173–194). New York, NY: Routledge.

Wyman, P. A., Brown, C. H., LoMurray, M., Schmeelk-Cone, K., Petrova, M., Yu, Q., & Wang, W. (2010). An outcome evaluation of the Sources of Strength suicide prevention program delivered by adolescent peer leaders in high schools. *American Journal of Public Health, 100*, 1653–1661.

18 Eating Disorders and Non-suicidal Self-Injury: From Primary Care to Inpatient Hospitalization

Jason J. Washburn, Denise M. Styer, Michelle Gebhardt, and Delia Aldridge

Abstract

Eating disorders (ED) and non-suicidal self-injury (NSSI) are serious, impairing, and potentially life-threatening conditions that typically require care across the continuum, from primary care to inpatient care. Primary care practitioners (PCPs) are critical to the treatment of ED and NSSI, playing important roles in identification and assessment. Numerous tools have been developed to facilitate PCPs' involvement in the continuum of care for ED. Although similar tools have not been fully developed or evaluated for NSSI, promising practices are available for PCPs to address NSSI. Recommendations are also available for determining the best level of care for ED and NSSI, including when to refer for inpatient treatment. Inpatient treatment for ED and NSSI is a critical part of the continuum of care for these conditions, especially in establishing safety, stabilizing symptoms, and beginning the process of recovery. Increased attention by researchers and providers to the role of PCPs and inpatient levels of care in the continuum of care for ED and NSSI will go far to improving our treatment of these complex conditions.

18.1 Introduction

Eating disorders and non-suicidal self-injury (NSSI) are serious, impairing, and potentially life-threatening conditions (Nock, 2010; Stice, Marti, & Rohde, 2012). People who suffer from eating disorders (ED) experience some of the highest rates of mortality of any psychiatric disorders (Arcelus, Mitchell, Wales, & Nielsen, 2011), and NSSI is recognized as a strong predictor of future suicide attempts (Asarnow et al., 2011; Klonsky, May, & Glenn, 2013; Whitlock et al., 2013). It is

J.J. Washburn (✉) • D.M. Styer • M. Gebhardt • D. Aldridge
Alexian Brothers Behavioral Health Hospital, Center for Evidence-Based Practice, 1650 Moon Lake Blvd., Hoffman Estates, IL 60169, USA
e-mail: jason.washburn@alexian.net

L. Claes and J.J. Muehlenkamp (eds.), *Non-Suicidal Self-Injury in Eating Disorders*, DOI 10.1007/978-3-642-40107-7_18, © Springer-Verlag Berlin Heidelberg 2014

critical that people who are at risk for either or both of these conditions be identified and treated as early as possible to prevent the potentially lethal progression of these disorders. Although many individuals with eating disorders and NSSI will be assessed and treated for their conditions by a mental health specialist (e.g., psychologist, psychiatrist, clinical social worker, psychiatric nurse), a good number of people will be missed and only come into contact with treatment providers when their conditions worsen and emergency care is required (Hart, Granillo, Jorm, & Paxton, 2011; Whitlock, Eckenrode, & Silverman, 2006).

In health systems with increasingly limited resources, it is critical that general practitioners know for whom treatment is or is not necessary. An estimated 25 % of college students who self-injure have only done so once in their lifetime (Whitlock et al., 2006) and are unlikely to need treatment. Further, abnormal eating behavior fluctuates over time and may not develop into an eating disorder (Steinhausen, Gavez, & Winkler Metzke, 2005). Unfortunately, the mental health specialists who are most skilled in determining who does and does not require treatment are often least likely to be in a position to identify these conditions at an early stage. Mental health specialists do not seek out people with ED or NSSI, relying instead on referrals from people who are not mental health specialists, such as primary care practitioners (PCPs) (Nicholls & Yi, 2012).

Mental disorders are increasingly identified and treated at the primary care level (Berger-Jenkins, Mccord, Gallagher, & Olfson, 2012; Cappelli et al., 2012; Nutting et al., 2005) so much so that primary care is often considered the de facto mental health system (Gray & Brody, 2005). As PCPs carry a greater burden in the treatment of common mental disorders, such as depression and anxiety, they become less likely to refer to mental health specialists for any condition (Faghri, Boisvert, & Faghri, 2010). This is concerning as PCPs have limited training in identifying complicated conditions such as ED and NSSI and may miss opportunities to identify and interrupt their progression (Bryant-Waugh, Lask, Shafran, & Fosson, 1992; Walsh, Wheat, & Freund, 2000).

This chapter focuses on the role of PCPs in the treatment of ED and NSSI. Practical guidance is provided for PCPs to identify and assess the severity of ED and NSSI, as well as determine the best level of care for someone with these complex conditions. Because PCPs are often in the position of determining if and when to refer a patient with ED or NSSI to inpatient treatment, we end with a discussion of this most costly level of care.

18.2 The Role of Primary Care in the Treatment of ED and NSSI

18.2.1 Initial Identification

PCPs, including physicians (i.e., family practice, internal medicine, pediatric, OB/GYNs), nurses, nurse practitioners, and physician assistants, are critical to the treatment of ED and NSSI because of their role in the initial identification of the problem behavior. PCPs have a unique relationship with their patients that make them particularly well positioned to identify ED and NSSI symptoms that are emerging or have previously gone unnoticed.

PCPs have several advantages over other providers in the initial detection of ED and NSSI. First, PCPs are the provider most people go to when experiencing any health-related problem (Faghri et al., 2010). For some insurance plans, PCPs act as a gatekeeper, with all care originating from and coordinated by the PCP (Forrest, 2003). Given that ED and NSSI are likely to be associated with increased somatic complaints and associated medical complications (e.g., wound care and infection, respiratory acidosis, tooth enamel erosion), it is likely that they will have contact with PCPs at early stages in the progression of their conditions (Lask et al., 2005). Further, people with ED and NSSI may come into contact with their PCPs through routine check-ups or acute care appointments, providing yet another opportunity for identification of ED and NSSI. Second, PCPs are likely to have a unique relationship with their patients that facilitates disclosure of the ED and NSSI behavior (Robinson & Roter, 1999). The trust patients place in their PCPs may make them more likely to disclose personal information that they may not disclose to others (Chen, 2008). Third, PCPs tend to interact with people during periods of distress in which they may be more inclined to disclose ED or NSSI. Finally, PCPs have unique access to the patient's body, which can be critical for identification of ED and NSSI symptoms. Through routine physical exams, PCPs can view parts of the body that may be kept hidden or obscured from family members, friends, and other professionals (Murray, Warm, & Fox, 2005; Trautmann, Worthy, & Lokken, 2007). Because physical examinations often entail a systematic checking of the body, usually from head to toe, it can be difficult for someone to conceal evidence of self-injury during such an exam.

In order to identify ED and NSSI, it is important for PCPs to be cognizant of the signs and symptoms of these conditions. Fortunately, much has been written about how to identify ED in the primary care context (Sim et al., 2010; Williams, Goodie, & Motsinger, 2008). Anorexia nervosa can be quickly identified through assessment of weight that is below ideal body weight (i.e., 85 %). In contrast, there is often not an obvious physical sign for other eating disorders, such as bulimia nervosa, binge eating disorder, or eating disorder not otherwise specified. As such, the American Academic of Pediatrics (Rosen, 2010) recommends PCPs to consider several findings on a physical exam as red flags for ED, such as sinus bradycardia and other cardiac arrhythmias or murmurs, orthostatic changes in pulse or blood pressure, hypothermia, cachexia, thinning or dry hair, sialadenitis, angular stomatitis, palatal scratches, oral ulcerations, dental anomalies (e.g., enamel erosion), dry, sallow skin, lanugo, signs of excessive exercise, delayed or interrupted pubertal developmental, and atrophic breasts and/or vaginitis.

In contrast to ED, very little has been published about the signs and symptoms of NSSI. Fortunately, NSSI can often be identified through a physical exam when wounds and scars are present or when injuries are a presenting problem (e.g., wounds requiring suturing, infected wounds, surgery for foreign body removal, broken bones). Wounds or scars can come from numerous different forms of self-injury, such as cuts, skin carving, severe scratching, bruises from head banging or punching, and burns. The following features of wounds or scars should raise concern about NSSI (Walsh, 2006; Whitlock, 2009): (1) numerous unexplained wounds or scars; (2) presenting for wound care on multiple occasions; (3) wounds or scars that are in various stages of healing; (4) wounds that are reopened or agitated; (5) wounds or scars within easy reach of the patient's dominate hand; (6) wounds or scares that are grouped or clustered together; and (7) wounds or scars that are linear, slightly curved, or otherwise patterned (e.g., similar shape and size, parallel, crisscross, symmetrical).

Wounds or scars, however, may not always be evident or available for exam by the PCP. Consequently, it is important for the PCP to also be aware of other signs or symptoms that may indicate NSSI, such as:

- Seeking treatment for numerous "accidents," especially when the explanation about the accident does not make sense or is unbelievable or the explanation is given too nonchalantly (e.g., "clumsy" or "accident prone").
- Becoming uncomfortable when talking about how a wound occurred or refusing to share what happened.
- Soft-tissue wounds in which an object is embedded in such a way that it does not appear accidental (Bennett, Shiels, Young, Lofthouse, & Mihalov, 2011).
- Refusing a physical examination or hiding or covering parts of the body.
- Refusing to wear a bathing suit or seeking a physician's excuse not to wear specific clothing or participate in sports.

PCPs should be careful to not jump to conclusions with regard to the above signs and symptoms for ED and NSSI. For example, some of these signs and symptoms for ED and NSSI are also signs and symptoms for physical or sexual abuse, and it may be prudent to inquire directly about abuse. While there may be numerous reasons behind these signs and symptoms, it is generally safe to assume that there is a larger problem of some kind when these signs and symptoms are present.

When a patient does not provide a reasonable explanation for these signs or symptoms or appears evasive, we recommend that PCPs directly inquire about ED and NSSI. If ED or NSSI is suspected, screening instruments can be helpful in determining if there is a need for a specialty care referral. For ED, numerous screening instruments are available, and some have been developed specifically for the PCP context. The SCOFF questionnaire is composed of the following five questions that are easy to remember, quick to administer, and simple to score (Hill, Reid, Morgan, & Lacey, 2010; Morgan, Reid, & Lacey, 1999): Do you make yourself Sick because you feel uncomfortably full? Do you worry you have lost Control over how much you eat? Have you recently lost more than One stone (14lbs) in a 3-month period? Do you believe yourself to be Fat when others say you are too thin? Would you say that Food dominates your life? An initial validation study found that an answer of "Yes" on two or more of the SCOFF questions was 100 % sensitive in identifying anorexia and bulimia nervosa, with only 12 % false positive rate (Morgan et al., 1999).

Because of concerns that the SCOFF is not as sensitive or selective as initially reported, the Eating disorder Screen for Primary care (ESP) was developed (Cotton, Ball, & Robinson, 2003). The ESP was found to have 100 % sensitivity in primary care settings when two or more of the following questions were answered abnormally: Are you satisfied with your eating patterns? Do you ever eat in secret? Does your weight affect the way you feel about yourself? Have any members of your family suffered with an eating disorder? Do you currently suffer with or have you ever suffered in the past with an eating disorder?

For NSSI, no screeners have been specifically designed and evaluated for PCPs. Although many assessments have been developed for NSSI (Klonsky & Weinberg, 2009), none of the available assessments are especially relevant or practical for the PCP; they either provide irrelevant information for a PCP (e.g., functions of NSSI) or do not provide the information necessary to make an appropriate referral. Drs. Patrick Kerr, Jennifer Muehlenkamp, and James Turner proposed a useful strategy to assess risk for NSSI in family medicine practice: the STOPS-FIRE guide (Kerr, Muehlenkamp, & Turner, 2010). The STOPS-FIRE guide involves an assessment of the following factors related to NSSI: Suicidal ideations, Number of Types of self-injury methods, Onset of self-injury, Place or location of the self-injury, Severity of tissue damage due to self-injury, Functions of self-injury, Intensity of the urge to self-injury, Repetition of self-injury, and Episodic frequency of self-injury in a given day.

Although the STOPS-FIRE guide is an excellent, *comprehensive* guide for NSSI risk, PCPs may not have the time to address all nine domains with the 20 min available in a typical office visit (Abbo, Zhang, Zelder, & Huang, 2008). Consequently, we recommend that PCPs use the following four probes to directly identify NSSI: "I notice that you have some wounds and scars..." (1) Can you tell me where these came from? (2) It looks like you are hurting yourself; can you tell me how you hurt yourself? (3) How often do you hurt yourself? (4) Where else do you have wounds or scars? These probes assume that self-injury is a likely cause of any suspect wounds and scars. Anecdotally, we find that this approach results in greater self-disclosure. It is critical, however, that PCPs use these probes in a nonjudgmental, matter-of-fact manner, just as they would with any other health risk. These probes can too easily come across as judgmental or shaming if delivered with the wrong tone or body language. Even though ED and NSSI behavior can be perplexing, seem illogical, or instill strong emotional reactions, PCPs must remember that the patient is suffering and needs someone who will acknowledge their pain and care for them. As such, the goal is not to "catch" a patient in a lie or to force them to acknowledge their ED or NSSI behavior, but instead to encourage a patient to seek help for these difficult and complex conditions.

18.2.2 Assessing Severity

Once ED or NSSI is identified, it is critical for the PCP to assess for severity. Although PCPs may be tempted to immediately refer away a patient once ED or NSSI is identified, an immediate referral may not always be appropriate, could be ill advised, and may be difficult to obtain (Trude & Stoddard, 2003). Indeed, immediate referrals may not actually be "immediate" given that access to mental health specialists, especially psychiatrists, is often limited (Merritt Hawkins, 2012). A recent study of 230 outpatient psychiatrists found that only 3 % offered immediate appointments, with wait times ranging from 4 to 55 days (Goldner, Jones, & Fang, 2011). Without conducting a brief assessment of severity, a PCP may put a patient on a waitlist for specialty mental health services when risk for serious injury or death is imminent. General emergency departments may also not be appropriate for referral because the average weight time for psychiatric complaints in the emergency room is 11.5 h (Weiss et al., 2012). As such, we recommend that PCPs, at a minimum, assess for suicidal risk before allowing a patient with ED or NSSI symptoms to leave their offices.

There are many ways to assess for suicide risk, but it is best for PCPs to directly ask about suicide, especially given that spontaneous disclosure of suicide risk is uncommon (Nutting et al., 2005). Probing or assessing about suicide is best achieved when it is integrated into the larger conversation. Framing suicide questions by relating them to issues already under discussion can be especially helpful in normalizing the questions (Vannoy et al., 2010). When already discussing ED and NSSI symptoms, framing can be accomplished easily (e.g., "has your ED/NSSI become so difficult to manage that you have thought about killing yourself?").

When assessing suicide risk, PCPs should use a stepwise approach (Mcdowell, Lineberry, & Bostwick, 2011) that assesses hopelessness, thoughts of death and suicide, history of suicide attempts, the presence of a plan, and, if present, the lethality of the plan, means to implement the plan, and intent to implement the plan. The American Psychiatric Association's (APA) *Practice Guideline for the Assessment and Treatment of Patients With Suicidal Behaviors* (http://focus.psychiatryonline.org/content.aspx?bookid=28§ionid=1663420) provides examples of questions that can be asked to obtain this information. The SAFE-T risk categorization scheme can also be used to categorize risk for suicide once the above information has been obtained (http://store.samhsa.gov/shin/content//SMA09-4432/SMA09-4432.pdf). PCPs may also benefit from using the Risk Assessment version of the Columbia Suicide Severity Rating Scale (http://www.cssrs.columbia.edu/) to structure their final determination of risk and/or the self-report version of this scale to supplement their probes.

When PCPs are unable to immediately refer a patient with identified ED or NSSI for assessment by a mental health specialist, it is necessary to obtain more detailed information to determine the best level of care for referral. For ED, numerous articles and guides have been published on how to assess ED severity in primary care (Kondo & Sokol, 2006; Sim et al., 2010; Williams et al., 2008). We believe, at a minimum, it is necessary for PCPs to assess the following factors when determining an appropriate level of care referral for ED: the patient's weight (including proportion of ideal body weight and recent patterns of weight loss or gain), the medical stability of the patient, and the extent of food restriction, exercise, and purging behavior. Although a physical exam and labs will provide necessary data about body weight and medical stability (e.g., heart rate, blood pressure, temperature, glucose, potassium, electrolytes, hydration, organ compromise, diabetes risk, and management), information on ED can be obtained either through probes or through interview or self-report measures, such as the Eating Disorder Examination Questionnaire (Cooper, Cooper, & Fairburn, 1989).

As with initial identification, much less guidance is available about the assessment of severity of NSSI in the primary care context. Although numerous assessments of NSSI are available (Klonsky & Weinberg, 2009), they were created for research, are limited to specific aspects of NSSI (e.g., functions for NSSI), or are too lengthy for PCPs. As such, we recommend that PCPs focus on obtaining the information necessary to determine the best level of care referral, such as risk for suicide, frequency and severity of self-injury, and degree of urge to self-injure. To determine the severity of self-injury, there are several preexisting, albeit complex ways to assess wound severity (e.g., Injury Severity Score, Abbreviated Injury Scale, New Injury Severity Score, Anatomic Profile, Modified Injury Severity Scale). To facilitate an efficient assessment of wound severity, we recommend the following parsimonious guide:

- *Minimal Severity*: The wound doesn't require medical attention beyond basic wound care (e.g., cleansing and bandaging).
- *Moderate Severity*: The wound is infected, opened, or has been reinjured.
- *High Severity*: The wound requires major medical attention (e.g., sutures, staples, surgery, etc...), the wound is on the face, neck, breasts, or genitals, or the self-injury involves swallowing objects or embedding objects in the body.

18.2.3 Referring to Specialized Mental Health Treatment

Assessment of severity of ED and NSSI is necessary for determining the best level of care for which a PCP will refer a specific patient. Determining the exact level of care can be challenging for PCPs. Although there is often disagreement about what criteria should determine what level of care (Olmsted et al., 2010), the APA has been clear about what criteria qualifies someone with an eating disorder for a specific level of care (see: Table 8, Level of Care Guidelines for Patients with Eating Disorders, http://psychiatryonline.org/content.aspx?bookid=28§ionid=1671334). The APA discusses five levels of care: weekly or monthly outpatient treatment, intensive outpatient treatment (generally 4 h per day), partial hospitalization or full-day outpatient treatment, residential treatment, and inpatient hospitalization. The appropriate level of care for someone with an ED is determined by evaluating a range of criteria, specifically medical stability, suicidal behavior, weight as percentage of healthy body weight, motivation to recover (cooperativeness, insight, ability to control obsessions), co-occurring disorders, level of structure needed for eating and weight gain, ability to control compulsive exercise, purging behavior or use of laxatives and diuretics, environmental stress, and geographic availability of the treatment programs (American Psychiatric Association, 2006).

Unfortunately, a similar level of care guideline is not available for NSSI. Given the lack of clear guidelines for determining level of care for NSSI, we created the Alexian Brothers Levels of Care Criteria (ABLCC) to assist treatment providers, including those with little to no experience with NSSI, in making appropriate level of care decisions. The ABLCC reflects over 10 years of clinical experience with thousands of patients evaluated for our Self-Injury Recovery Services treatment programs. The ABLCC is based on the APA level of care criteria developed for the treatment of Eating Disorders, providing criteria for the five levels of care described above, as well as a version with only inpatient, residential and outpatient levels of care (available from first authors by request). The following factors are included in the ABLCC to assist with determining the appropriate level of care for individuals with NSSI: suicide risk, features of NSSI (frequency and severity, urge to self-injure), motivation to change, cooperation with treatment providers and agreement with the treatment plan, functional impairment, environmental support, and treatment availability. We've found that these factors, when considered together in a matrix similar to the grid proposed by APA for eating disorders, are helpful in guiding decisions about the least restrictive necessary level of care for NSSI. By isolating where an individual with NSSI falls on this matrix of factors, the clinician can determine which of the five levels of care are necessary for a specific individual.

An important caveat when referring to an outpatient level of care for ED and NSSI is that referrals should be made to licensed clinicians who provide psychotherapy (e.g., clinical psychologist, clinical social worker, master's level licensed therapist) as well as to a psychiatrist or psychiatric nurse practitioner. Although psychotherapy may only be required for mild cases of ED or NSSI, in our experience, medication evaluation and management are typically necessary for moderate to severe cases of ED or NSSI. Ideally, referrals should be made to clinicians who specialize in these conditions. We recognize, however, that specialists in ED and NSSI are limited, and therefore PCPs should seek out clinicians who are willing to learn how to best treat patients with these conditions.

18.2.4 Brief Interventions

It is important to acknowledge that referrals may not be sufficient for a patient with ED or NSSI. These are complex conditions that involve dangerous behaviors that the patient may be less than willing to change. As such, PCPs should consider learning brief interventions for behavioral change. Brief interventions, sometimes referred to as "brief advice," are physician-led interventions designed to help reduce harm associated with a behavioral or mental health problem in their patients and to increase motivation to address the problem. Brief interventions were developed initially to address alcohol abuse among patients in a primary care setting and have been shown to be effective at reducing alcohol use as well as alcohol-related problems, such as accidents and mortality (Bertholet, Daeppen, Wietlisbach, Fleming, & Burnand, 2005; Cuijpers, Riper, & Lemmers, 2004).

Brief interventions are based on physician-advice and motivational interviewing models (Miller & Rollnick, 1991) and integrate psychoeducation and cognitive-behavioral strategies. Brief interventions involve brief (15 min) one-to-one counseling from 1 to 4 sessions in which the PCP focuses on motivating the patient for change using psychoeducation and nonjudgmental and empathic weighing of the facts. Although brief interventions have not been evaluated specifically for self-injury, physicians can easily modify the brief intervention approach developed for alcohol abuse. Michael Fleming's brief intervention for alcohol abuse (Fleming & Manwell, 1999) provides verbal scripts that physicians can modify to conduct the four steps involved in the brief intervention: Direct Feedback, Negotiation and Goal Setting, Commitment to Behavior Change, and Follow-up and Reinforcement.

18.2.5 Ongoing Involvement in Treatment

After a referral is made and specialty treatment begins, PCPs should remain involved with the patient. It is critical for the PCP to determine if a patient followed through with a referral for specialty mental health treatment. We recommend that PCPs contact patients within 1 week of making a referral. A quick check-in over the phone can motivate the patient to follow through with the referral and address any barriers with the referral. We also recommend that PCPs schedule an initial monthly follow-up with a patient after the start of specialty mental health treatment. This initial follow-up appointment serves three purposes. First, it demonstrates to the patient that the PCP is taking their ED and NSSI seriously and that the PCP cares about their health and safety. Second, it allows the PCP to double-check that the patient has followed through with specialty mental health treatment and that the specialty care is appropriate and acceptable to the patient and provides an opportunity to obtain any necessary consents for release of information with the specialty provider. Finally, it provides an opportunity for the PCP to monitor weight, exam previously identified wounds, and/or to identify any new health concerns or wounds through a body check. The body check should be introduced not as a means of "catching" additional ED or NSSI behaviors, but as a means of making sure that any additional health problems or injuries are appropriately treated to maintain safety.

After the initial monthly follow-up appointment, the PCP should continue to monitor the patient's physical health (e.g., body weight, wound/injury status) until symptoms have sufficiently improved. The frequency of the visits will depend on severity and progress in mental health treatment. Some patients may only need occasional appointments throughout a year, whereas other patients may need monthly check-ups. We recommend that PCPs work directly with the mental health provider to determine how frequent the patient should have a PCP appointment.

18.3 The Role of Emergency Department Practitioner in the Treatment of ED and NSSI

PCPs provide an excellent opportunity to identify and intervene with ED and NSSI because in theory they see the general population; in reality, however, a large minority of people does not use their PCP for their healthcare needs. There has been a substantial shift in where people seek care for new concerns from primary care and to the emergency department (Pitts, Carrier, Rich, & Kellermann, 2010), and barriers to receiving timely care from a PCP, especially financial or insurance-based barriers, may motivate some people to seek nonurgent care in the emergency department (Cheung, Wiler, Lowe, & Ginde, 2012). Further, people with ED and NSSI may be more likely to use the emergency department due to the urgent health needs often associated with these conditions (Dooley-Hash, Lipson, Walton, & Cunningham, 2012). As such, the Emergency Department Practitioner (EDP) is often in a similar role of the PCPs when it comes to identifying and addressing ED and NSSI symptoms.

When treating or evaluating people with ED or NSSI, EDPs must be cognizant of the fact that the emergency department is an open environment, often with only a thin curtain separating the patient from other providers or patients. Patients with ED and NSSI often feel shame and embarrassment about their conditions, and EDPs must demonstrate sensitivity by speaking quietly when inquiring about ED or NSSI. EDPs also should be careful about how they talk to other professionals about patients with ED or NSSI. Many of our patients have reported that they have felt disrespected, belittled, or shamed when they overheard comments from EDPs, such as “We have a cutter in room 6” or “Someone’s starving themselves again.” For NSSI specifically, it is also important for EDPs to recognize that even though a patient may self-injure to feel pain, people that self-injure should receive the same care as any other patient, including the provision of analgesics for painful procedures.

18.4 The Role of the Inpatient Unit in the Treatment of ED and NSSI

PCPs often struggle with determining if a patient with ED or NSSI requires inpatient care. Although there is a growing body of literature for the outpatient treatment of ED and NSSI, relatively little information is available for treatment at the inpatient level of care, especially for NSSI. Despite the little information available for inpatient treatment for ED and NSSI, it is likely that PCPs will at some point need to refer a patient to this most acute level of care (Olmsted et al., 2010).

18.4.1 Goals of Inpatient Treatment

Inpatient treatment is an intensive, restrictive, and costly form of a treatment; as such, it is extremely time limited and should be reserved for only those individuals who cannot be successfully or safely treated in other contexts (American Psychiatric Association, 2003). As such, the ultimate goal of inpatient treatment is to treat or manage symptoms to a point that it is safe and effective to transfer to a less intensive level of care. Although the ultimate goal of any treatment for ED and NSSI is to desist from pathological behaviors and to restore psychological, emotional, and physical health, these are not realistic goals for inpatient treatment. It is counter-productive for people that self-injure and their families and providers to expect that inpatient treatment will achieve these goals independently. Instead, the goals of inpatient treatment for ED and NSSI should include establishing and maintaining safety, stabilizing symptoms, and beginning the process of recovery from ED and NSSI.

18.4.2 Establishing and Maintaining Safety

Inpatient treatment is typically reserved for when risk to life, either the patients or another's life, is the paramount concern. As such, establishing and maintaining safety is the primary concern for all inpatient psychiatric treatments (Kanerva, Lammintakanen, & Kivinen, 2013). In contrast to other disorders, an *enhanced* environment of safety is necessary for inpatient treatment of individuals with ED and NSSI. Because ED and NSSI can be easily engaged in during an inpatient visit, we recommend that ED and NSSI be *continuously* monitored by inpatient professionals. We recommend that patients with ED and NSSI be discouraged from being alone in their rooms, be visible at all times when in the therapeutic milieu of the inpatient unit, and that observation be enhanced during times of rest or sleep in their rooms. Enhanced observation should include at least 15-min checks when sleeping or otherwise alone. Although 15-min checks are unlikely to be helpful in preventing suicide (Jayaram, Sporney, & Perticone, 2010), we have found them be helpful in preventing ED behavior (e.g., purging, exercise) and low-lethality NSSI. For patients at high risk for suicide, significant underweight or malnutrition, or high risk for potentially lethal NSSI (e.g., drawing blood, embedding or swallowing objects, injuries focused on the head, genitals, or internal organs), we recommend continuous (24/7) observation.

It is also important to enhance standard belongings searches and body checks for patients with NSSI. Body checks allow for documentation of scars, identification of current wounds, and an evaluation of risk for infection and/or more severe damage or harm that requires medical intervention. Belongings searches must be done carefully to make certain that the patient not only is precluded from bringing anything that could be used for a suicide attempt (standard inpatient protocol) but also anything that could be used for self-injury by anyone on the unit.

In addition to securing inpatients' belongings, inpatient professionals must evaluate the objects they use every day on the unit. These everyday objects, such as paperclips, erasers, pens/pencils, staples, bottles, mirrors, CDs/DVDs, may be repurposed as low-lethality self-injury tools. Although it is possible to restrict easy access to specific types of objects that contain metal, glass, or potentially breakable hard plastic, it is not possible to remove all potential self-injury tools from a unit (indeed, patients will always have access to their finger nails and teeth). It is tempting for inpatient professionals to have a "zero tolerance" policy around ED and NSSI behavior; however, this will likely result in an increase in physical interventions (e.g., holds, restraints, seclusion rooms) for nonlethal behavior. Further, for some patients with NSSI, the act of self-injuring can prevent or reduce suicidal urges. As such, we strongly recommend only physically intervening in ED or NSSI behavior when it is imminently life threatening and instead relying on therapeutic strategies to interrupt the ED or NSSI behavior. By using therapeutic strategies instead of physical interventions, patients can be provided with numerous opportunities to practice these strategies and reinforce the need to develop alternative affective or interpersonal skills.

18.4.3 Stabilizing Symptoms

After establishing and maintaining safety, the second priority of inpatient hospitalization treatment for ED and NSSI is stabilizing priority symptoms. Although individuals with ED and NSSI present with numerous potential treatment targets, symptoms that are most likely to keep a patient at the inpatient level of care should be considered priority symptoms. Common priority symptoms include suicidal behavior, substantial underweight (<85 % ideal body weight), pathological eating behaviors (dietary restraint, binging, and purging), and NSSI that is frequent and/or severe. Stabilization of these symptoms is best achieved through a combination of program structure and milieu (e.g., risk precautions), psychotherapeutic techniques (e.g., cognitive-behavioral therapy, dialectical behavior therapy), psychotropic medication, and other medical interventions (e.g., re-feeding protocols and structured eating).

For underweight patients, weight gain will always be the primary target symptom as weight gain is associated with improved short-term outcomes after discharge (Lund et al., 2009). It is critical to acknowledge, however, that the effectiveness of current re-feeding protocols are increasingly being questioned in the literature, especially given that weight gain is highly variable across patients (Hart, Abraham, Franklin, & Russell, 2010). There is growing evidence suggesting that standard re-feeding protocols, which are calorically conservative due to concerns with hypophosphatemia (re-feeding syndrome), should be more aggressive. Several recent studies have found that re-feeding protocols that start with higher calorie diets are associated with faster weight gain and shorter hospitalization (Garber, Michihata, Hetnal, Shafer, & Moscicki, 2012; Whitelaw, Gilbertson, Lam, & Sawyer, 2010). Although concern for hypophosphatemia remains with more aggressive re-feeding protocols, the condition may be more manageable and less of a threat than previously thought (Whitelaw et al., 2010). Weight gain, however, shouldn't be the only focus of treatment for underweight patients, as psychological and emotional improvements (e.g., distress, body image, coping skills) may also be necessary for long-term improvement of ED (Long, Fitzgerald, & Hollin, 2012).

For both ED and NSSI inpatients, the application of psychotherapeutic strategies should be provided with care, as some strategies may need to be modified for an inpatient environment. For example, ED and NSSI behaviors are often so engrained in individuals who make it to an inpatient level of care that they may not even be aware that they are engaging in the pathological behavior. In these instances, it is important to acknowledge that self-monitoring may not be successful, and inpatient professionals may be necessary to assist in developing awareness of ED and NSSI behavior and to provide external monitoring until self-monitoring skills develop. Further, inpatient professionals should be mindful of the cognitive demand required by certain strategies, especially for patients who are experiencing cognitive difficulties due to distress or underweight. For example, behavioral strategies may be more effective than more complex cognitive strategies for some patients. Although we believe that certain psychotherapeutic strategies must be adopted to fit individuals at the inpatient level of care, inpatient professionals should also be careful not to drift away from therapeutic techniques with demonstrated efficacy (Waller, Stringer, & Meyer, 2012).

The goal of these structural, pharmacologic, medical, and therapeutic interventions is to stabilize primary symptoms, not to fully treat these symptoms. For example, for many patients with NSSI, the goal may be to decrease the severity and/or frequency of injury to a degree that they can be transferred to a lower level of care, not to fully desist from self-injury. Indeed, it is not uncommon for a patient to transfer to a lower level of care even with strong urges to self-injure or engage in DE. In our experience, the urge to engage in ED or NSSI may actually be higher at the time of discharge than at the time of admission for some patients because they are actively avoiding the use of unhealthy albeit immediately effective forms of affective and behavioral regulation (i.e., ED or NSSI). At the inpatient level of care, stabilization of symptoms may be achieved when high-risk ED and NSSI behavioral patterns are interrupted and stopped from escalating, with outpatient treatment carrying on the goal of eventually desisting from these unhealthy behaviors.

Inpatient professionals must also be careful not to interpret dramatic changes on the inpatient unit as indicative of long-lasting change. Some patients will fully abstain from ED and NSSI behaviors almost immediately upon entry onto the unit. In our experience, this abstinence is always temporary and is often associated with clinical perfectionism (e.g., being the "perfect patient") or is an attempt to get discharged sooner. Although a brief respite from ED and NSSI behavior is often an excellent opportunity to build skills and develop new behavioral patterns, inpatient professionals often must work extra hard to help these patients develop the skills and strategies they need to succeed at a lower level of care (Phillips et al., 2010).

18.4.4 Beginning the Process of Recovery from ED and NSSI

We believe it is not enough to just stabilize individuals with ED and NSSI and move them to the next level of care. The inpatient level of care also provides an excellent opportunity to *begin* to address contributing emotional and psychological factors to ED and NSSI symptoms (Long et al., 2012). For example, because many individuals may not be fully motivated to change their ED or NSSI behavior (Wade, Frayne, Edwards, Robertson, & Gilchrist, 2009), inpatient professionals can begin to address cognitive, emotional, and behavioral factors that may improve long-term motivation and commitment to change (Kress & Hoffman, 2008). Although motivation enhancement as a single module or pretreatment may not be effective with these complex disorders (Allen et al., 2012), we can begin the process of continuously addressing motivation and commitment to behavior change at the inpatient level (Waller, 2012).

Another important preparatory role for inpatient professionals is to collaborate with the patient to develop a comprehensive case formulation (Hunter, Gardner, Wilkniss, & Silverstein, 2008). The inpatient environment provides an opportunity to gather rich clinical data that can be used to develop an understanding of changeable contributing and maintaining factors to ED and NSSI. The formulation then becomes a treatment roadmap for the patient after they leave the unit and proceed with lower levels of care. Several theoretical formulations are available to guide ED inpatient professionals in what are the most important factors to evaluate with their patients, such as the transdiagnostic cognitive-behavior formulation for ED (Fairburn et al., 2009) and the integrated theoretical model of NSSI (Nock & Cha, 2009).

Psychoeducation plays an important role in preparing inpatients for a lower level of care. As a general strategy, psychoeducation has been shown to improve knowledge (Mueser et al., 2002) and, as a more specific strategy, may be associated with improved outcomes (Storch, Keller, Weber, Spindler, & Milos, 2011; Wiseman, Sunday, Klapper, Klein, & Halmi, 2002). Psychoeducation is also necessary for both motivation (e.g., understanding consequences of ED and NSSI) and formulation (understanding factors that maintain ED and NSSI).

Engaging the family with inpatient treatment can be especially important for the treatment of ED and NSSI, especially given the complex family systems associated with these conditions (Di Pierro, Sarno, Perego, Gallucci, & Madeddu, 2012; Sim et al., 2009). Family involvement at the inpatient level of care has been shown to be helpful in addressing caregiver stress in group or individual formats (Whitney et al., 2012). Family involvement at the inpatient level of care should, at a minimum, involve psychoeducation about ED and NSSI, a discussion of expectations and goals for inpatient treatment, and how best to support their loved one through treatment. It is also important to involve the family in the implementation of safety plans after discharge from inpatient treatment (Stanley & Brown, 2012). When possible, inpatient professionals can also work with families to begin to address emotional and psychological contributions to ED and NSSI, such as identifying concerns with family communication, behavioral management, and structure (Godart et al., 2012).

Condition-specific interventions, some of which may have begun at the symptoms stabilization level, may also be built upon during the inpatient level of care to help patients get started on a path to recovery. For example, for ED, beginning to address body image and satisfaction, overvaluation of shape and weight, nutrition interventions, and clinical perfectionism may result in better overall outcomes (Danielsen & Ro, 2012; Grilo, White, Gueorguieva, Wilson, & Masheb, 2012; Halmi et al., 2000; Lock, Williams, Bamford, & Lacey, 2012; Vansteelandt, Pieters, Vanderlinden, & Probst, 2010). Much less is known empirically about NSSI-specific interventions that may help with treatment at lower levels of care. In our experience, however, it is important to help patients with NSSI to begin to address factors that contribute to and maintain their NSSI behavior (Nock & Cha, 2009), such as understanding the functions of NSSI (Klonsky, 2007), identifying triggers for NSSI, and developing alternative affect regulation skills (Storch et al., 2011).

18.4.5 Managing the Milieu and Social Contagion on the Inpatient Unit

Management of the clinical milieu is critical to successful treatment of ED and NSSI at the inpatient level of care. Indeed, the therapeutic milieu of an inpatient unit—and group treatment of any kind—introduces the potential for social learning and reinforcement of ED and NSSI behaviors, often referred to as social or peer contagion (Walsh & Doerfler, 2009). For example, in our experience, it is common for inpatients to report that they experience a strong urge to engage in ED or NSSI behavior when they either witness or hear about ED or NSSI behavior from another patient. We have found that even discussion of stressful events, expression of emotion, or interpersonal conflict within a group or milieu setting can create an urge to engage in ED or NSSI behaviors for some patients. Social contagion can also operate by decreasing motivation for changing ED or NSSI behavior by prompting permission-giving thoughts, such as "If she's doing it, why can't I?" Inpatients may also actively encourage each other to engage in ED or NSSI (Whitlock, Powers, & Eckenrode, 2006). A pernicious form of social contagion we have observed is the ED or NSSI "competition," in which patients attempt to "out do" each other, either through telling progressively more severe "war stories" about ED or NSSI experiences, by weight loss and dietary restriction contests, or by engaging in progressively more lethal NSSI. Finally, social contagion can also result in learning new ED and NSSI behaviors, either through observation and social learning, or by patients directly teaching each other (Whitlock, Powers, & Eckenrode, 2006).

It is important to note that the empirical literature on social or peer contagion with ED is lacking, with no clear systematic evidence (Vandereycken, 2011). There is some evidence that people will trade "tips" for ED behavior (Murray, 2002) and the multitude of Web sites that promote eating disorders suggest a clear vehicle by which social or peer contagion works over the internet (Jett, Laporte, & Wanchisn, 2010). Anecdotally, we have experienced ED patients engage in competitions on the inpatient unit, such as attempting to choose foods with the least caloric value, eating less food than another patient, seeing who can curl up smaller in their chair, and who can shake their leg faster or get out of their chair the most times in an attempt to burn calories.

Inpatient professionals must be aware of the risk for social contagion and actively work to mitigate the potential (Richardson, Surmitis, & Hyldahl, 2012). For example, we actively prevent the sharing of "war stories" or descriptions of specific ED or NSSI behaviors because these may trigger other patients or result in a competition. We also have patients cover wounds and scars by large bandages and clothing. We also do not allow patients with ED to know their weight. Through strictly enforced milieu or group rules, as well as redirecting or separating patients when necessary, social contagion can be actively managed on an inpatient unit to minimize triggering of or competition with ED and NSSI behavior.

18.4.6 The Efficacy of Inpatient Treatment

Most clinicians agree that the inpatient level of care is necessary and critical for those individuals whose ED and NSSI symptoms have escalated to a point that they are facing imminent and serious health risks (Gowers, 2012). Despite general agreement about the need for care at the inpatient level, few studies have specifically examined the efficacy of inpatient treatment (Lock, 2011) and no studies have evaluated inpatient treatment of NSSI. A few cohort studies of ED suggest some support for inpatient hospitalization (Collin, Power, Karatzias, Grierson, & Yellowlees, 2010) and partial hospitalization treatment (Ben-Porath, Wisniewski, & Warren, 2010; Willinge, Touyz, & Thornton, 2010), yet findings are mixed. For example, one study of 43 individuals with bulimia nervosa found that approximately one third evidenced complete remission, one third evidenced partial remission, and one third still met diagnostic criteria 3 years after inpatient or partial hospitalization treatment (Zeeck, Weber, Sandholz, Joos, & Hartmann, 2011). Another study of 57 adolescents with anorexia nervosa found that only 28 % remitted 1 year after discharge from an inpatient unit (Salbach-Andrae et al., 2009).

Determination of the efficacy of inpatient treatment depends on the outcomes being examined. If the goal of inpatient treatment is remission of ED or NSSI, there is limited support for inpatient versus outpatient treatment (Lock, 2011). We believe that inpatient treatment, however, is not intended as a stand-alone treatment for ED and NSSI, and the goals of inpatient treatment do not include remission of ED or NSSI. Inpatient treatment is only one point in a continuum of care and is designed to stabilize an individual with ED and NSSI so he or she can be treated at a lower level of care. Indeed, remission of ED and NSSI is likely to depend on the quality and continuity of the outpatient treatment that follows inpatient treatment, rather than inpatient treatment per se (Long et al., 2012). Determination of the efficacy of inpatient treatment must include an examination of outcomes that match the goals of inpatient treatment. For example, a meta-analysis of 2,273 individuals with anorexia nervosa found that weight gain is faster for inpatient than outpatient treatment (Hartmann, Weber, Herpertz, & Zeeck, 2011), supporting the inpatient goal of symptom stabilization for ED. More research, however, needs to examine appropriate outcomes for inpatient treatment before a determination can be made regarding the efficacy of this level of care within a continuum of treatment for ED and NSSI.

18.5 Summary

Eating disorders and NSSI are complex and challenging disorders that typically require participation of multiple providers in multiple contexts across the continuum of care. Primary care providers are critical partners in the identification and treatment of ED and NSSI, especially at the beginning stage of treatment, but also as people obtain specialty mental health treatments. More research is needed to understand how best to maximize the ability of PCPs to facilitate the identification and treatment of ED and NSSI. More research is also needed to better understand the role of inpatient care in the continuum of care for ED and NSSI and to maximize the benefits of this costly level of care.

References

Abbo, E. D., Zhang, Q., Zelder, M., & Huang, E. S. (2008). The increasing number of clinical items addressed during the time of adult primary care visits. *Journal of General Internal Medicine, 23*(12), 2058–2065. doi:10.1007/s11606-008-0805-8.

Allen, K. L., Fursland, A., Raykos, B., Steele, A., Watson, H., & Byrne, S. M. (2012). Motivation-focused treatment for eating disorders: A sequential trial of enhanced cognitive behaviour therapy with and without preceding motivation-focused therapy. *European Eating Disorders Review, 20*(3), 232–239. doi:10.1002/erv.1131.

American Psychiatric Association. (2003). Practice guideline for the assessment and treatment of patients with suicidal behaviors. *The American Journal of Psychiatry, 160*(11 Suppl), 1–60.

American Psychiatric Association. (2006). *Practice guidelines for the treatment of patients with eating disorders* (3rd ed.). Washington, DC: American Psychiatric Association.

Arcelus, J., Mitchell, A. J., Wales, J., & Nielsen, S. (2011). Mortality rates in patients with anorexia nervosa and other eating disorders. A meta-analysis of 36 studies. *Archives of General Psychiatry, 68*(7), 724–731. doi:10.1001/archgenpsychiatry.2011.74.

Asarnow, J. R., Porta, G., Spirito, A., Emslie, G., Clarke, G., Wagner, K. D., et al. (2011). Suicide attempts and nonsuicidal self-injury in the treatment of resistant depression in adolescents: Findings from the tordia study. *Journal of the American Academy of Child and Adolescent Psychiatry, 50*(8), 772–781.

Bennett, G. H., Shiels, W. E., 2nd, Young, A. S., Lofthouse, N., & Mihalov, L. (2011). Self-embedding behavior: A new primary care challenge. *Pediatrics, 127*(6), e1386–e1391. doi:10.1542/peds.2010-2877.

Ben-Porath, D. D., Wisniewski, L., & Warren, M. (2010). Outcomes of a day treatment program for eating disorders using clinical and statistical significance. *Journal of Contemporary Psychotherapy, 40*(2), 115–123.

Berger-Jenkins, E., Mccord, M., Gallagher, T., & Olfson, M. (2012). Effect of routine mental health screening in a low-resource pediatric primary care population. *Clinical Pediatrics, 51*(4), 359–365. doi:10.1177/0009922811427582.

Bertholet, N., Daeppen, J. B., Wietlisbach, V., Fleming, M., & Burnand, B. (2005). Reduction of alcohol consumption by brief alcohol intervention in primary care: Systematic review and meta-analysis. *Archives of Internal Medicine, 165*(9), 986–995. doi:10.1001/archinte.165.9.986.

Bryant-Waugh, R. J., Lask, B. D., Shafran, R. L., & Fosson, A. R. (1992). Do doctors recognise eating disorders in children? *Archives of Disease in Childhood, 67*(1), 103–105.

Cappelli, M., Gray, C., Zemek, R., Cloutier, P., Kennedy, A., Glennie, E., et al. (2012). The heads-Ed: A rapid mental health screening tool for pediatric patients in the emergency department. *Pediatrics, 130*(2), e321–e327. doi:10.1542/peds.2011-3798.

Chen, P. E. (2008). Do patients trust doctors too much? *The New York Times*. Retrieved from http://www.nytimes.com/2008/12/19/health/18chen.html

Cheung, P. T., Wiler, J. L., Lowe, R. A., & Ginde, A. A. (2012). National study of barriers to timely primary care and emergency department utilization among Medicaid beneficiaries. *Annals of Emergency Medicine, 60*(1), 4–10.e12. doi:10.1016/j.annemergmed.2012.01.035.

Collin, P., Power, K., Karatzias, T., Grierson, D., & Yellowlees, A. (2010). The effectiveness of, and predictors of response to, inpatient treatment of anorexia nervosa. *European Eating Disorders Review, 18*(6), 464–474. doi:10.1002/erv.1026.

Cooper, Z., Cooper, P. J., & Fairburn, C. G. (1989). The validity of the eating disorder examination and its subscales. *The British Journal of Psychiatry, 154*, 807–812.

Cotton, M. A., Ball, C., & Robinson, P. (2003). Four simple questions can help screen for eating disorders. *Journal of General Internal Medicine, 18*(1), 53–56.

Cuijpers, P., Riper, H., & Lemmers, L. (2004). The effects on mortality of brief interventions for problem drinking: A meta-analysis. *Addiction, 99*(7), 839–845. doi:10.1111/j.1360-0443.2004.00778.x.

Danielsen, M., & Ro, O. (2012). Changes in body image during inpatient treatment for eating disorders predict outcome. *Eating Disorders, 20*(4), 261–275. doi:10.1080/10640266.2012.689205.

Di Pierro, R., Sarno, I., Perego, S., Gallucci, M., & Madeddu, F. (2012). Adolescent nonsuicidal self-injury: The effects of personality traits, family relationships and maltreatment on the presence and severity of behaviours. *European Child and Adolescent Psychiatry, 21*(9), 511–520. doi:10.1007/s00787-012-0289-2.

Dooley-Hash, S., Lipson, S. K., Walton, M. A., & Cunningham, R. M. (2012). Increased emergency department use by adolescents and young adults with eating disorders. *International Journal of Eating Disorders*. doi:10.1002/eat.22070.

Faghri, N. M. A., Boisvert, C. M., & Faghri, S. (2010). Understanding the expanding role of primary care physicians (PCPs) to primary psychiatric care physicians (PPCPs): enhancing the assessment and treatment of psychiatric conditions. *Mental Health in Family Medicine, 7*(1), 17–25.

Fairburn, C. G., Cooper, Z., Doll, H. A., O'connor, M. E., Bohn, K., Hawker, D. M., et al. (2009). Transdiagnostic cognitive-behavioral therapy for patients with eating disorders: A two-site trial with 60-week follow-up. *The American Journal of Psychiatry, 166*(3), 311–319. doi:10.1176/appi.ajp.2008.08040608.

Fleming, M., & Manwell, L. B. (1999). Brief intervention in primary care settings. A primary treatment method for at-risk, problem, and dependent drinkers. *Alcohol Research & Health, 23*(2), 128–137.

Forrest, C. B. (2003). Primary care in the united states: Primary care gatekeeping and referrals: Effective filter or failed experiment? *BMJ, 326*(7391), 692–695. doi:10.1136/bmj.326.7391.692.

Garber, A. K., Michihata, N., Hetnal, K., Shafer, M. A., & Moscicki, A. B. (2012). A prospective examination of weight gain in hospitalized adolescents with anorexia nervosa on a recommended refeeding protocol. *Journal of Adolescent Health, 50*(1), 24–29. doi:10.1016/j.jadohealth.2011.06.011.

Godart, N., Berthoz, S., Curt, F., Perdereau, F., Rein, Z., Wallier, J., et al. (2012). A randomized controlled trial of adjunctive family therapy and treatment as usual following inpatient treatment for anorexia nervosa adolescents. *PLoS One, 7*(1), e28249. doi:10.1371/journal.pone.0028249.

Goldner, E. M., Jones, W., & Fang, M. L. (2011). Access to and waiting time for psychiatrist services in a Canadian urban area: A study in real time. *Canadian Journal of Psychiatry. Revue Canadienne de Psychiatrie, 56*(8), 474–480.

Gowers, S. G. (2012). Developmental considerations in choosing treatment settings for child and adolescent eating disorders. In J. Lock (Ed.), *The oxford handbook of child and adolescent eating disorders: Developmental perspectives* (pp. 185–197). New York, NY: Oxford University Press.

Gray, G. V., & Brody, D. S. (2005). The evolution of behavioral primary care. *Professional Psychology: Research and Practice, 36*(2), 123–129.

Grilo, C. M., White, M. A., Gueorguieva, R., Wilson, G. T., & Masheb, R. M. (2012). Predictive significance of the overvaluation of shape/weight in obese patients with binge eating disorder: Findings from a randomized controlled trial with 12-month follow-up. *Psychological Medicine, 43*(6), 1335–1344. doi:10.1017/S0033291712002097.

Halmi, K. A., Sunday, S. R., Strober, M., Kaplan, A., Woodside, D. B., Fichter, M., et al. (2000). Perfectionism in anorexia nervosa: Variation by clinical subtype, obsessionality, and pathological eating behavior. *The American Journal of Psychiatry, 157*(11), 1799–1805.

Hart, S., Abraham, S., Franklin, R., & Russell, J. (2010). Weight changes during inpatient refeeding of underweight eating disorder patients. *European Eating Disorders Review*. doi:10.1002/erv.1052.

Hart, L. M., Granillo, M. T., Jorm, A. F., & Paxton, S. J. (2011). Unmet need for treatment in the eating disorders: A systematic review of eating disorder specific treatment seeking among community cases. *Clinical Psychology Review, 31*(5), 727–735. doi:10.1016/j.cpr.2011.03.004.

Hartmann, A., Weber, S., Herpertz, S., & Zeeck, A. (2011). Psychological treatment for anorexia nervosa: A meta-analysis of standardized mean change. *Psychotherapy and Psychosomatics, 80*(4), 216–226. doi:10.1159/000322360.

Hill, L. S., Reid, F., Morgan, J. F., & Lacey, J. H. (2010). Scoff, the development of an eating disorder screening questionnaire. *International Journal of Eating Disorders, 43*(4), 344–351. doi:10.1002/eat.20679.

Hunter, R. H., Gardner, W. I., Wilkniss, S., & Silverstein, S. M. (2008). The multimodal functional model–advancing case formulation beyond the "diagnose and treat" paradigm: Improving outcomes and reducing aggression and the use of control procedures in psychiatric care. *Psychological Services, 5*(1), 11–25.

Jayaram, G., Sporney, H., & Perticone, P. (2010). The utility and effectiveness of 15-minute checks in inpatient settings. *Psychiatry (Edgmont), 7*(8), 46–49.

Jett, S., Laporte, D. J., & Wanchisn, J. (2010). Impact of exposure to pro-eating disorder websites on eating behaviour in college women. *European Eating Disorders Review, 18*(5), 410–416. doi:10.1002/erv.1009.

Kanerva, A., Lammintakanen, J., & Kivinen, T. (2013). Patient Safety in Psychiatric Inpatient Care: A Literature Review. *Journal of Psychiatric and Mental Health Nursing, 20*(6), 541–548. doi:10.1111/j.1365-2850.2012.01949.x.

Kerr, P. L., Muehlenkamp, J. J., & Turner, J. M. (2010). Nonsuicidal self-injury: A review of current research for family medicine and primary care physicians. *Journal of the American Board of Family Medicine, 23*(2), 240–259. doi:10.3122/jabfm.2010.02.090110.

Klonsky, E. D. (2007). The functions of deliberate self-injury: A review of the evidence. *Clinical Psychology Review, 27*(2), 226–239.

Klonsky, E. D., May, A. M., & Glenn, C. R. (2013). The relationship between nonsuicidal self-injury and attempted suicide: Converging evidence from four samples. *Journal of Abnormal Psychology, 122*(1), 231–237.

Klonsky, E. D., & Weinberg, A. (2009). Assessment of nonsuicidal self-injury. In M. K. Nock (Ed.), *Understanding nonsuicidal self-injury: Origins, assessment, and treatment* (pp. 183–199). Washington, DC: American Psychological Association.

Kondo, D. G., & Sokol, M. S. (2006). Eating disorders in primary care. A guide to identification and treatment. *Postgraduate Medicine, 119*(3), 59–65.

Kress, V. E., & Hoffman, R. M. (2008). Non-suicidal self-injury and motivational interviewing: Enhancing readiness for change. *Journal of Mental Health Counseling, 30*(4), 311–329.

Lask, B., Bryant-Waugh, R., Wright, F., Campbell, M., Willoughby, K., & Waller, G. (2005). Family physician consultation patterns indicate high risk for early-onset anorexia nervosa. *International Journal of Eating Disorders, 38*(3), 269–272. doi:10.1002/eat.20163.

Lock, J. (2011). Family treatment for eating disorders in youth and adolescents. *Psychiatric Annals, 41*(11), 547–551.

Lock, L., Williams, H., Bamford, B., & Lacey, J. H. (2012). The St George's eating disorders service meal preparation group for inpatients and day patients pursuing full recovery: A pilot study. *European Eating Disorders Review, 20*(3), 218–224. doi:10.1002/erv.1134.

Long, C. G., Fitzgerald, K. A., & Hollin, C. R. (2012). Treatment of chronic anorexia nervosa: A 4-year follow-up of adult patients treated in an acute inpatient setting. *Clinical Psychology & Psychotherapy, 19*(1), 1–13. doi:10.1002/cpp.738.

Lund, B. C., Hernandez, E. R., Yates, W. R., Mitchell, J. R., Mckee, P. A., & Johnson, C. L. (2009). Rate of inpatient weight restoration predicts outcome in anorexia nervosa. *International Journal of Eating Disorders, 42*(4), 301–305. doi:10.1002/eat.20634.

Mcdowell, A. K., Lineberry, T. W., & Bostwick, J. M. (2011). Practical suicide-risk management for the busy primary care physician. *Mayo Clinic Proceedings, 86*(8), 792–800. doi:10.4065/mcp.2011.0076.

Merritt Hawkins. (2012). *2012 review of physician recruiting incentives*. Retrieved from http://www.merritthawkins.com/uploadedFiles/MerrittHawkins/pdf/mha2012survpreview.pdf

Miller, W. R., & Rollnick, S. (1991). *Motivational interviewing*. New York, NY: Guilford.

Morgan, J. F., Reid, F., & Lacey, J. H. (1999). The scoff questionnaire: Assessment of a new screening tool for eating disorders. *BMJ, 319*(7223), 1467–1468.

Mueser, K. T., Corrigan, P. W., Hilton, D. W., Tanzman, B., Schaub, A., Gingerich, S., et al. (2002). Illness management and recovery: A review of the research. *Psychiatric Services, 53* (10), 1272–1284.

Murray, B. (2002). "Partners in illness": Patients trading thinness tips. *Monitor on Psychology, 33* (42–43).

Murray, C. D., Warm, A., & Fox, J. (2005). An internet survey of adolescent self-injurers. *Advances in Mental Health, 4*(1), 1–9.

Nicholls, D. E., & Yi, I. (2012). Early intervention in eating disorders: A parent group approach. *Early Intervention in Psychiatry, 6*(4), 357–367. doi:10.1111/j.1751-7893.2012.00373.x.

Nock, M. K. (2010). Self-injury. *Annual Review of Clinical Psychology, 6*, 339–363. doi:10.1146/annurev.clinpsy.121208.131258.

Nock, M. K., & Cha, C. B. (2009). Psychological models of nonsuicidal self-injury. In M. K. Nock (Ed.), *Understanding nonsuicidal self-injury: Origins, assessment, and treatment* (pp. 65–77). Washington, DC: American Psychological Association.

Nutting, P. A., Dickinson, L., Rubenstein, L. V., Keeley, R. D., Smith, J. L., & Elliott, C. E. (2005). Improving detection of suicidal ideation among depressed patients in primary care. *Annals of Family Medicine, 3*(6), 529–536.

Olmsted, M. P., Mcfarlane, T. L., Carter, J. C., Trottier, K., Woodside, D. B., & Dimitropoulos, G. (2010). Inpatient and day hospital treatment for anorexia nervosa. In C. M. Grilo & J. E. Mitchell (Eds.), *The treatment of eating disorders: A clinical handbook* (pp. 198–211). New York, NY: Guilford.

Phillips, R., Stewart, S. M., Presnell, K., Simmons, A., Kennard, B. D., Liss, D., et al. (2010). Psychological variables impacting weight gain rapidity in adolescents hospitalized for eating disorders. *European Eating Disorders Review, 18*(5), 376–384. doi:10.1002/erv.998.

Pitts, S. R., Carrier, E. R., Rich, E. C., & Kellermann, A. L. (2010). Where Americans get acute care: Increasingly, It's not at their doctor's office. *Health Affairs, 29*(9), 1620–1629. doi:10.1377/hlthaff.2009.1026.

Richardson, B. G., Surmitis, K. A., & Hyldahl, R. S. (2012). Minimizing social contagion in adolescents who self-injure: Considerations for group work, residential treatment, and the internet. *Journal of Mental Health Counseling, 34*(2), 121–132.

Robinson, J. W., & Roter, D. L. (1999). Psychosocial problem disclosure by primary care patients. *Social Science and Medicine, 48*(10), 1353–1362.

Rosen, D. S. (2010). Identification and management of eating disorders in children and adolescents. *Pediatrics, 126*(6), 1240–1253. doi:10.1542/peds.2010-2821.

Salbach-Andrae, H., Schneider, N., Seifert, K., Pfeiffer, E., Lenz, K., Lehmkuhl, U., et al. (2009). Short-term outcome of anorexia nervosa in adolescents after inpatient treatment: A prospective study. *European Child and Adolescent Psychiatry, 18*(11), 701–704. doi:10.1007/s00787-009-0024-9.

Sim, L. A., Homme, J. H., Lteif, A. N., Vande Voort, J. L., Schak, K. M., & Ellingson, J. (2009). Family functioning and maternal distress in adolescent girls with anorexia nervosa. *International Journal of Eating Disorders, 42*(6), 531–539. doi:10.1002/eat.20654.

Sim, L. A., Mcalpine, D. E., Grothe, K. B., Himes, S. M., Cockerill, R. G., & Clark, M. M. (2010). Identification and treatment of eating disorders in the primary care setting. *Mayo Clinic Proceedings, 85*(8), 746–751. doi:10.4065/mcp.2010.0070.

Stanley, B., & Brown, G. K. (2012). Safety planning intervention: A brief intervention to mitigate suicide risk. *Cognitive and Behavioral Practice, 19*(2), 256–264.

Steinhausen, H. C., Gavez, S., & Winkler Metzke, C. (2005). Psychosocial correlates, outcome, and stability of abnormal adolescent eating behavior in community samples of young people. *International Journal of Eating Disorders, 37*(2), 119–126. doi:10.1002/eat.20077.

Stice, E., Marti, C. N., & Rohde, P. (2012). Prevalence, incidence, impairment, and course of the proposed DSM-5 eating disorder diagnoses in an 8-year prospective community study of young women. *Journal of Abnormal Psychology*. doi:10.1037/a0030679.

Storch, M., Keller, F., Weber, J., Spindler, A., & Milos, G. (2011). Psychoeducation in affect regulation for patients with eating disorders: A randomized controlled feasibility study. *American Journal of Psychotherapy, 65*(1), 81–93.

Trautmann, J., Worthy, S. L., & Lokken, K. L. (2007). Body dissatisfaction, bulimic symptoms, and clothing practices among college women. *Journal of Psychology, 141*(5), 485–498. doi:10.3200/JRLP.141.5.485-498.

Trude, S., & Stoddard, J. J. (2003). Referral gridlock: Primary care physicians and mental health services. *Journal of General Internal Medicine, 18*(6), 442–449.

Vandereycken, W. (2011). Can eating disorders become 'contagious' in group therapy and specialized inpatient care? *European Eating Disorders Review, 19*(4), 289–295.

Vannoy, S. D., Fancher, T., Meltvedt, C., Unutzer, J., Duberstein, P., & Kravitz, R. L. (2010). Suicide inquiry in primary care: Creating context, inquiring, and following up. *Annals of Family Medicine, 8*(1), 33–39. doi:10.1370/afm.1036.

Vansteelandt, K., Pieters, G., Vanderlinden, J., & Probst, M. (2010). Body dissatisfaction moderates weight curves in the inpatient treatment of anorexia nervosa. *International Journal of Eating Disorders, 43*(8), 694–700. doi:10.1002/eat.20763.

Wade, T. D., Frayne, A., Edwards, S. A., Robertson, T., & Gilchrist, P. (2009). Motivational change in an inpatient anorexia nervosa population and implications for treatment. *The Australian and New Zealand Journal of Psychiatry, 43*(3), 235–243. doi:10.1080/00048670802653356.

Waller, G. (2012). The myths of motivation: Time for a fresh look at some received wisdom in the eating disorders? *International Journal of Eating Disorders, 45*(1), 1–16. doi:10.1002/eat.20900.

Waller, G., Stringer, H., & Meyer, C. (2012). What cognitive behavioral techniques do therapists report using when delivering cognitive behavioral therapy for the eating disorders? *Journal of Consulting and Clinical Psychology, 80*(1), 171–175. doi:10.1037/a0026559.

Walsh, B. W. (2006). *Treating self-injury: A practical guide*. New York, NY: Guilford.

Walsh, B., & Doerfler, L. A. (2009). Residential treatment of nonsuicidal self-injury. In M. K. Nock (Ed.), *Understanding nonsuicidal self-injury: Origins, assessment, and treatment* (pp. 271–290). Washington, DC: American Psychological Association.

Walsh, J. M., Wheat, M. E., & Freund, K. (2000). Detection, evaluation, and treatment of eating disorders the role of the primary care physician. *Journal of General Internal Medicine, 15*(8), 577–590.

Weiss, A. P., Chang, G., Rauch, S. L., Smallwood, J. A., Schechter, M., Kosowsky, J., et al. (2012). Patient- and practice-related determinants of emergency department length of stay for patients with psychiatric illness. *Annals of Emergency Medicine, 60*(2), 162–171.e165. doi:10.1016/j.annemergmed.2012.01.037.

Whitelaw, M., Gilbertson, H., Lam, P. Y., & Sawyer, S. M. (2010). Does aggressive refeeding in hospitalized adolescents with anorexia nervosa result in increased hypophosphatemia? *Journal of Adolescent Health, 46*(6), 577–582. doi:10.1016/j.jadohealth.2009.11.207.

Whitlock, J. (2009). *The cutting edge: non-suicidal self-injury in adolescence. Research fACTs and findings*. Ithaca, NY: ACT for Youth Center of Excellence.

Whitlock, J., Eckenrode, J., & Silverman, D. (2006). Self-injurious behaviors in a college population. *Pediatrics, 117*(6), 1939–1948.

Whitlock, J., Muehlenkamp, J., Eckenrode, J., Purington, A., Baral Abrams, G., Barreira, P., et al. (2013). Nonsuicidal self-injury as a gateway to suicide in young adults. *Journal of Adolescent Health, 52*(4), 486–492. doi:10.1016/j.jadohealth.2012.09.010.

Whitlock, J. L., Powers, J. L., & Eckenrode, J. (2006). The virtual cutting edge: The internet and adolescent self-injury. *Developmental Psychology, 42*(3), 407–417. doi:10.1037/0012-1649.42.3.407.

Whitney, J., Murphy, T., Landau, S., Gavan, K., Todd, G., Whitaker, W., et al. (2012). A practical comparison of two types of family intervention: An exploratory RCT of family day workshops and individual family work as a supplement to inpatient care for adults with anorexia nervosa. *European Eating Disorders Review, 20*(2), 142–150. doi:10.1002/erv.1076.

Williams, P. M., Goodie, J., & Motsinger, C. D. (2008). Treating eating disorders in primary care. *American Family Physician, 77*(2), 187–195.

Willinge, A. C., Touyz, S. W., & Thornton, C. (2010). An evaluation of the effectiveness and short-term stability of an innovative Australian day patient programme for eating disorders. *European Eating Disorders Review, 18*(3), 220–233. doi:10.1002/erv.997.

Wiseman, C. V., Sunday, S. R., Klapper, F., Klein, M., & Halmi, K. A. (2002). Short-term group CBT versus psycho-education on an inpatient eating disorder unit. *Eating Disorders, 10*(4), 313–320. doi:10.1080/10640260214504.

Zeeck, A., Weber, S., Sandholz, A., Joos, A., & Hartmann, A. (2011). Stability of long-term outcome in bulimia nervosa: A 3-year follow-Up. *Journal of Clinical Psychology, 67*(3), 318–327. doi:10.1002/jclp.20766.

19 Males with Non-suicidal Self-Injury and Eating Disorder: A Unique Approach

Fernando Fernández-Aranda, Susana Jimenez-Murcia, Isabel Sánchez, Mohammed Anisul Islam, and José M. Menchón

19.1 Introduction

Although in general population research, the variable gender has been considered in many studies, in mental disorders NSSI has basically been studied in female patients and more in those individuals with comorbid Axis II disorders (Nitkowski & Petermann, 2011). In ED literature, males have frequently been neglected due to low prevalence rates (Núñez-Navarro et al., 2012; Claes et al., 2012; Tchanturia et al., 2012).

19.2 NSSI and Gender Characteristics in General Population

Research shows that NSSI is 1.5–3 times more prevalent in the female population than in males as supported by several literature review studies (Muehlenkamp, Claes, Havertape, & Plener, 2012; Yates, 2004). In a Hong Kong study (Cheung et al., 2013), a higher prevalence rate of NSSI was found in adolescent females (19.7 %) compared to males (13.4 %). This is further supported by other studies (Kuentzel, Arble, Boutros, Chugani, & Barnett, 2012; Zetterqvist, Lundh, Dahlström, & Svedin, 2013).

Young men and women differ significantly in age of onset, degree of medical injury, and NSSI methods (Andover et al., 2010). Among the school-going children (ages 7–16) with NSSI (Barrocas, Hankin, Young, & Abela, 2012), girls showed NSSI earlier than boys (in the nineth grade school, 19 % and 5 %, respectively), and it was found that, whereas girls engaged in cutting the skin more often, boys reported hitting themselves more frequently. An explanation of this difference may be compliance to the norms of gender roles such as emotional control, resistance to pain, toughness, and aggression which may play a part in NSSI in males (Andover et al., 2010).

F. Fernández-Aranda (✉) • S. Jimenez-Murcia • I. Sánchez • M.A. Islam • J.M. Menchón
Department of Psychiatry, University Hospital of Bellvitge-IDIBELL and CIBEROBN, Barcelona, Spain
e-mail: ffernandez@bellvitgehospital.cat

L. Claes and J.J. Muehlenkamp (eds.), *Non-Suicidal Self-Injury in Eating Disorders*,
DOI 10.1007/978-3-642-40107-7_19, © Springer-Verlag Berlin Heidelberg 2014

Several other factors have been found to play a part in the distinction of NSSI in gender. Childhood abuse was strongly associated with the development of NSSI in both genders, but in females this could have been partly mediated by dissociation, alexithymia, and self-blame and in males by dissociation and self-blame (Swannell et al., 2012). Factors like sexual orientation and Axis I comorbidity have also been strongly associated with NSSI, especially in females (Hintikka et al., 2009; Whitlock et al., 2011).

However, besides general psychopathology, several studies in male inmates and forensic inpatients showed that NSSI in men co-occurred with other symptoms, such as aggression and addictive behavior (Hillbrand, Krystal, Sharpe, & Foster, 1994). More males with NSSI showed more antisocial traits compared to females (Claes, Vandereycken, & Vertommen, 2007).

19.3 NSSI in Males with a Psychiatric Disorder

Claes et al. (2007)'s paper is one among the very few studies that primarily focused on gender differences in NSSI in psychiatric patients. In their sample of 399 patients (265 females and 134 males), more females with NSSI displayed scratching, bruising, cutting, and nail-biting and were involved in an abusive relationship compared to males, starving and laxative abuse. Males showed higher scores on burning oneself, alcohol abuse, driving recklessly, and sexual promiscuity. However, males reported feeling more pain during the NSSI. In addition, females took care of their injuries and hid their wounds more often than males (Claes et al., 2007). Furthermore men reported a higher frequency of NSSI episodes per day. More females reported avoiding negative feelings and painful memories, getting into a numb state, making oneself unattractive, suppressing suicidal thoughts, and punishing oneself as their motivation behind their self-destructive action (Claes et al., 2007).

Many studies have shown NSSI to be closely related to impulsivity (McCloskey, Look, Chen, Pajoumand, & Berman, 2012). To explain the co-occurrence of NSSI and other impulse-control problems, several authors (e.g., Glenn & Klonsky, 2010) considered dysfunctional personality traits, such as higher impulsiveness, novelty seeking, and harm avoidance, as possible explanatory factors of NSSI. Research has shown a strong link between NSSI and other psychiatric disorders, such as borderline personality disorder (Andover & Gibb, 2010; You, Leung, Lai, & Fu, 2012), other personality disorders (Cawood & Huprich, 2011), anxiety disorders (Chartrand, Sareen, Toews, & Bolton, 2012), posttraumatic stress disorder (Weierich & Nock, 2008), attention deficit hyperactivity disorder (Hurtig, Taanila, Moilanen, Nordström, & Ebeling, 2012), bipolar disorder (Esposito-Smythers et al., 2010), affective disorders (Dougherty et al., 2009; Fliege, Lee, Grimm, & Klapp, 2009; Hintikka et al., 2009), and alcohol and drug abuse (Fliege et al., 2009; Hasking, Momeni, Swannell, & Chia, 2008) in both males and females (Table 19.1).

Table 19.1 Recent studies about NSSI in males with psychiatric disorder

Authors	Year	Sample	Diagnosis	Results
You	2012	4,782 students	BPD	BPD symptoms were significantly associated with NSSI
Chatrand	2012	85 (of 20,130) adult patients	Anxiety	Anxiety disorders were associated with NSSI
Muehlenkamp	2011	441 adolescent patients	BPD	Two BPD symptoms exhibit distinct relationships to NSSI but not strong variation in their relationship to BPD
Hurtig	2012	457 of 9,432 patients	ADHD	NSSI in ADHD group > NSSI in control
Asarnow	2011	327 adolescents	Depression	NSSI (38 %) > Suicide attempt (23 %) in depression
Cawood and Huprich	2011	302 college students	PD	NSSI correlated with PD
Esposito-Smythers	2010	432 patients	Bipolar disorder	34 % of BD children and 37 % of BD adolescents reported at least one incident of NSSI
Dougherty	2009	56 adolescents	Depressive symptoms and impulsivity	NSSI (who had attempted suicide) patients reported worse depression, hopelessness, and impulsivity compared to NSSI patients
Fliege	2009	74 patients	Axis I disorders	Self-harmers more frequently diagnosed with anxiety, depressive, substance abuse/dependence, or eating disorders than those without self-destructive behavior

Note: *BPD* Borderline Personality Disorder, *ADHD* Attention Deficit Hyperactivity Disorder, *PD* Personality Disorder

19.4 Prevalence and Characteristics of NSSI in Male ED Patients

Whereas the prevalence of NSSI in female ED patients is high (Claes, Vandereycken, & Vertommen, 2003; Favaro & Santonastaso, 1998; Paul, Schroeter, Dahme, & Nutzinger, 2002), ranging between 13 and 68 % (Svirko & Hawton, 2007), the reported NSSI prevalence in ED males is much lower, 21 % (Claes et al., 2012). Along the last 12 years, from an unselected sample of 2158 ED referrals who were sought and assessed consecutively in the specialized Unit at the University Hospital of Bellvitge (Barcelona, Spain), those with NSSI without suicidal attempts were selected. As expected, average prevalence of NSSI in females (22.9 %) was higher than in males (17.7 %). Although some variations have been observed in specific years, the scores and distribution over time were maintained. Barrocas et al. (2012) found that compared to adolescent males (5.1 %), the rate of females was more than three times higher (18.9 %).

In males, NSSI have mainly been developed simultaneously with their ED (Claes et al., 2012; Paul et al., 2002), and no significant differences were found in the prevalence of NSSI among ED subtypes when considering AN, BN, and EDNOS (Claes et al., 2012; Paul et al., 2002), although there was a tendency towards more NSSI in bulimic patients, similarly as reported in female ED (Svirko & Hawton, 2007). The few studies investigating the association in males between NSSI and ED and general psychopathology found that males engaging in NSSI showed significantly more severity of eating disorder (Claes et al., 2012; Ross, Heath, & Toste, 2009;), higher general psychopathology, and more impulsive behaviors (Claes & Vandereycken, 2007; Claes et al., 2012). As shown in a previously conducted collaborative study by our group (Claes et al., 2012), male ED patients with NSSI showed higher harm avoidance and a tendency to lower scores on the TCI-R scale self-directedness.

From 156 consecutively admitted male ED patients, we compared clinical and psychopathological features among those patients who presented only NSSI ($N = 21$; 13.5 %), those who presented NSSI + suicidal attempts ($N = 21$; 13.5 %) vs. those without NSSI/suicidal attempts ($N = 114$; 73.0 %) (Fig. 19.1).

Regarding *age of ED onset*, in accordance with previous reports (Claes et al., 2012), no significant differences were obtained among the groups. Concerning *psychopathological symptoms* (namely, lifetime impulse-related disorders and addictive behaviors), as shown in Table 19.2, both groups NSSI and NSSI + suicidal attempts were those who presented more lifetime alcohol abuse/dependence (23.8 % and 33.3 %, respectively) and stealing behavior (28.6 % and 14.3 %, respectively). Both groups were also those who showed current higher general psychopathology measured by means of total average scores in the SCL-90-R scale (Derogatis, 1990) [NSSI: $M = 1.77$ (SD = 0.65); NSSI/Suicide attempts: $M = 1.71$ (SD = 0.91); without NSSI/Suicidal attempts: $M = 1.13$ (SD = 0.75)].

As expected, the NSSI/Suicide attempts group presented the higher lifetime suicidal ideation (81 %), followed by the NSSI group (57.1 %). Although there were no significant differences among the groups on some impulse-control disorders (namely pathological gambling and kleptomania), as reported in other studies (Fernandez-Aranda et al., 2008; Fernández-Aranda et al., 2006; Jimenez-Murcia et al., 2013, in press), they were clearly gender associated.

19.5 NSSI in ED Males and Therapy Approach

One of the core components related to NSSI is impulsivity and lack of emotional-regulation skills (Claes, Klonsky, Muehlenkamp, Kuppens, & Vandereycken, 2010). These factors are even more relevant in ED with NSSI (male and female) than in ED without NSSI. Due to the limited positive effects of traditional therapies to improve impulsiveness and emotional regulation in ED (Agüera et al., 2012), several attempts have been developed to address those in a specific way with limited evidence (Gonzales & Bergstrom, 2013).

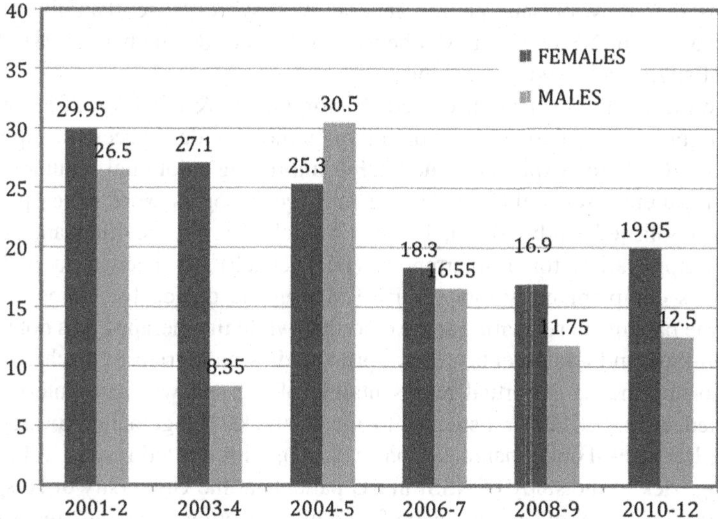

Fig. 19.1 Percentage of NSSI in 1.720 eating disorders consecutive patients assessed, between 2001 and 2012, among females and males

Table 19.2 Lifetime impulsive behaviors and impulse-related disorders among 156 ED males (21 NSSI; 21 NSSI/Suicide attempters; 114 without NSSI/Suicide attempts)

	NSSI	NSSI/ Suicide attempts	Without NSSI/ Suicide attempts	*p*
Alcohol abuse/dependence	23.8 %	33.3 %	10.6 %	<0.016
Drug abuse/dependence	28.6 %	28.6 %	13.3 %	ns
Pathological gambling	4.8 %	14.3 %	7.1 %	ns
Stealing behavior	28.6 %	14.3 %	7 %	<0.012
Kleptomania	4.8 %	0 %	1.8 %	ns

Note: NSSI (Non-suicidal self-injury group; $N = 21$); NSSI/Suicide attempts ($N = 21$); Without NSSI/Suicide attempts ($N = 114$); ns = not statistically significant

The few reports describing new or improved therapy strategies to deal with NSSI (Gonzales & Bergstrom, 2013; Hawton et al., 1998; Linehan et al., 2006; Muehlenkamp, 2006; Slee, Garnefski, van der Leeden, Arensman, & Spinhoven, 2008; Washburn et al., 2012) (e.g., dialectical behavior therapy, interpersonal psychotherapy, trans-diagnostic cognitive-behavior therapy, emotion-focused therapy) in general psychiatric patients are mainly focusing on techniques such as self-regulation skills, emotional awareness, stress management, and self-control strategies. As suggested by some authors (Swannell et al., 2012), improving their capacity for regulating emotions and changing their attribution style may contribute to reduction of NSSI. However, when considering the current ED literature, there is a lack of empirically supported therapies. Regarding ED males, although it is to be expected that they present poorer general therapy response than their female counterparts with NSSI (Chen, Matthews, Allen, Kuo, & Linehan, 2008), there is a lack of studies addressing this topic.

Some recent studies have discussed (Victor, Glenn, & Klonsky, 2012) whether NSSI might be an addictive behavior, although more evidence seem to support the emotional-regulation explicatory model. For improving emotional-regulation skills in NSSI patients, some therapies using new technologies were developed. In a recently published study (Rizvi, Dimeff, Skutch, Carroll, & Linehan, 2011), a software application for a smartphone (DBT coach) has been used with BPD patients as complementary tool for BDT. Using the device for almost 2 weeks helped the patients in regulating some emotions while the therapist was not present. With children and adolescents, several pilot studies have tried to teach emotional regulation by means of virtual representation of the self with computerized task (Wrzesien et al., 2012) or listening to music tracks (Stegemann, Brüggemann-Etchart, Badorrek-Hinkelmann, & Romer, 2010), with limited results so far.

Going back to the study of NSSI in ED patients at the University of Hospital in Bellvitge, significant differences were found in *motivation to change* (measured by means of a 0–8 lineal scale, as described somewhere; Casasnovas et al., 2007). The NSSI male ED patients were those who showed the lower subjective desire for treatment (NSSI: $M = 3.2$ (SD = 3.3); NSSI + Suicide attempts: $M = 7$ (SD = 1.3); Without NSSI/Suicidal attempts: $M = 5.3$ (SD = 2.7)). In contrast, the reported worry of the family (externally driven motivation) was high among all the groups [NSSI: $M = 6.6$ (SD = 1.5); NSSI + Suicide attempts: $M = 7.3$ (SD = 1.1); Without NSSI/Suicidal attempts: $M = 6.4$ (SD = 2.2)).

As reported previously in the literature (Muehlenkamp et al., 2009; Vansteenkiste, Claes, Soenens, & Verstuyf, 2013), a more externally driven motivation might be associated with their own resistance to change, but also to individual processes. In this sense, automatic negative reinforcement (e.g., to escape from negative emotions) and family dynamics (e.g., social positive and negative reinforcement) might be acting as relevant maintaining factors (Robertson, Miskey, Mitchell, & Nelson-Gray, 2013).

At the University Hospital of Bellvitge, since 2009 a specific designed video-game has been developed for treating patients with impulse-related disorders (namely, eating disorders and impulse-control disorders), many of whom had engaged in NSSI. This new technological platform is a complementary approach to the usual CBT applied at our Center (Fernández-Aranda et al., 2009; Peñas-Lledó et al., 2010), trying to address impulsiveness and emotional-regulation skills (Fernandez-Aranda et al., 2012).

As described in previous studies (Fernandez-Aranda et al., 2012), while the patient is playing the videogame (named "Islands") during 20 min, several biosensors and complementary devices (camera and microphone) are detecting the emotional expression (facial and speech anger–joy emotions) and physiological reactivity of the patient while confronted with specific game situations and the triggered emotions. Physiological reactivity and emotional recognition will continuously track the emotional state of the player along the video game, while the game

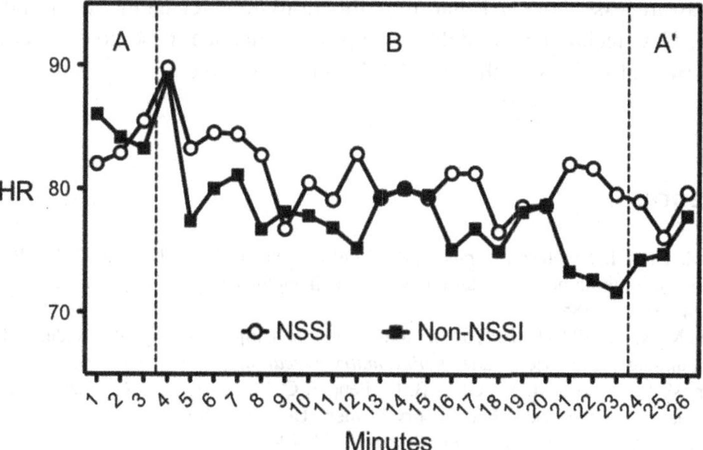

Fig. 19.2 Heart Rate in two ED patients (with and without NSSI), during a session of emotional-regulation videogame (Islands), following A-B-A' design

will automatically respond in return by modifying aspects of the game play difficulty, in a closed loop. The final objective is not to win, in a classical game manner, but to achieve a greater capacity of self-control. At all times, the patient will receive feedback regarding his/her achievements. In ED, some results have already been published after using with 23 ED and 11 HC, with promising findings. The complete procedure and component details of Island Videogame are further detailed in Fernandez-Aranda et al. (2012) and Jimenez-Murcia et al. (2009)'s articles. As shown in Fig. 19.2, ABA design procedure was followed in each single session, and physiological measurements were taken from baseline (phase A: 3 min), during the game (phase B: 20 min) and post-game (phase A': 3 min). In this graph, the performance of two patients (with and without NSSI) on Heart Rate (HR) is shown.

Conclusion

NSSI has more frequently been observed among females than males in adolescents and the general adult population. In ED, NSSI has been associated with higher symptomatology and psychopathology, but also with impulsive behavior and personality traits. Whereas the prevalence of NSSI in female ED patients is high (rate 13–68 %), the reported NSSI prevalence in ED males is much lower (around 20 %). In males, NSSI has mainly been developed simultaneously with the ED and is associated with greater general psychopathology, harm avoidant personality traits, and with lower internal motivation. No significant prevalence differences are described between ED subtypes. There is a lack of empirically supported therapies for ED patients with NSSI. Besides stabilizing their mood and increasing own motivation to change, targets for a therapy should be improving their capacity for regulating emotions, increasing self-awareness about self-harming functions, and changing their attribution style. New technologies might be helpful to enhance those goals as additional therapy tool with usual therapy (DBT, enhanced CBT).

References

Agüera, Z., Krug, I., Sánchez, I., Granero, R., Penelo, E., Peñas-Lledó, E., et al. (2012). Personality changes in bulimia nervosa after a cognitive behaviour therapy. *European Eating Disorders Review, 20*, 379–385.

Andover, M. S., & Gibb, B. E. (2010). Non-suicidal self-injury, attempted suicide, and suicidal intent among psychiatric inpatients. *Psychiatry Research, 30*(178), 101–105.

Andover, M. S., Primack, J. M., Gibb, B. E., Pepper, C. M., Baetens, I., & Claes, L. (2010). An examination of non-suicidal self-injury in men: Do men differ from women in basic NSSI characteristics? *Archives of Suicide Research, 14*, 79–88.

Barrocas, A. L., Hankin, B. L., Young, J. F., & Abela, J. R. (2012). Rates of nonsuicidal self-injury in youth: Age, sex, and behavioral methods in a community sample. *Pediatrics, 130*, 39–45.

Casasnovas, C., Fernández-Aranda, F., Granero, R., Krug, I., Jiménez-Murcia, S., Bulik, C. M., et al. (2007). Motivation to change in eating disorders: Clinical and therapeutic implications. *European Eating Disorders Review, 15*, 449–456.

Cawood, C. D., & Huprich, S. K. (2011). Late adolescent nonsuicidal self-injury: The roles of coping style, self-esteem, and personality pathology. *Journal of Personality Disorders, 25*, 765–781.

Chartrand, H., Sareen, J., Toews, M., & Bolton, J. M. (2012). Suicide attempts versus nonsuicidal self-injury among individuals with anxiety disorders in a nationally representative sample. *Depression and Anxiety, 29*, 172–179.

Chen, E. Y., Matthews, L., Allen, C., Kuo, J. R., & Linehan, M. M. (2008). Dialectical behavior therapy for clients with binge-eating disorder or bulimia nervosa and borderline personality disorder. *International Journal of Eating Disorders, 41*, 505–512.

Cheung, Y. T., Wong, P. W., Lee, A. M., Lam, T. H., Fan, Y. S., & Yip, P. S. (2013). Non-suicidal self-injury and suicidal behavior: Prevalence, co-occurrence, and correlates of suicide among adolescents in Hong Kong. *Social Psychiatry and Psychiatric Epidemiology, 48*(7), 1133–1144.

Claes, L., Jiménez-Murcia, S., Agüera, Z., Castro, R., Sánchez, I., Menchón, J. M., et al. (2012). Male eating disorder patients with and without non-suicidal self-injury: A comparison of psychopathological and personalityfeatures. *European Eating Disorders Review, 20*, 335–338.

Claes, L., Klonsky, E. D., Muehlenkamp, W., Kuppens, P., & Vandereycken, W. (2010). The affect-regulation function of non-suicidal self-injury in eating- disordered patients: Which affect states are regulated? *Comprehensive Psychiatry, 51*, 386–392.

Claes, L., & Vandereycken, W. (2007). Self-injurious behaviour: Differential diagnosis and - functional differentiation. *Comprehensive Psychiatry, 48*, 137–144.

Claes, L., Vandereycken, W., & Vertommen, H. (2003). Eating-disordered patients with and without self-injurious behaviours: A comparison of psychopathological features. *European Eating Disorders Review, 11*, 379–396.

Claes, L., Vandereycken, W., & Vertommen, H. (2007). Self-injury in female versus male psychiatric patients: A comparison of characteristics, psychopathology and aggression regulation. *Personality and Individual Differences, 42*, 611–621.

Derogatis, L. R. (1990). *SCL-90-R. Administration, scoring and procedures manual*. Baltimore, MD: Clinical Psychometric Research.

Dougherty, D. M., Mathias, C. W., Marsh-Richard, D. M., Prevette, K. N., Dawes, M. A., Hatzis, E. S., et al. (2009). Impulsivity and clinical symptoms among adolescents with non-suicidal self-injury with or without attempted suicide. *Psychiatry research, 169*, 22–27.

Esposito-Smythers, C., Goldstein, T., Birmaher, B., Goldstein, B., Hunt, J., Ryan, N., et al. (2010). Clinical and psychosocial correlates of non-suicidal self-injury within a sample of children and adolescents with bipolar disorder. *Journal of Affective Disorders, 125*(1–3), 89–97.

Favaro, A., & Santonastaso, P. (1998). Impulsive and compulsive self-injurious behaviour in bulimia nervosa: Prevalence and psychological correlates. *The Journal of Nervous and Mental Disease, 186*, 157–165.

Fernández-Aranda, F., Jiménez-Murcia, S., Álvarez, E., Granero, R., Vallejo, J., & Bulik, C. M. (2006). Impulse control disorders in eating disorders: Clinical and therapeutic implications. *Comprehensive Psychiatry, 47*, 482–488.

Fernandez-Aranda, F., Jimenez-Murcia, S., Santamaria, J. J., Gunnard, K., Soto, A., Kalapanidas, E., et al. (2012). Video games as a complementary tool in mental disorders: Playmancer a European multicenter study. *Journal of Mental Health, 21*, 364–374.

Fernández-Aranda, F., Martínez, C., Álvarez-Moya, E., Núñez, A., Sánchez, I., Granero, R., et al. (2009). Predictors of early change in bulimia nervosa after a brief psycho-educational therapy. *Appetite, 52*, 805–808.

Fernandez-Aranda, F., Poyastro Pinheiro, A., Thornton, L. M., Berrettini, W. H., Crow, S., Fichter, M. M., et al. (2008). Impulse control disorders in women with eating disorders. *Psychiatry Research, 157*, 147–157.

Fliege, H., Lee, J. R., Grimm, A., & Klapp, B. F. (2009). Risk factors and correlates of deliberate self-harm behavior: A systematic review. *Journal of Psychosomatic Research, 66*, 477–493.

Glenn, C. R., & Klonsky, E. D. (2010). A multimethod analysis of impulsivity in nonsuicidal self-injury. *Personality Disorders, 1*, 67–75.

Gonzales, A. H., & Bergstrom, L. (2013). Adolescent non-suicidal self-injury (NSSI) interventions. *Journal of Child and Adolescent Psychiatric Nursing, 26*, 124–130.

Hasking, P., Momeni, R., Swannell, S., & Chia, S. (2008). The nature and extent of non-suicidal self-injury in a non-clinical sample of young adults. *Archives of Suicide Research, 12*, 208–218.

Hawton, K., Arensman, E., Townsend, E., Bremner, S., Feldman, E., Goldney, R., et al. (1998). Deliberate self harm: Systematic review of efficacy of psychosocial and pharmacological treatments in preventing repetition. *British Medical Journal, 317*, 441–447.

Hillbrand, M., Krystal, J. H., Sharpe, K. S., & Foster, H. G. (1994). Clinical predictors of self-mutilation in hospitalized forensic patients. *The Journal of Nervous and Mental Disease, 182*, 9–13.

Hintikka, J., Tolmunen, T., Rissanen, M. L., Honkalampi, K., Kylmä, J., & Laukkanen, E. (2009). Mental disorders in self-cutting adolescents. *Journal of Adolescent Health, 44*, 464–467.

Hurtig, T., Taanila, A., Moilanen, I., Nordström, T., & Ebeling, H. (2012). Suicidal and self-harm behaviour associated with adolescent attention deficit hyperactivity disorder-a study in the Northern Finland Birth Cohort 1986. *Nordic Journal of Psychiatry, 66*, 320–328.

Jimenez-Murcia, S., Fernández-Aranda, F., Kalpanidas, E., Konstantas, D., Ganchev, T., Kocsis, O., et al. (2009). Playmancer project: A serious videogame as an additional therapy tool for eating and impulse control disorders. *Studies in Health Technology and Informatics, 144*, 163–166.

Jiménez-Murcia, S., Steiger, H., Isräel, M., Granero, R., Prat, R., Santamaría, J. J, et al. (2013, in press). Pathological gambling in eating disorders: Prevalence and clinical implications. *Comprehensive Psychiatry*. doi:10.1016/j.comppsych.2013.04.014.

Kuentzel, J. G., Arble, E., Boutros, N., Chugani, D., & Barnett, D. (2012). Nonsuicidal self-injury in an ethnically diverse college sample. *The American Journal of Orthopsychiatry, 82*, 291–297.

Linehan, M. M., Comtois, K. A., Murray, A. M., Brown, M. Z., Gallop, R. J., Heard, H. L., et al. (2006). Two-year randomized controlled trial and follow-up of dialectical behavior therapy vs. therapy by experts for suicidal behaviors and borderline personality disorder. *Archives of General Psychiatry, 63*, 757–766.

McCloskey, M. S., Look, A. E., Chen, E. Y., Pajoumand, G., & Berman, M. E. (2012). Nonsuicidal self-injury: Relationship to behavioral and self-rating measures of impulsivity and self-aggression. *Suicide & Life-Threatening Behavior, 42*, 197–209.

Muehlenkamp, J. J. (2006). Empirically supported treatments and general therapy guidelines for non-suicidal self-injury. *Journal of Mental Health Counseling, 28*, 166–185.

Muehlenkamp, J. J., Claes, L., Havertape, L., & Plener, P. L. (2012). International prevalence of adolescent non-suicidal self-injury and deliberate self-harm. *Child and Adolescent Psychiatry and Mental Health, 6*, 2–9.

Muehlenkamp, J. J., Engel, S. G., Wadeson, A., Crosby, R. D., Wonderlich, S. A., Simonich, H., et al. (2009). Emotional states preceding and following acts of non-suicidal self-injury in bulimia nervosa patients. *Behavior Research and Therapy, 47*, 83–87.

Muehlenkamp, J. J., Ertelt, T. W., Miller, A. L., & Claes, L. (2011). Borderline personality symptoms differentiate non-suicidal and suicidal self-injury in ethnically diverse adolescent outpatients. *Journal of Child Psychology and Psychiatry, 52*, 148–155.

Nitkowski, D., & Petermann, F. (2011). Non-suicidal self-injury and comorbid mental disorders: A review. *Fortschritte der Neurologie-Psychiatrie, 79*, 9–20.

Núñez-Navarro, A., Agüera, Z., Krug, I., Jiménez-Murcia, S., Sánchez, I., Araguz, N., et al. (2012). Do men with eating disorders differ from women in clinics, psychopathology and personality? *European Eating Disorders Review, 20*, 23–31.

Paul, T., Schroeter, K., Dahme, B., & Nutzinger, D. O. (2002). Self-injurious behavior in women with eating disorders. *The American Journal of Psychiatry, 159*, 408–411.

Peñas-Lledó, E., Agüera, Z., Sánchez, I., Gunnard, K., Jiménez-Murcia, S., & Fernández-Aranda, F. (2013). Differences in cognitive behavioral therapy dropout rates between bulimia nervosa subtypes based on drive for thinness and depression. *Psychotherapy and Psychosomatics, 82*(2), 125–126. doi:10.1159/000339620.

Rizvi, S. L., Dimeff, L. A., Skutch, J., Carroll, D., & Linehan, M. M. (2011). A pilot study of the DBT coach: An interactive mobile phone application for individuals with borderline personality disorder and substance use disorder. *Behavior Therapy, 42*, 589–600.

Robertson, C. D., Miskey, H., Mitchell, J., & Nelson-Gray, R. (2013). Variety of self-injury: Is the number of different methods of non-suicidal self-injury related to personality, psychopathology, or functions of self-injury? *Archives of Suicide Research, 17*, 33–40.

Ross, S., Heath, N. L., & Toste, J. R. (2009). Non-suicidal self-injury and eating pathology in high school students. *The American Journal of Orthopsychiatry, 79*, 83–92.

Slee, N., Garnefski, N., van der Leeden, R., Arensman, E., & Spinhoven, P. (2008). Cognitive-behavioural intervention for self-harm: Randomised controlled trial. *The British Journal of Psychiatry, 192*, 202–211.

Stegemann, T., Brüggemann-Etchart, A., Badorrek-Hinkelmann, A., & Romer, G. (2010). The function of music in the context of non-suicidal self-injury. *Praxis der Kinderpsychologie und Kinderpsychiatrie, 59*, 810–830.

Svirko, E., & Hawton, K. (2007). Self-injurious behavior and eating disorders: The extent and nature of the association. *Suicide and Life Threatening Behavior, 37*, 409–421.

Swannell, S., Martin, G., Page, A., Hasking, P., Hazell, P., Taylor, A., et al. (2012). Child maltreatment, subsequent non-suicidal self-injury and the mediating roles of dissociation, alexithymia and self-blame. *Child Abuse & Neglect, 36*, 572–584.

Tchanturia, K., Liao, P. C., Forcano, L., Fernández-Aranda, F., Uher, R., Treasure, J., et al. (2012). Poor decision making in male patients with anorexia nervosa. *European Eating Disorders Review, 20*, 169–173.

Vansteenkiste, M., Claes, L., Soenens, B., & Verstuyf, J. (2013). Motivational dynamics among eating-disordered patients with and without nonsuicidal self-injury: A self-determination theory approach. *European Eating Disorders Review, 21*, 209–214.

Victor, S. E., Glenn, C. R., & Klonsky, E. D. (2012). Is non-suicidal self-injury an "addiction"? A comparison of craving in substance use and non-suicidal self-injury. *Psychiatry Research, 197*, 73–77.

Washburn, J. J., Richardt, S. L., Styer, D. M., Gebhardt, M., Juzwin, K. R., Yourek, A., et al. (2012). Psychotherapeutic approaches to non-suicidal self-injury in adolescents. *Child and Adolescent Psychiatry and Mental Health, 6*, 14.

Weierich, M. R., & Nock, M. K. (2008). Posttraumatic stress symptoms mediate the relation between childhood sexual abuse and nonsuicidal self-injury. *Journal of Consulting and Clinical Psychology, 76*, 39–44.

Whitlock, J., Muehlenkamp, J., Purington, A., Eckenrode, J., Barreira, P., Baral Abrams, G., et al. (2011). Nonsuicidal self-injury in a college population: General trends and sex differences. *Journal of American College Health, 59*, 691–698.

Wrzesien, M., Rey, B., Alcañiz, M., Baños, R., Martínez, M. G., Pérez-López, D., et al. (2012). Virtual representations of the self: Engaging teenagers in emotional regulation strategies learning. *Studies in Health Technologies and Informatics, 181*, 248–252.

Yates, T. M. (2004). The developmental psychopathology of self-injurious behavior: Compensatory regulation in posttraumatic adaptation. *Clinical Psychology Review, 24*, 35–74.

You, J., Leung, F., Lai, C. M., & Fu, K. (2012). The associations between non-suicidal self-injury and borderline personality disorder features among Chinese adolescents. *Journal of Personality Disorders, 26*, 226–237.

Zetterqvist, M., Lundh, L. G., Dahlström, O., & Svedin, C. G. (2013). Prevalence and function of Non-Suicidal Self-Injury (NSSI) in a community sample of adolescents, using suggested DSM-5 criteria for a potential NSSI disorder. *Journal of Abnormal Child Psychology, 41*(5), 759–773.

Index

L. Claes and J.J. Muehlenkamp (eds.), *Non-Suicidal Self-Injury in Eating Disorders*,
DOI 10.1007/978-3-642-40107-7, © Springer-Verlag Berlin Heidelberg 2014

R

S

Printed in the United States
By Bookmasters